Raqs in th

Also by Heather D. Ward
and from McFarland

Egyptian Belly Dance in Transition:
The Raqs Sharqi Revolution, 1890–1930 (2018)

Raqs in the City

The Belly Dance Landscape of Cairo

HEATHER D. WARD

McFarland & Company, Inc., Publishers
Jefferson, North Carolina

This book has undergone peer review.

Library of Congress Cataloging-in-Publication Data

Names: Ward, Heather D., author.
Title: Raqs in the city : the belly dance landscape of Cairo / Heather D. Ward.
Description: Jefferson, North Carolina : McFarland & Company, Inc., Publishers, 2024. | Includes bibliographical references and index.
Identifiers: LCCN 2024023041 | ISBN 9781476690308 (paperback : acid free paper) ♾ ISBN 9781476653488 (ebook)
Subjects: LCSH: Belly dance—Egypt—Cairo—History. | Belly dance—Social aspects—Egypt—Cairo. | Neighborhoods—Egypt—Cairo—History. | Cairo (Egypt)—Historical geography.
Classification: LCC GV1798.5 .W373 2024 | DDC 793.3—dc23/eng/20240606
LC record available at https://lccn.loc.gov/2024023041

British Library cataloguing data are available

ISBN (print) 978-1-4766-9030-8
ISBN (ebook) 978-1-4766-5348-8

Front cover images: *left to right:* A khawal or jink of the mid- to late nineteenth century (Délié and Béchard carte de visite, circa 1870s, Getty Research Institute, Los Angeles [2008.R.3]); Turn-of-the-century Azbakīyah, looking east along the street today known as ʿAlī al- Kassār Street (postcard, circa 1900); An advertisement for the ʿawālim Anīsah al-Miṣrīyah and Nabawīyah (Nabawīyah Muṣṭafa, who eventually transitioned to dancing in films), indicating their business address on Muḥammad ʿAlī Street; Dancers onstage at Cairo's El Dorado entertainment hall (Lichtenstern and Harari postcard, postmarked 1905); *background:* Map of early nineteenth century Cairo (Dufour, 1838).

Printed in the United States of America

McFarland & Company, Inc., Publishers
Box 611, Jefferson, North Carolina 28640
www.mcfarlandpub.com

Table of Contents

Preface

Every time I visit Cairo, there's a pilgrimage that I am sure to make. It starts by exiting the bustling Cairo Metro at the chaotic 'Atabah station, and then navigating toward the correct exit—if I get it wrong, I'll stumble out into the maze of the Azbakīyah book market and lose my bearings entirely. The exit that I want opens onto 26 Yūliyū Street (26 July Street) and the west end of what remains of Cairo's Azbakīyah Gardens. From here, I can easily get to all my special places.

Usually, I begin the pilgrimage by walking northward, then hanging a right onto 'Alī al- Kassār Street. This route takes me to the heart of Azbakīyah—for centuries, a vibrant center of popular entertainment; today, a busy but somewhat decrepit locus of working-class commerce. It's hard to believe that this dusty, overcrowded city neighborhood was once the site of a massive lake. I picture the brightly-decorated pleasure craft of Cairo's medieval elites sailing on the still waters, while popular entertainers ply their trades among the common people picnicking on the shore. The image fades as a car horn sounds and I dodge an oncoming taxi.

I walk along the north side of what used to be Azbakīyah Gardens—the formal pleasure gardens that were laid out many decades after the lake was drained—and glance up at the Belle Époque arcaded buildings that loom to my left. At Khazindār Square, I turn left, and here, I pause for a moment, imagining the streets and alleys of Azbakīyah at the dawn of the twentieth century. The sounds of music, song, and laughter spill forth from the open door of every café, bar, and music hall. Women beckon passers-by to come see a dance show—or, perhaps, to enjoy more private entertainments. Under the light of the gas lamps, both locals and foreigners crowd through in search of an evening's pleasure. In the midst of this heady atmosphere, the frequent glimpse of a British military uniform is a harsh reminder to the locals of a brutal occupation that shows no sign of ending. I stroll west on Najīb al-Rīḥānī Street, cut left down the tiny Bāb al-Baḥrī Street, and find myself back on ʻAlī al- Kassār Street. From here, I return to my starting point.

Back in front of the ʻAtabah station exit, this time I head west onto 26 July Street. Before the time of Khedive Ismāʻīl, this was the westernmost extent of the Ottoman city. Now, this street leads me towards the heart of Cairo's "new" downtown. I turn right onto ʻImād al-Dīn Street, the Broadway of Cairo. The street's glory days have long since faded, but the surviving cinemas and theaters make them easier to imagine than Azbakīyah's long-vanished music halls. I walk the length of the street, and think of all the Egyptian celebrities of the twentieth century who got their start here. Circling back, I stop in at the old Alfi Bey Restaurant for a snack and a rest. Located on what was once the site of a popular theater known as the Printania, the restaurant was one of the filming locations for *Carioca*, a television series about the remarkable life of Taḥīyah Carioca, the belly dancer and actress who got her start in the Ṣālat Badīʻah Maṣābnī, just up the street on ʻImād al-Dīn. That establishment was one of many that was owned and operated by Badīʻah Maṣābnī, the legendary artist and entrepreneur and a star maker of early-to-mid twentieth-century Cairo. I take a last sip of Nescafé and return to ʻAtabah station.

Sometimes, my pilgrimage begins by walking southward toward Opera Square, also known as Ibrāhīm Bāshā Square, after the massive sculpture that watches over it. Cairo's original opera house once graced this square, until it was destroyed by fire in 1971. This square was also the site of the grand Casino Opera, Badīʻah Maṣābnī's final entertainment venture before she retired to Lebanon in 1950. Now a multi-story shopping mall stands in its place. At Opera Square, I take up a position near the swarming traffic so that I can flag down one of the passing microbuses, the easiest and cheapest way—aside from walking—to get to the area around the al-Azhar and Ḥusayn mosques. The process is simple: as soon as a microbus pulls up, I ask, "Ḥusayn?" If the driver answers in the affirmative, I hop in, and then we're off, careening around the square and then along the al-Azhar Bridge towards the beating heart of the Fatimid city. While I fish around for a few pound coins to pass up to the driver, I glance out at the masses of people below—there is no more striking reminder of the vitality this city than to witness the throbbing pulse of life that spreads out from ʻAtabah Square and along the al-Mūskī Street.

Tumbling out of the microbus, I begin to wander the narrow lanes and alleys of the old city. It's not difficult to walk the entire length of the Fatimid city. Sometimes, I begin at Bāb al-Futūḥ and follow the path of the original *qaṣabah*, the main north-south thoroughfare of the old city core, all the way south to Bāb Zuwaylah. At the latter's imposing twin minarets, I turn right, following the southern boundary of the Fatimid city until I reach Būr Sa'īd Street. Most present-day Cairenes don't realize that Būr Sa'īd Street occupies the bed of a former canal, the Khalīj al-Miṣrī, once the western boundary of the city and a defining feature of Cairo's social and spatial reality. A short walk south on Būr Sa'īd Street leads me to its intersection with Muḥammad 'Alī Street. For over a century, this street was a hub for Cairo's singers, dancers, and musicians, as well as for a range of other businesses connected to the entertainment trades. Today, the street is mostly home to furniture stores. Nevertheless, walking along this street, I can still spot the occasional music shop. I follow the street until I arrive back at 'Atabah, my mind swirling with images of Cairo now, and imaginings of Cairo in the past.

For many Egyptians, my fascination with these particular spaces is confusing and a source of consternation. They simply can't understand why I would want to go to places like 'Atabah, Azbakīyah, and Muḥammad 'Alī Street. When I announce to well-intentioned friends that I am once again headed to "Ḥusayn"—shorthand for the old city—they ask, "Why don't you go somewhere nice this time, like Sharm or Hurghada?"* If I mention to Egyptians outside the entertainment trades that I plan to visit Muḥammad 'Alī Street, I am met with looks of bemusement or concern.

These reactions can be partially explained by social class. In general, the places I visit on my pilgrimage are now "low class" areas: the majority of the people who live and work in these spaces belong to the lower and lower-middle classes of Cairene society, and the more well-to-do view these locations as undesirable and potentially dangerous. However, I find that social class alone is insufficient to explain the complex perceptions attached to these spaces.

My earliest engagement with these places came while researching and writing my previous book, *Egyptian Belly Dance in Transition: The Raqs Sharqi Revolution, 1890–1930*. The streets and alleys around the old Azbakīyah Gardens, nearby 'Imād al-Dīn Street, and Muḥammad 'Alī Street were the staging grounds for the developments in Egyptian belly dance that I explored in the book. In the course of my research, I came to realize that all of these spaces bore strong historic associations with belly dance, belly dancers, and professional entertainment in general. They were also spaces of moral ambiguity, where the norms of Egyptian society were blurred, challenged, and occasionally upended. In some cases, the association with professional entertainment has persisted into the present day; such is the case with Muḥammad 'Alī Street, which remains firmly linked to music, song, and dance, in spite of the current realities of the

* Two popular tourist resorts on the Red Sea.

street. In others, such as Azbakīyah, the direct connection to the entertainment trades has faded, but ambivalent attitudes persist in the popular imagination.

My fascination with these spaces persisted long after the completion of the book, and I continued to explore their histories. I soon realized that the ties binding these spaces to professional entertainment and entertainers extended much deeper than the turn of the nineteenth and twentieth centuries. For example, the area that would become the Azbakīyah Gardens carried its associations with entertainment, recreation, and leisure since the era of the Fatimids a thousand years ago. Near the intersection of Muḥammad ʿAlī Street with Fatimid Cairo's southern boundary, there was a market for musical instruments fully five hundred years before Muḥammad ʿAlī Street was even constructed, indicating a long historic connection between this space and professional entertainment. I also discovered that other spaces in the geography of urban Cairo have historic associations with entertainment and leisure, including, surprisingly, the city's massive cemeteries.

The long-lasting associations between certain Cairo spaces and professional entertainment and entertainers intrigued me, and I began to wonder about the precise nature of the relationship between these spaces and professional belly dancers. Just as the aforementioned spaces have been viewed as ambiguous and morally suspect, belly dancers exist as liminal and ambiguous figures in Egyptian society. They are socially marginal: they routinely engage in behaviors that violate normative gender roles, and because dance is generally viewed as a low-status and undesirable occupation, many belly dancers hail from lower-class backgrounds. Notably, the marginality of belly dancers is also shaped by the settings in which they perform: each setting—popular festival, wedding, cabaret, five-star hotel, and so on—produces a unique web of social and cultural meanings, further informed by the issues of gender and class, which bind the fortunes of the dancers who perform within them. Nevertheless, in spite of their marginality, professional belly dancers are considered vital to many events and celebrations, with the result that these marginal figures frequently intrude into the daily social and spatial reality of Egyptian life.

The presence of belly dance and its professional practitioners in certain Cairo spaces such as Azbakīyah, ʿImād al-Dīn Street, and Muḥammad ʿAlī Street, together with the importance of space in meaningfully framing and shaping dance and dancer, challenged me to dig deeper into the historic interconnection between dance spaces and dance practitioners. I wanted to understand the nature of the relationship between belly dance space and belly dancer in the Cairo landscape, how this relationship developed, and how it has impacted the position of belly dance and its professional practitioners in Egyptian society. I also wondered about the implications of this relationship for belly dance in the current moment, as well as for the future trajectories of the dance. With these issues in mind, I began researching and writing this book.

As an independent researcher, operating without the support of an academic institution, I have frequently questioned my own sanity in taking on a project of this magnitude. I am grateful to so many individuals for their support, moral and otherwise, without which I would not have been able to bring this book to completion. I cannot possibly offer a complete accounting of everyone here, and I beg to apologize to anyone whose name has slipped from my memory while writing these acknowledgments.

I would first like to thank Christine Sahin for being a sounding board when this project was in its infancy, for pointing me in the direction of a number of useful resources, and most importantly, for providing invaluable feedback on an early draft of this manuscript. I am also grateful to George Dimitri Sawa for always taking the time to answer my out-of-the-blue research questions. I wish to express my sincere appreciation to Layla Milholen and to McFarland & Company, Inc., for taking a chance on another of my belly dance projects, as well as for their patience and guidance. I am indebted to my permissions researcher, Margaret Gaston, for her invaluable assistance. Many thanks to the Smithsonian Institution, the Getty Research Institute, and Dr. Edouard Lambelet for granting permission to use images from their collections.

I am deeply grateful to each and every individual who has assisted with my research on-site in Egypt. In particular, I wish to thank the traditional entertainers from whom I have learned so much, including but not limited to Khayrīyah Māzin of Luxor, Umm Hāshim of Abū Shūshah, and Riḍā and Sayyid Ḥankish of Muḥammad ʿAlī Street. I also wish to thank my friend Saʿd Ḥassan, who has assisted me in Upper Egypt, and my friend Khālid Manṣūr and his sons Bijād and Ziyād, who have helped me in Cairo. I wish to extend my sincere thanks to my Arabic tutor, Eva Adel, whose excellent and patient instruction has empowered me during my research in Egypt. In addition to these individuals, I would be remiss if I did not express my deep appreciation to members of the Jābr family for facilitating my stays in Cairo.

I am extremely grateful to all the aficionados of Egyptian dance who have supported my research over the last several years, whether by reading my writing, listening to my lectures, attending my classes and workshops, or subscribing to my Patreon. Your interest and enthusiasm have given me the motivation and the determination that I need to keep doing this work.

Lastly, there are three people to whom I owe the deepest debt of gratitude: Kenneth Ward, Dianne Ward, and Mousa Salameh. Your love and support have given me the strength and confidence that I can never seem to muster on my own. Words fail me here; anything I write will be insufficient to capture the depth of my love and appreciation.

Notes on Transcription and Translation

In general, I followed the ALA-LC (American Library Association and Library of Congress) system when transcribing Arabic terms, including the names of individuals and places. I used the anglicized spellings of well-known place names, such as Alexandria and Cairo, and of certain well-known individuals from recent Egyptian history, such as Gamal Abdel Nasser and Anwar Sadat. I also used the anglicized spellings of the names of individuals who regularly employ an anglicized spelling of their own names. In quotations, I followed the transcription system of the quoted author.

Translation of Arabic sources was accomplished with the invaluable assistance of Mr. Mousa Salameh. I translated European-language sources myself.

Introduction

What Is Belly Dance?

In the English language, the term "belly dance" is often used in a very broad sense to refer to an array of similar, but distinct, dance forms from the Middle East, North Africa, and parts of Central Asia. The dances that are gathered together under the "belly dance" moniker are characterized by torso-focused movement vocabulary and generally involve solo improvisation by individual practitioners. The term "belly dance" emerged as a literal translation of *danse du ventre*, the French designation for this collection of dances (Carlton 1994, Hawthorn 2019). Hawthorn (2019) has documented the usage of *danse du ventre* in reference to Middle Eastern and North African dance forms as early as the 1860s. While the English translation "belly dance" is often attributed to Sol Bloom, entrepreneur and manager of the Midway Plaisance at the 1893 Columbian Exposition in Chicago, Hawthorn demonstrates that "belly dance" was used as the English-language equivalent of *danse du ventre* as early as 1889 (Hawthorn 2019: 7).

The term "belly dance" is also used quite liberally to refer to a variety of dance styles originating outside of the Middle East. Many of these were created in North America, including Fat Chance Belly Dance Style (formerly American Tribal Style) created by Carolena Nericcio, the Tribal Fusion styles popularized by dancers such as Jill Parker and Rachel Brice, and Improvisational Team Synchronization (formerly Improvisational Tribal Style) created by Amy Sigil. These dance styles, while deriving a great deal of their foundational movements from the aforementioned dances of the Middle East, North Africa, and Asia, differ profoundly from the source dances in aesthetic, musical accompaniment, and costuming.

The colonial origins of this term, and the present-day ambiguity of its usage, raise questions regarding the term's utility and appropriateness, and challenge its continued use in discourse around actual Middle Eastern and North African dance styles. Nevertheless, for a number of reasons, "belly dance" is difficult to discard, at least in the present moment. The term continues to be widely used, not only in primarily English-language contexts, but even among Arabic-speaking dance practitioners and entrepreneurs within Egypt.* For studies like the present one, it is challenging to find a workable alternative in the English language. For example, "Egyptian dance" is too broad, necessarily encompassing an array of traditional Egyptian folk dance forms beyond the specific dance of interest in the current text. On the other hand, terms like *raqṣ sharqī* and *raqṣ baladī* are too specific, excluding other related Egyptian dance forms that are not truly captured by these terms.

Consequently, I have chosen to retain the term, but with clear definition. The term "belly dance" is used as a shorthand for a collective of related Egyptian dance forms, including the dances of the traditional entertainers known as the *'awālim* and the *ghawāzī* (and their predecessors), as well as the concert dance form known as *raqṣ sharqī* (literally, "eastern dance," often rendered as "Oriental dance" in English). These dance forms are united by a fundamental technique of torso-based movements such as articulated hip and shoulder movements, circles and "figure eights" of the pelvis, and abdominal undulations. Beyond the movement vocabulary, these dances share an aesthetic centered on effective musical interpretation: a skilled performer must embody the rhythmic structure, melodic phrasing, and feeling of her musical accompaniment. Notably, until rather recently, most professional practitioners of these dance styles could also sing (see Van Nieuwkerk 1995: 14, 59, 208).

There are definite stylistic distinctions among these dance forms. For example, *raqṣ sharqī* includes a range of steps and turns—some of which were introduced from non-Egyptian sources—that are not present in the *'awālim* and *ghawāzī* repertoires. Upper Egyptian *ghawāzī* technique depends upon a distinctive and heavy style of footwork that is entirely absent from Lower Egyptian *ghawāzī* and urban *'awālim* and *raqṣ sharqī* styles. Appropriate musical accompaniment varies tremendously from region to region and from urban to rural settings. Yet, there is a core unity of technique and aesthetic among these styles. They are branches of the same tree, and the trunk of that tree is *raqṣ baladī* ("indigenous dance"), the informal social form of belly dance.† *Raqṣ baladī* is performed by

* For example, some present-day Cairo discos and nightclubs targeted at Egyptian clientele sometimes use "belly dance" and "belly dancer" in their advertising copy; often these English words are mingled with Arabic text in the same advertisements.

† It is worth noting here that ordinary Egyptians generally do not make the fine terminological distinctions that I am making here. That is, Egyptians often use the terms *raqṣ sharqī* and *raqṣ baladī* interchangeably, regardless of whether they are referring to social or professional variants of the dance. Nevertheless, I find these distinctions necessary for clarity in the context of the current discussion.

ordinary Egyptians, regardless of age or gender, among family and friends in social settings, particularly at festive events like weddings. The fundamental torso-based movements of professional belly dance emerge from the essential technique of this traditional social dance.

Historically, both social and professional variants of belly dance have been a vital part of events and celebrations that mark momentous occasions. This includes events that commemorate or celebrate significant transitions in the life cycles of individuals, such as circumcisions and weddings. It also includes events that punctuate the life cycle of the calendar year, such as the periodic saint's day festivals known as *mawālid* (singular, *mūlid*). On such occasions, ordinary people dance socially with friends and relatives, while professional dancers are frequently hired to enhance the festive atmosphere.

Professional belly dance has also become popular outside of these traditional social contexts. At the dawn of the twentieth century, *raqṣ sharqī* emerged within the context of the music halls and theaters of Cairo and Alexandria (Ward 2018). In these venues, whose sole *raison d'être* was the presentation of arts and entertainment, professional belly dance was detached from the traditional social occasions that had previously justified its performance. Within a few decades, this theatrical version of belly dance would become accessible to a broader public through its inclusion in Egyptian film and television. More recently, Egyptians have *raqṣ sharqī* literally at their fingertips thanks to the Internet, social media, and the widespread availability of cell phones in Egypt. Through these new media, Egyptians can easily watch and copy their favorite dancers, incorporating their signature movements into their personal *raqṣ baladī* styles.

Yet, in spite of the underlying similarities in basic technique and aesthetic, *raqṣ baladī* is separated from professional belly dance by a seemingly unbridgeable divide in public perception. *Raqṣ baladī*, performed informally for personal enjoyment, is widely accepted in Egyptian society. The various forms of professional belly dance, which involve paid performance for the entertainment of strangers, occupy a much more tenuous and ambiguous position in the culture, and the professional practitioners of belly dance find themselves marginalized in a society that has long considered them an essential part of important social events and celebrations.

Professional Belly Dance in Egyptian Social Context

Both historically and in the present day, the overwhelming majority of the dance's professional performers have been female. The *'awālim* and the *ghawāzī* are female dancers, and most practitioners of *raqṣ sharqī* have been female as well. The most famous of these women have become household names among Egyptians: Taḥīyah Carioca, Sāmiyah Jamāl, Fifi 'Abduh, Dīnā Ṭal'at.

However, it is important to note that professional belly dance in Egypt has included both male and female practitioners throughout its history. In the early nineteenth century, Edward Lane documented two categories of male professional belly dancer in Egypt: the *khawal* and the *jink* (Lane 1860: 381–382, Lane 2005 [1836]: 376–377). Though it has been suggested that these dancers only succeeded due to the temporary suppression of female dancers, Karayanni effectively disputes this, arguing that male dancers were a longstanding part of popular entertainment throughout the Middle East and Central Asia (Karayanni 2004: 67–97). Indeed, over a century before Lane, Aḥmad al-Damurdāshī describes how Ismā'īl Bāshā, the Ottoman governor of Egypt from 1695 to 1697, hired male dancers and their troupes to perform at the lavish celebration for the circumcision of his two sons (al-Damurdāshī 1991: 64–67).

In fact, male dancers appear to have been commonplace in Egypt in the Ottoman period and into the Khedivial era, perhaps reflecting the popularity of male dancers in the broader Ottoman Empire. Centuries earlier, one finds occasional mention of *mukhannathūn* (singular *mukhannath*), male entertainers who assumed female mannerisms and dress, performing in Egypt (see, for example, al-Maqrīzī 1906–1908, volume 1: 110, in an account from the Mamluk period). McPherson, documenting *mawālid* in the early decades of the twentieth century, describes a famous male dancer named Ḥusayn Fu'ād (McPherson 1941: 84–85). In the present day, well-known Egyptian male professional belly dancers include Tito Seif, Khaled Mahmoud, and Tommy King (also known as Hatem Hamdi).

For centuries, professional practitioners of belly dance—whether male or female—have faced social stigmatization due to their profession. Though some dancers have been able to attain impressive wealth and celebrity, their success has generally come at a great social cost. In the present day, professional belly dancers at all levels of the trade—from the poorest street wedding performers to the most famous stars of stage and screen—frequently find themselves not only stigmatized and stereotyped by the society at large, but also rejected and even abused by their own families and loved ones. The social challenges faced by these entertainers have been vividly recounted in a number of recent documentaries, including *The Bellydancers of Cairo* (2006), *Dancers* (2007), *La Nuit, Elles Dansent* (2011), and *In Our Own Words: The Cairo Dance Scene Explained* (2020). In these films, Egyptian dancers from all levels of the trade describe the abuses that they have endured, ranging from insults to threats to actual physical violence. The experiences of these entertainers affirm that in

Egypt, professional belly dancers, regardless of their degree of wealth or fame, face a marginal existence in society.

The social opprobrium meted out to Egypt's professional belly dancers begs further analysis. In recent decades, academic researchers have begun to problematize the complex and conflicted relationship between Egyptians and professional belly dance and to examine how Egyptians' ambivalence toward their native dance and its professional performers embodies social discourse on issues such as gender and class. Of particular note for purposes of the current study are the scholarly investigations of Karin Van Nieuwkerk, Noha Roushdy, and Christine Sahin.

Karin Van Nieuwkerk's study of female singers and dancers in Egypt remains a landmark in exploring the complicated position of these women in Egyptian society (Van Nieuwkerk 1995). Van Nieuwkerk conducted her fieldwork in Egypt in 1989 and 1990, focusing on entertainers from the traditional circuit of weddings and saints' day festivals, as well as nightclub entertainers. Noting what she describes as the "tainted reputation of female entertainers" (Van Nieuwkerk 1995: 2–3), she set out to determine whether these women are condemned because of their trade, or because they are female practitioners of the trade.

Indeed, Van Nieuwkerk's research affirms that female professional entertainers tend to be judged more harshly than their male counterparts. To explain this disparity, she investigates how cultural constructions of male *versus* female bodies inform Egyptian expectations regarding proper feminine behavior, and how female entertainers routinely violate these normative expectations (see Van Nieuwkerk 1995: 141–157). Drawing on the work of Fatema Mernissi, Van Nieuwkerk explains that within Egyptian gender constructs, the female body is *by definition* sexual. That is, while the male body is seen as multi-dimensional and productive, the female body is defined exclusively by its sexual aspect. Moreover, the sexuality of the female body is seen as powerful, necessitating that it be contained within the proper context (marriage) and rendering practices such as veiling and seclusion necessary not only to protect women's modesty, but to protect men from women's powerful sexuality.

Female professional entertainers, counter to social expectations regarding proper feminine behavior, deploy their sexual bodies outside of socially-sanctioned contexts (e.g., in the sanctity of the marital union), thus earning a negative reputation. As Van Nieuwkerk (1995: 154) notes:

> Female entertainers' main instrument for making money consists of their *'awra* [shameful thing], their sexual bodies and voices. Female entertainers thus use the female power to seduce to secure a living. They profit from the cultural construction of the female body as seductive but pay for it in terms of status and respect.

Male professional entertainers, because their bodies are not viewed as inherently exciting and arousing, are judged differently. In the case of male dancers (Van Nieuwkerk 1995: 132):

> They are not highly esteemed, yet this is not account of their immorality but because they do "women's work." ...I once asked a sheikh why male dancing is not *ḥarâm* [taboo]. The answer was easy: "A man's body is not shameful [*'awra*]," and regardless of how it moves and shakes, "it cannot excite."

It is telling that when female professional entertainers were temporarily banned from performing publicly in the 1830s, contemporary male dancers were unaffected and were able to fill the void (see Clot-Bey 1840: 94–95). It is also noteworthy that male entertainers can be adversely impacted by their association with females in the trade. In a more recent work exploring Egyptian masculinity through the life and experiences of the well-known Muḥammad 'Alī Street musician Sayyid Ḥankish, Van Nieuwkerk notes that that the problematic reputations of female entertainers cast a pall over the careers and reputations of the male musicians who perform with them (Van Nieuwkerk 2019: 59–63, 121, 145). Notably, one of Sayyid's conditions for marrying his wife was that she retire from the trade (*ibid.*, 97–98).

Nevertheless, it is important to note that male belly dancers have also faced stigmatization in Egyptian society. This point is not really addressed by Van Nieuwkerk, though her lack of attention to this issue is likely due to the fact that her fieldwork researching the song/dance trade predated the recent resurgence of male belly dancers in Egypt.* The often negative perceptions of male belly dancers appear to be rooted in something more complex than merely a disdain for men doing "women's work." Comments by Egyptians—both dancer and non-dancer alike—suggest that the negative attitudes derive from a discomfort with men engaging in behaviors deemed "effeminate" and thus raising the specter of homosexuality, a taboo in Egyptian society (see, for example, Madkour 2008, *The New York Times* 2008, el-Sharkawy 2017). Male dancers frequently distance themselves from effeminacy and, by implication, homosexuality. For example, Egyptian dancer Tito Seif states: "I don't believe that a male belly dancer should imitate a woman.... We should not forget that we are men, and dance in a manly way" (*The New York Times* 2008). Similarly, male dancer Khalil Khalil asserts that male belly dance costuming should never imitate female costuming (el-Sharkawy 2017).

In essence, male dancers, like their female counterparts, are viewed

* Van Nieuwkerk (1995: 132) writes: "There are no male belly dancers anymore—only male folk dancers in theaters and in wedding processions exist." This was likely true at the time of her research, but certainly does not hold true today.

as transgressing gender norms, but in different ways. That is, while female dancers violate gender norms by failing to contain and regulate their sexual bodies, male dancers do so by assuming female behaviors and attire. Statements like those by Tito Seif and Khalil Khalil suggest the strategies that male dancers must employ in order to navigate their perceived violation of social norms. Unfortunately, an in-depth ethnographic analysis of these men akin to Van Nieuwkerk's study of female entertainers—something which would shed a great deal more light on the current situation of male professional belly dancers in Egypt—has yet to be undertaken.

Importantly, Van Nieuwkerk also demonstrates that gender-informed perceptions of professional entertainers are mediated through the lens of social class (see, for example, Van Nieuwkerk 1995: 106–115). In general, dance is considered an extremely low-status occupation in Egypt (Van Nieuwkerk 1995: 187–192). Many professional entertainers in Egypt, particularly the entertainers who form the primary focus of Van Nieuwkerk's research, hail from the lower and lower-middle classes of Egyptian society. Such work is undesirable to higher-class individuals, but accessible to lower-class men and women who lack the skills, education, or connections to secure other kinds of employment.

Members of the lower and lower-middle classes—the "significant others," in Van Nieuwkerk's words, of her research subjects—tend to be more accepting of entertainers than members of the upper and upper-middle classes. The latter tend to dismiss entertainers based on their lower-class origins. Further, although they are prone to judge female entertainers more harshly, lower and lower-middle class Egyptians are more likely to tolerate women working in the entertainment trade, if their financial circumstances necessitate it. Nevertheless, among all strata of Egyptian society, the entertainment trades are seen as disrespectable for women, and female professional entertainers are viewed as morally suspect.

Beyond issues of gender and class, Van Nieuwkerk's research also reveals the impact of performance context on the status of professional entertainers (see, for example, Van Nieuwkerk 1995: 122–129). Importantly, performers working in traditional settings, such as weddings, tend to be viewed more favorably than those working in nightclub settings. She notes: "Whereas weddings are joyful celebrations and can be defined as the context of happiness, nightclubs are considered the domain of greediness, excitement, and sexuality" (Van Nieuwkerk 1995: 180). The divergent attitudes toward these different performance contexts then inform perceptions of entertainers' behavior within each setting. For female professional entertainers, in particular, behaviors that are viewed as "all in good fun" in the context of a traditional celebration such as a wedding are seen in an entirely different light in a nightclub setting:

> At weddings, for instance, a dancer occasionally performs in front of the couple and puts their hands on her belly and breasts while she rolls her belly and moves her breasts. I expected this to be considered outrageous behavior. Yet several people explained that it was innocent merriment and fun (*farfasha*). A nightclub dancer who exhibited the same behavior, lacking the context of a happy occasion and working in an atmosphere of sexual excitement, would be considered prostituting herself to earn money [Van Nieuwkerk 1995: 128–129].

Even in the socially-sanctioned context of a wedding, the female dancer exists as a marginal persona, and her behaviors are transgressive of normative expectations regarding proper feminine behavior. However, in the wedding, she is regarded as necessary to enhance the festive atmosphere of the celebration, and her marginality is tolerated.

While Van Nieuwerk's analysis focuses on female professional entertainers from the traditional circuit, Noha Roushdy's (2009) examination of Egyptian belly dance takes into account the perspectives of both professional and non-professional practitioners, and expands her analysis to include professional dancers from a broader range of social backgrounds and work settings. Nevertheless, like Van Nieuwkerk, Roushdy focuses exclusively on female practitioners. Roushdy studies how belly dance operates within Egyptian society as a challenge to normative discourses regarding proper femininity. She approaches belly dance as "...a form of symbolic inversion of the dominant culture, through which the dominant repertoire of femininity and proper personhood that it inverts can be elucidated" (Roushdy 2009: 13).

As Roushdy notes, the social practice of *raqṣ baladī*, particularly by women, is governed by unspoken rules of propriety and decorum, including the avoidance of any behaviors that would suggest emulation of the professional forms of the dance. For example, social dancers generally avoid extended eye contact with spectators or with other dancers, rather choosing to focus their gaze on their own hips or waist. Individuals often require gentle persuasion by friends and family before agreeing to dance. The parameters of propriety and decorum vary in different contexts, and social dancers must develop strategies to navigate each setting while preserving their modesty and reputations:

> How an individual woman reacts in different contexts where dancing is taking place depends on her relationship to others present, to the host or hostess, her familiarity with the surrounding environment, and her personal disposition.... When a woman does participate, the appropriateness of her performance is usually conditioned by her compliance with the decorum that is expected of her in the particular context in which she is dancing [Roushdy 2009: 54–55].

Roushdy, as a native Egyptian woman, is bound by these parameters as well. She notes that while conducting her research, she found it necessary to downplay her personal interest in belly dance and "not to attempt to disturb the boundary that has been placed between 'ordinary' Egyptian women—who occupy the center and who may or may not dance for pleasure—and those 'other' women, who make money out of it" (*ibid.*, 93).

Those "other" women continue to play a significant role in Egyptian society, and "ordinary" Egyptians regularly encounter their dancing in weddings, nightclubs, films, and television. Yet, female professional belly dancers exist as marginal figures: in Roushdy's words, they are "betwixt and between" figures who embody the tension between proper and improper feminine behavior. She writes: "The professional dancer ... can also be likened to a liminal persona, as an occasional intruder into the dominant culture and everyday life, a marginal figure who, in spite of her centrality, occupies the lowest rungs of society" (*ibid.*, 14). The professional dancer exists as a paradox—an individual who is both desired and disdained in Egyptian society—and individual dancers struggle to negotiate their marginal status. Roushdy notes that "...the self-representation of individual dancers reveals individually tailored discourses that reflect a unanimous attempt on the part of dancers to physically and discursively negotiate their marginalization in Egyptian society" (*ibid.*, 85). Professional dancers attempt to evade or moderate their stigmatization and marginalization by choosing performance contexts that align with their self-representation (*ibid.*, 84–89).

Complementing the work of Van Nieuwkerk and Roushdy, Christine Sahin (2018) explores dancing bodies and performance contexts as sites of discourse on issues such as gender, sexuality, nationality and class in post-2011 Cairo. Sahin's intersectional and multi-sited approach combines observations of dance shows in a variety of differently-classed performance settings in Cairo with direct interviews of professional dancers, audience members, and others involved with the dance industry. She considers both dance and non-dance bodies in her analysis, noting that:

> A multiplicity of fluid meanings is constantly negotiated within a dance event, but solely spotlighting the dancer misses out on critical nuances and other meanings being constructed and transmitted from other bodies, particularly other marginalized bodies such as non-dance laboring and spectating bodies. This is also related to the caution of highlighting the dancer's experience at the expense of seriously considering the power dynamics and semiotics circulating between the variety of bodies making up the larger dance event [Sahin 2018: 43–44].

In essence, meanings are constructed, negotiated, and contested across multiple bodies within the dance space, necessitating a holistic consideration of all participants.

The pervasive importance of class in Egyptian society is a recurring theme in Sahin's work. As she notes, social mobility is extremely challenging in Egypt (Sahin 2018: 149–151). Even if an individual of lower-class origins attains great wealth, that individual remains tied to his or her class origins. As has already been noted, dance is a low-status occupation in Egypt, and many professional belly dancers hail from lower-class backgrounds. While it is possible for dancers to transcend their class origins in terms of wealth and celebrity, it is much more challenging for them to escape the perception of belonging to the lower echelons of Egyptian society. As a consequence, many dancers, once they achieve success in higher-class settings, deny any associations with lower-class performance contexts. Nevertheless, even the most successful dancers appear unable to escape their marginality, since the trade itself is so poorly esteemed. Sahin recounts how Egyptian dancer Randa Kamel, a popular star on the international dance workshop circuit, worried over the negative impact of her chosen career on her son's marriage prospects; this is a widespread concern among Egypt's professional belly dancers (Sahin 2018: 145).

Sahin's analysis is especially effective in showcasing the tactics that professional dancers employ within their performances in order to challenge and reframe their marginal status. Sahin offers her observations of Amina, a working-class cabaret dancer hired to dance in a five-star hotel nightclub. In spite of being hired at such an elite venue, and despite employing techniques and staging comparable to those of "higher-class" performers, signifiers such as posture and costuming immediately transmitted her lower-class status to her audience members, and for the bulk of her performance:

> The combination of her class, nationality, and cabaret work origins worked to overshadow the actuality of her laboring body in an air of suspicion, greed, and distrust. It was a notable contradiction, first, that despite working in a five-star hotel, her body was still marked as "working class" and "cabaret." Furthermore, that her working-class "cabaret" body was more heavily policed within the elite space, despite the fact that her class-border crossing was the pinnacle reason that capital was being exchanged and accumulated within the Empress [nightclub] [Sahin 2018: 239].

Yet, in closing her show with a performance to a *taqsīm baladī*, a form of structured improvisation with strong attachments to urban lower-class culture, Amina embraced and celebrated her lower-class affiliation, thus challenging and disrupting the elite space:

> As Amina stands with her hands on her hips, *mandil* [tissue] still in hand, looking out upon her spectators with a smoldering glance, she daringly demands a foremost focus on cultivating her complex redefinition of *asil* [authentic] relationalities; where bodies that bear the often polished-over and invisiblized labor, marginalization, and sometimes violence of dominant discourses are instead centralized and given space to become centralized in their full creative and commanding potential [Sahin 2018: 252].

As with Van Nieuwkerk and Roushdy, male belly dancers are outside of the scope of Sahin's analysis, and it is worth noting again that there has been no ethnographic analysis of male professional belly dancers in Egypt comparable to the works just described. There have been some scholarly treatments of male dancers in Egypt, most notably the work of Shay (2014) and Karayanni (2004). Shay's broad-ranging 2014 study of public performers in the Middle East, North Africa, Central Asia, and the Mediterranean confronts social definitions of masculinity, femininity, and effeminacy, and how these inform attitudes toward male entertainers (Shay 2014). However, Shay's work does not offer a specific and targeted analysis of Egypt's male entertainers, particularly those working in the present day.

Karayanni's 2004 study examines how colonial discourses on sex, gender, race, and national identity intersect on the Middle Eastern dancing body. He challenges colonial narratives regarding Middle Eastern dance by demonstrating the longstanding presence of male entertainers in popular entertainment throughout the Middle East and Central Asia, while giving particular attention to some of the nineteenth-century male dancers described in European travel narratives (Karayanni 2004: 67–97). However, Karayanni's work is primarily focused on identifying, examining, and challenging the colonial gaze rather than on detailing the history of male dancers within an Egyptian social context. As noted earlier, male professional belly dancers face stigmatization and marginalization in Egyptian society, and their marginal status appears to be rooted in their transgression of gender norms (although a different sort of transgression than that of their female counterparts). Yet, a comprehensive ethnographic analysis of male professional belly dancers in Egypt has yet to be done.

Several themes emerge from the previous discussion. First, the marginality of professional belly dancers within Egyptian society is informed by notions of gender. Belly dancers routinely engage in behaviors that violate normative gender roles. Female dancers disrupt the social order by deploying their sexual bodies outside of socially sanctioned contexts. Their male counterparts, on the other hand, challenge normative gender expectations with behaviors and attire that are perceived as effeminate. In essence, both male and female dancers exist outside the gender norms of Egyptian society.

Second, the marginality of dancers is tied to notions of class. In Egypt, dance is generally viewed as a low-status and undesirable occupation, and many professional belly dancers hail from lower-class backgrounds. Among their lower-class peers, these dancers tend to be judged less harshly than by members of the higher classes of Egyptian society. Yet, dancers from lower-class origins who attain great wealth and celebrity find it challenging to transcend their class background. Even the most successful dancers find themselves unable to overcome their marginal status in Egyptian society, since the trade itself is held in such low esteem. Their occupation excludes them from higher-class affiliation.

For these reasons, professional belly dancers are perceived as existing outside of the mainstream of Egyptian society. Yet, in spite of their marginality, dancers are considered vital to many events and celebrations, with the result that ordinary Egyptians frequently encounter and share spaces with these marginal figures. Indeed, at times, the dancer is admitted into the most private and intimate of settings. In Celame Barge's *Dancers* (2007), there is a scene in which the young dancer Chams, prior to her performance at a local wedding, is invited into the home with the couple's female relatives, where they serve her food and mend her costume. The dancer's importance to these festive occasions enables her to cross into spaces from which she might otherwise be excluded. Lorius (1996) describes how the celebrity dancer Fifi 'Abduh, in spite of her urban lower-class (*baladī*) affiliations, was frequently hired to entertain at elite weddings, and how she leveraged her background both to support and subvert her elite audience's perceptions. In essence, the professional belly dancer exists as an ambiguous and liminal figure in Egyptian society: socially marginal, yet frequently present—at times even central—within the social and spatial realities of Egyptian life.

Professional Belly Dance in Egyptian Spatial *Context*

The issue of space requires further consideration. Each of the important analyses just described allude to the role of the performance context—the *space* of performance—in framing and shaping not only the dance performance, but also the perceptions and the behaviors of both performers and spectators. As discussed earlier, Van Nieuwkerk points out that Egyptians hold conflicting attitudes toward traditional *versus* nightclub settings, and she describes how these attitudes inform public perceptions of the dancers who perform in these spaces. Further, she illustrates that both professional entertainers and Egyptians in general make important distinctions not only *between* the traditional performance circuit (weddings and *mawālid*) and the nightclub circuit, but also *within* each circuit. For example, she notes how some traditional entertainers view the *mawālid* as less prestigious than the context of popular weddings, and as a consequence, refuse to work in these settings (Van Nieuwkerk 2019: 52, 60). Van Nieuwkerk also describes the differently classed nightclub venues in Cairo (Van Nieuwkerk 1995: 87–89).

However, Sahin delves much further into the nightclub circuit, detailing the disparities—both subtle and overt—in clientele, in performer and audience behaviors, and in the ebb and flow of the dance performance, among the nightclubs of the Nile cruise boats, the Haram Street cabarets, and the prestigious five-star hotels. As Sahin notes, some dancers who start their careers in the cabarets will deny their experience in these settings once they have achieved success in more prestigious venues (Sahin 2018: 151). This aligns with Roushdy's observation that professional dancers negotiate their marginality by attempting to choose and control the contexts of their performances (Roushdy 2009: 84). In short, each performance setting—*mūlid*, wedding, cabaret, five-star hotel—produces a unique web of social and cultural meanings. Professional belly dancers develop strategies for navigating within these meaningful spaces: choosing or avoiding certain spaces, adjusting technique and style, carefully selecting appropriate costuming.

Indeed, so crucial is the space of performance, that it has impacted not only the choices of individual performers, but the broader stylistic evolution of belly dance as a whole. In my own work, I have described how the emergence of new performance venues in Egypt's urban centers in the late nineteenth century facilitated transformations in the traditional dance styles of the *ʿawālim* and the *ghawāzī*, leading to the emergence of an entirely new genre of professional belly dance (Ward 2018). Within the theaters and music halls of turn-of-the-century Cairo and Alexandria, Egyptian artists and entertainers were actively and creatively negotiating the tensions between tradition and modernity and between indigenous* interests and foreign influences. These creative spaces enabled the hybridization of foreign and indigenous elements within Egyptian belly dance, ultimately giving rise to theatrical *raqṣ sharqī*, today the most widely recognized incarnation of professional belly dance.

---

* It is important to note here that Egyptian identity has been defined in different ways throughout Egyptian history, rendering the meaning of terms like "indigenous" and "native" somewhat variable. In general, when I use terms like "indigenous Egyptian" or "native Egyptian," I am referring to the locally born and locally residing popular classes of Egyptian society, as opposed to foreign occupiers and ruling elites. However, this distinction becomes significantly muddied during the British Occupation, when even some members of Egypt's Turco-Circassian ruling elite began to embrace the budding Egyptian nationalist movement (e.g., Khedive ʿAbbās Ḥilmī).

Less directly addressed in prior research is the manner in which professional belly dancers impact and shape the spaces they occupy. Sahin's work comes closest to confronting this issue. She notes that, while the dance space is critical in shaping meaning, the bodies within the space are active in creating meanings of their own. In other words, researchers must attend not only to "how space shapes meanings but how bodies moving within such spaces choreograph significant weight in what semiotics are created, deconstructed, and exchanged" (Sahin 2018: 127–128). Moreover, individual dancers navigate spaces in unique ways, creating meaning in personal ways: "Although dance's form and structure are shaped by the space it occurs within, it is the bodies within those spaces that have the ultimate power in creating meanings. Thus, different dancers create different shows with differing semiotics even while sharing the same stage space" (Sahin 2018: 199–200).

However, while Sahin's work addresses how dancers construct and negotiate meanings within the spaces of performance, it does not fully address how *the space itself* is imparted with meaning due to the presence of the dancer. Importantly, professional belly dancers occupy certain spaces within the Cairene landscape, and the perception of these spaces appears to be tied, at least in part, to the presence of professional entertainers. Of interest in this regard are not only the spaces of professional performance, but also the spaces that entertainers inhabit when they are not on stage. In the massive metropolis of Cairo, there are spaces that carry deep historical attachments to professional entertainers. Sites such as Azbakīyah, 'Imād al-Dīn Street, Muḥammad 'Alī Street, and Haram Street have been linked to professional entertainers and to the entertainment trades for generations, and their images in the Egyptian public imagination appear to have been molded by their association with professional entertainers, particularly belly dancers.

The enduring image of Muḥammad 'Alī Street as Cairo's *Shāri' al-Fann*, or Street of Art, illustrates the deep connection between professional entertainers and certain Cairo spaces. This broad boulevard, extending from 'Atabah Square southeast to the Citadel, was constructed during the reign of Khedive Ismā'īl (r. 1863–1879) (Abu-Lughod 1971: 95–97, 112–113). The street was conceived under his grandfather, Muḥammad 'Alī Bāshā (r. 1805–1848), as a means to connect the latter's palaces at Azbakīyah and the Citadel. Under Ismā'īl, Muḥammad 'Alī Street joined the Khedive's newly-developed downtown to the historic seat of his dynasty's power.

From its earliest days, Muḥammad 'Alī Street was home to Cairo's musicians, singers, and dancers, many of whom found work in the weddings of the urban lower and middle classes, or else in the entertainment halls that were emerging in nearby Azbakīyah and 'Imād al-Dīn Street.

The street also became home to a range of businesses connected to the entertainment industry, including costumers, musical instrument manufacturers, record producers, and more. Interestingly, a market for musical instruments existed in this part of the city *centuries before* the construction of Muḥammad ʿAlī Street, and popular lore tied the area's questionable reputation to this market and to the entertainers who patronized it. The area's prior connections to professional entertainment indicate that it was not a coincidence that the newly-constructed street became a draw for people in the entertainment trade, and they demand a deeper analysis of precisely when and how these connections developed.

The golden age of Muḥammad ʿAlī Street was in the early-to-mid twentieth century, when the street was lined with shops selling musical instruments and with cafés where male musicians and singers would sit, sip tea, and smoke shisha while waiting to be hired for parties (Puig 2001, 2006). The female singer/dancers known as *ʿawālim* resided there, as well as in the smaller streets and alleys near the main street (Van Nieuwkerk 1995: 50). Famous *ʿawālim* hung signs outside of their homes to advertise their availability for weddings and parties; they conducted meetings with clients in their downstairs offices or else in the local cafés. The reputation of the street was well-known. Katherine Zirbel (2000: 124) writes:

> As home to families of musicians, dancers, actors, singers, and circus performers, it was a neighborhood that gained quasi-bohemian associations with its intersection of working-class identification and popular arts, along with stories of licentious living, prostitution, and drugs.

Beginning in the 1970s, however, the role of Muḥammad ʿAlī Street as a center for the entertainment industry declined precipitously (Puig 2001, 2006; Van Nieuwkerk 1995: 55–60). Gradually, most of the music shops were replaced by furniture stores, and nearly all of the entertainers' cafes closed their doors. In spite of this decline, the association of Muḥammad ʿAlī Street with entertainment and professional entertainers has endured. In the early 1990s, even as the real Muḥammad ʿAlī Street was overtaken by furniture shops, the beloved Egyptian actress Sharīhān sang and danced her way through a vibrant neighborhood of popular entertainers in the stage musical *Shāriʿ Muḥammad ʿAlī*. The street's somewhat risqué and dangerous reputation has persisted as well. In my own experience, if I mentioned my visits to Muḥammad ʿAlī Street to Egyptians outside the entertainment trades, I was generally met with reactions ranging from incredulity to concern for my safety.

The meaningful presence of belly dance and its professional practitioners in Cairo spaces such as Muḥammad ʿAlī Street, together with the undeniable importance of space in meaningfully framing and shaping both dance and dancer, demand a more in-depth investigation of the interconnection between dance spaces and dance practitioners. What is the nature of the relationship between belly dance space and belly dancer in the Cairo landscape? What role has this relationship played in positioning dance and dancer in Egyptian society through the course of Cairo's history?

A Theoretical Framework for Examining the Relationship Between Dancer and Dance Space

In recent decades, space and place have emerged as important avenues of inquiry in fields as varied as anthropology, history, human geography, philosophy, and sociology (Lawrence and Low 1990, Low and Lawrence-Zúñiga 2003). A great deal of recent scholarship has been focused on the process by which space, the physical and ambient dimension of human experience, is transformed into place, sites that are invested with cultural and social meanings (Aucoin 2017: 396–397). Aucoin (2017: 397) writes: "Those cultural activities in which people engage in order to render spaces meaningful, whether these spaces are built, worked over, lived in, or part of a space imaginary, are place-making practices." In essence, the actions of human agents imbue spaces with meaning. On the other hand, meaningful spaces frame and shape the world—physical and social—of the individuals who act within them. In short, to understand space and place requires an awareness of the impact of individual agency on the production and reproduction of space/place, while conversely, to understand the motivations and choices of individual actors requires a cognizance of the predispositions generated within the spatial milieu.

Here it is critical to turn to the work of Pierre Bourdieu and his theory of practice, as it provides an overall framework for examining the relationship between meaningful spaces and human agents. Bourdieu's monumental contribution to understanding human societies is in reconciling structuralist and phenomenological approaches by framing the relationship between subjectivity and objectivity as dialectical and mutually constituting. In other words, social structures are constituted by the actions of individual agents, while on the other hand, the perceptions and choices of individual actors are unconsciously informed by social structures. Central to Bourdieu's theoretical framework is the concept of *habitus*, defined as:

> Systems of durable, transposable *dispositions*, structured structures predisposed to function as structuring structures, that is, as principles of the

> generation and structuring of practices and representations which can be objectively "regulated" and "regular" without in any way being the product of obedience to rules, objectively adapted to their goals without presupposing a conscious aiming at ends or an express mastery of the operations necessary to attain them and, being all this, collectively orchestrated without being the product of the orchestrating action of a conductor [Bourdieu 1977: 72].

Habitus is the unconscious disposition of individuals toward certain routine actions and representations. Yet, engaging in routine practice unconsciously reinforces the social order which generates the dispositions of the individual actor. In other words, habitus consists of systems of dispositions that are informed by the social structure which habitus itself generates.

In essence, the social order is produced—and reproduced—through the collective practice of individual agents, each informed by his or her own habitus. Even the most mundane day-to-day activities are integral to the process of social production/reproduction, for it is through ordinary practice, predisposed by habitus, that the social order is both normalized and reified:

> Habitus is both a system of schemes of production of practices and a system of perception and appreciation of practices. And, in both of these dimensions, its operation expresses the social position in which it was elaborated [Bourdieu 1989: 19].

Critically, for the individual agent, habitus creates the normal world, "...a world of common sense, a world that seems self-evident."

Bourdieu long recognized the role of physical space in the formation of habitus and the process of social production/reproduction. This is well illustrated in his landmark study of the Kabyle house (Bourdieu 2003). In the structure of the Kabyle house, Bourdieu finds the spatial embodiment of Kabyle social structure. The physical layout of the house embodies a fundamental male-female opposition in Kabyle social reality that manifests in analogous oppositions of high-low, dry-wet, light-dark, etc. As Fogle (2011: 46) notes, the association between these oppositions is arbitrary; that is, "the very opposition of their terms is the mediating factor that creates the analogy." The house itself exists in opposition to the outside world: the house is the female domain, and the external world is the male domain. Thus, the internal organization of the house exists as an inversion or mirror image of the organization of the outside world. In Bourdieu's (2003: 140) words: "The house is an empire within an empire, but one which always remains subordinate because, even though it presents all the properties and all the relations which define the archetypal world, it remains a reversed world, an inverted reflection." In essence, the

Kabyle physical world presents a complex array of nested oppositions, all of which embody the fundamental male-female opposition.

What is important in Bourdieu's analysis, though, is not simply the elucidation of gender dynamics in Kabyle society. Rather, Bourdieu's examination of the Kabyle house is groundbreaking in revealing the critical role of physical space in the production and reproduction of the social order. As individuals move through and act within the Kabyle house, a space which is pregnant with social meanings, they are unconsciously invoking and reifying these meanings. Bourdieu writes:

> But it is in the dialectical relationship between the body and a space structured according to the mythico-ritual oppositions that one finds the form par excellence of the structural apprenticeship which leads to the em-bodying of the structures of the world, that is, the appropriating by the world of a body thus enabled to appropriate the world [Bourdieu 1977: 89].

That is, body and space are engaged in a dialectical relationship in which each imparts meaning upon the other: the body inscribes meanings onto physical space, while the meanings embedded in the structure of physical space are constantly re-experienced by the body as it exists and acts within that space.

Bourdieu's concern with space was elaborated upon in his later works. For Bourdieu, physical space and what he termed social space were interconnected (Bourdieu 1989, 1996, 2018). With the concept of social space, Bourdieu approached the structural analysis of social hierarchies and power dynamics in spatial terms:

> Just as physical space is defined by the mutual externality of parts, social space is defined by the mutual exclusion (or distinction) of positions which constitute it, that is, as a structure of juxtaposition of social positions. Social agents, but also things as they are appropriated by agents and thus constituted as properties, are situated in a location in social space which can be characterized by its position relative to other locations (as standing above, below or in between them) and by the distance which separates them [Bourdieu 1996: 12].

Bourdieu saw in physical space a "retranslation" of the relationships present in social space, and, conversely, the reification of the physical spatial order in the structure of social space. The actions of the body, predisposed by habitus, become the intersecting point between physical space and social space:

> The progressive inscription into bodies of the structures of the social order is perhaps accomplished, for the most part, *via moves and movements of the body, via the bodily poses and postures* that these social structures reconverted into physical structures—organize and qualify socially as in rive or decline,

> entry (inclusion) or exit (exclusion), bringing together or distancing in relation to central and valued site [Bourdieu 1996: 16].

These points are elaborated upon by Nikolaus Fogle, who builds on Bourdieu's work by integrating social space and physical space into an overarching theoretical framework (Fogle 2011). For Fogle, social space and physical space are engaged in a process of dialectical interaction, with habitus as mediating force and "analogical operator." Fogle's model is not a simple dialectic between social space and physical space, with habitus "translating" between them. Rather, Fogle stresses the subjective and objective dimensions of each of the three components, noting the dialectical interchange between physical space and habitus, as well as between social space and habitus.

In Bourdieu's formulation of social space, he suggests that proximity in social space typically implies proximity in physical space, and *vice versa* (see, for example, Bourdieu 1996: 13). He writes:

> The model thus defines distances that are *predictive* of encounters, affinities, sympathies, or even desires: concretely, this means that people located at the top of the space have little chance of marrying people located toward the bottom, first because they have little chance of meeting them physically (except in what are called "bad places," i.e., at the cost of a transgression of the social limits which reflect the spatial distances); then because, if they do meet them on some occasion, accidentally, they will not get on together, will not really understand each other, will not appeal to one another. On the other hand, proximity in social space predisposes to closer relations: people who are inscribed in a confined sector of space will be both closer (in their properties and in their dispositions, *their tastes*) and more disposed to get closer, as well as being easier to bring together, to mobilize [Bourdieu 1996: 19].

While he acknowledges that there are circumstances wherein individuals who are socially distant may be physically close, he tends toward the conclusion that socially distant individuals abhor sharing physical space with one another:

> We are thus led to question the belief that spatial closeness or, more precisely, the cohabitation of agents very distant in social space can, by itself, have an effect of social rapprochement or, if one prefers, of desegregation. In point of fact, nothing is further removed, and more intolerable, than people socially distant who happen to come close in physical space [Bourdieu 2018: 111].

This aspect of Bourdieu's work on social space is problematic, as it does not adequately account for the social heterogeneity that can exist *within* certain physical spaces. Indeed, throughout the history of Cairo, it is easy to find examples of spaces where socially-distant individuals mingle freely and deliberately. They include the many public entertainment spaces that have defined the Cairene landscape: the canals and ponds of the pre-nineteenth-century suburbs, the Azbakīyah Gardens, the city cemeteries, and the festive spaces centered on local shrines and tombs. In these spaces, social groups that were normally segregated were brought into close proximity, both spatially and socially: men and women, elite and poor, Christian and Muslim. Behaviors that were frowned upon in other spaces were ignored or even accepted. In essence, these were spaces within which the social order was challenged, even upended.

Here it is useful to turn to Michel Foucault's notion of heterotopia. Foucault envisioned a heterotopia as a space that both reflects and distorts other spaces, variously representing, reinforcing, challenging, or subverting the latter. In Foucault's words:

> There are also, probably in every culture, in every civilization, real places—places that do exist and that are formed in the very founding of society—which are something like counter-sites, a kind of effectively enacted utopia in which the real sites, all the other real sites that can be found within the culture, are simultaneously represented, contested, and inverted. Places of this kind are outside of all places, even though it may be possible to indicate their location in reality. Because these places are absolutely different from all the sites that they reflect and speak about, I shall call them, by way of contrast to utopias, heterotopias [Foucault 1986: 24].

Foucault uses the mirror as a metaphor for understanding the nature of the heterotopia. In one sense, the mirror is a utopia, a placeless place: "In the mirror, I see myself there where I am not, in an unreal, virtual space that opens up behind the surface" (*ibid.*). Yet, the mirror itself *does* exist in reality, where it challenges the latter with its reflected image. In this sense, the mirror is a heterotopia:

> It makes this place that I occupy at the moment when I look at myself in the glass at once absolutely real, connected with all the space that surrounds it, and absolutely unreal, since in order to be perceived it has to pass through this virtual point which is over there [*ibid.*].

In much the same manner, the heterotopia functions in relation to all other space, either by creating a space of illusion that exposes (and potentially challenges or subverts) real space, or else by creating an alternative to real space, a space of compensation.

Foucault argues that heterotopias are universal; that is, they exist in every human society. However, the function of a heterotopia is embedded in social and historical context. Accordingly, the function and the meaning of a single heterotopia may change as the surrounding social and historical circumstances change. To illustrate this, Foucault uses the example of the cemetery in the context of Western cultures. According to Foucault, though the cemetery persists as a heterotopic space throughout Western history, its heterotopic nature has transformed in accordance with changing attitudes regarding death. From the dawn of the nineteenth century, as death and the dead came to be associated with illness, the cemetery changed from a physical manifestation of resurrection and the afterlife positioned in the midst of the living, "the sacred and immortal heart of the city," to a space associated with illness and contagion pushed outside the boundaries of the city and the domain of the living.

Foucault also argues that several potentially incompatible spaces can be juxtaposed within the single space of a heterotopia, and that heterotopias are linked to breaks from traditional time. Using the example of the theater, Foucault points out how multiple diverse spaces can be brought together within the theatrical space: "The theater brings onto the rectangle of the stage, one after the other, a whole series of places that are foreign to one another." Following this logic, the theater also illustrates how the heterotopia breaks from traditional time: within the temporal bounds of the theatrical performance, time can be sped up or slowed down, and multiple times can be contained within the time of the show, as days, nights, months, and even years are played out on the stage.

Lastly in Foucault's formulation, heterotopias are defined by systems of opening and closing that isolate them from other spaces, yet also make them penetrable. That is, there must be something that separates and isolates the heterotopia from "normal" space and time. Foucault describes heterotopic sites where entry is compulsory, such as prison, and sites where certain behaviors are required for entry, such as public baths. He also describes heterotopias that seem open and free to all, but which actually carry hidden exclusions.

After introducing heterotopia in the late 1960s, Foucault never elucidated the concept further, with the result that it is both tantalizingly relevant and frustratingly ambiguous to researchers of space and place. Indeed, it has been suggested that the notion of heterotopia is so broad and so ambiguous as to be virtually useless as a theoretical concept. Foucault described a dizzying array of spaces as heterotopias: brothels, cemeteries, fairgrounds, prisons, and many others, leaving one wondering which spaces are *not* heterotopias.

Yet, it is precisely the ambiguity inherent within the concept that makes it so useful in examining socially heterogeneous and ambiguous spaces such as those that form the focus of the current analysis. Heynen (2008: 321–322) writes:

> Foucault's heterotopias ... are spatio-temporal constellations that are marked by a fundamental ambiguity. They might harbour liberating practices, but one should question whether the liberation applies to everyone who is involved.

> They might provide places for transgression and excess, but it seems very well possible that what is transgression for one actor means oppression and domination for another. Indeed heterotopias seem to be the spaces where the interplay between normative disciplining and liberating transgression manifests itself most clearly.

Heynen's last statement is key. For Foucault, heterotopias exist at the interface of normative and counter-normative discourses: they may simultaneously reinforce and challenge the social order.

It is perhaps more useful to focus on the heterotopic qualities of certain spaces rather than to label these spaces strictly as heterotopias. Returning to Foucault's initial definition, a space that is heterotopic is a space that is distinguishable—spatially and temporally—from other spaces, and that variously serves to represent, reinforce, challenge, or subvert aspects of those other spaces. Heterotopic spaces, as spaces that exist, in Foucault's words, "outside of all places," enable the disruption and inversion of the normal social order. As such, heterotopic spaces are strongly evocative of Mikhail Bakhtin's notion of the carnivalesque (Bakhtin 1984, 1998).

Bakhtin's writings on carnival and the carnivalesque revolve around his historical analysis of the Medieval European carnival, an event which:

> Celebrated temporary liberation from the prevailing truth and from the established order; it marked the suspension of all hierarchical rank, privileges, norms, and prohibitions. Carnival was the true feast of time, the feast of becoming, change, and renewal. It was hostile to all that was immortalized and completed [Bakhtin 1984: 10].

The carnival was a "second world" or "second life," one that existed outside of the bounds of the ordinary. In the carnival, social hierarchies were disrupted, enabling the free and familiar association of normally socially distant individuals. Social norms were suspended, and behaviors that would be considered eccentric or inappropriate during "non-carnival" time were permitted or even encouraged. Things earthly and body-based were celebrated rather than condemned. The carnival enabled what Bakhtin termed *carnivalistic mésalliances*: "All things that were once self-enclosed, disunified, distanced from one another by a noncarnivalistic hierarchical worldview are drawn into carnivalistic contacts and combinations" (Bakhtin 1998: 251).

The parallels here with Foucault's heterotopia are evident. In fact, I argue that these two concepts necessarily complement one another. Heterotopia provides the spatial dimension to the carnivalesque; that is, heterotopic spaces are spaces that embody the carnivalesque. Bakhtin himself remarked upon the spatial dimension of carnival, noting that the public square was the "main arena" for the carnival, and that in carnivalesque literature:

> The carnival square—the square of carnival acts—acquired an additional symbolic overtone that broadened and deepened it. In carnivalized literature the square, as a setting for the action of the plot, becomes two-leveled and ambivalent: it is as if there glimmered through the actual square the carnival square of free familiar contact and communal performances of crowning and decrowning. Other places of action as well ... can, if they become meeting- and contact-points for heterogeneous people—streets, taverns, roads, bathhouses, docks of ships, and so on—take on this additional carnival-square significance [Bakhtin 1998: 255–256].

Here, Bakhtin only accords this "symbolic overtone" to the carnival square in literature. That is, he recognizes the symbolic weight of the carnival space, but only in its literary incarnation. Going a step further, I argue that the "carnival square," or more broadly, the space that hosts the carnivalesque, becomes "two-leveled and ambivalent" *in actuality.* In other words, the space takes on the ambivalence and ambiguity of the action occurring within it: the space becomes heterotopic. This returns us to the work of Bourdieu, as it is practice—that is, the action of human agents—that inscribes meanings into physical space, and that is the mechanism by which human actors re-experience these meanings. Practice, predisposed by habitus, become the intersecting point between the spatial world and the social world, and the means by which the social order is produced.

There have been a few efforts to apply the concept of heterotopia to the Cairene landscape, most notably the works of Lucie Ryzova (2015) and Farha Ghannam (2016). Both have both relied on the notion of heterotopia in their examinations of certain spaces in present-day Cairo. Ryzova (2015: 5) approaches Cairo's downtown as a heterotopic space:

> It is a heterogeneous urban space, a space where everyone is a stranger *de passage*. This social porousness invites nonhegemonic forms of behaviour and is in turn constructed by them. It is also a symbolic location that is crucial—first by its absence and then by its presence—to Egyptian national imagery, and thus the site of competing claims on social order that extend well beyond its spatial boundaries.

Ryzova examines how diverse publics—artistic bohemians from the 1970s through 2000s, post–2011 revolutionary youth activists and sympathizers, and low-income boys and young men—produce and reproduce downtown Cairo through their practice. Simultaneously, she explores the historical and temporal dimension of downtown's heterotopic nature, noting how downtown has been variously constructed and contested throughout its history, as well as during particular times such as evenings, weekends, and popular holidays.

Farha Ghannam (2016) approaches Cairo's Taḥrīr Square, the flashpoint of the 2011 revolution, as a heterotopic space, "a 'counter arrangement,' which forcefully articulated an alternative understanding of order, citizenship, and civic responsibility that sharply contrasted with the corruption and injustice the protestors sought to transform." For Ghannam, the focus is on how the heterotopic space of Taḥrīr was re-appropriated and redefined by a variety of sociopolitical actors in the wake of the revolution. In her analysis, Ghannam comes to the conclusion that no space is inherently heterotopic: rather, it is the use of the space—that is, the practice of actors within the space—that give it its heterotopic qualities.

Importantly, in the works of both Ryzova and Ghannam, the discussion leads back to practice: the manner in which the collective action of individual agents imparts meanings within a space, and conversely, how actors re-experience those meanings while moving and acting within that space. Ryzova's discussion of Cairo's downtown illustrates how the varied publics of her analysis have each contributed to the inscription of meaning onto this space merely by their presence: socializing, "hanging out," strolling the downtown boulevards, "performing" political and social identities. Simultaneously, while moving through downtown, they are actively experiencing these embedded meanings. Cairo's downtown heterotopia is constantly and actively produced, and simultaneously experienced, by these diverse agents. As Ghannam (2016) explicitly states:

> Rather than a permanent quality or a fixed feature, it is the use of a particular space that makes it heterotopic. In this sense, no space is inherently, continuously, or fully heterotopia. For a space to be heterotopic, it must be used, I argue, in ways that materialize an alternative vision of society (or parts of it) that contrasts with the present, and that actualize a potential substitute for an existing system, or set of relationships.

In other words, while heterotopia offers a critical tool for conceptualizing the complexity and heterogeneity of particular spaces, it is practice that provides the overarching framework for understanding the mutually constituting relationship between these meaningful spaces and the human actors within them.

In essence, practice/habitus is necessary to explain how the spaces of interest in the current discussion came to be imbued with heterotopic qualities, and how these spaces retained these qualities for centuries, even in the face of changes to the physical landscape. These spaces played host to behaviors and activities that deviated from mainstream norms in this Muslim-majority city, and they enabled the mingling of normally discrete social groups—that is, carnivalesque behaviors and interactions. Practice provides the mechanism by which ambivalence and transgression were inscribed and re-inscribed into these spaces, allowing the abnormal to exist as a normal part of Cairo's social and spatial reality.

Dancer and Dance Space in the Cairo Landscape

In this work, I rely on the theoretical perspectives just outlined to examine the relationship between belly dance space and belly dancer in the Cairo landscape over the course of the city's history, from the establishment of al-Qāhirah in 969 AD until the present moment. Following Pierre Bourdieu, I approach the relationship between these spaces and the Egyptians existing and acting within them as dialectical and mutually constituting: individuals have inscribed meanings onto physical spaces in the Cairo landscape, while these meanings have been constantly re-experienced and reified by individuals as they have moved and acted within these spaces. In addition to leveraging Bourdieu's theory of practice, I draw upon Michel Foucault's concept of heterotopia and Mikhail Bakhtin's notion of the carnivalesque to accommodate the social heterogeneity and ambiguity that typifies so many of the Cairo spaces associated with professional entertainment and entertainers. I approach practice/habitus as the means by which ambivalence and transgression were inscribed and re-inscribed within certain Cairene spaces—that is, how carnivalesque behavior and interactions came to be embodied as heterotopic spaces. Taken together, these theoretical perspectives provide a robust framework for examining the relationship between belly dance spaces and belly dance practitioners in the Cairo landscape, and they help to explain why and how certain Cairo spaces have retained centuries-long historical associations with dance and dancers.

Over the course of the following chapters, I explore the dialectical interplay between professional belly dancers and the spaces of entertainment within the Cairo landscape, illustrating how the evolution of Cairo's entertainment landscape from the Fatimid era until the present day has been deeply interwoven with the evolving roles of dance and dancers in Egyptian society. The routine practice of individual dancers, alongside the routine practice of their accompanying musicians, their audiences, and others, have contributed to the production of meaningful spaces in the Cairo landscape. Meanwhile, those meaningful spaces have predisposed the individuals moving within them toward certain perceptions and actions; that is, those spaces have informed each individual's habitus. In this manner, the Cairo landscape has been embedded with meanings pertaining to dance and dancers that have been re-inscribed as agents have moved and acted within it. The entertainment landscape of Cairo has emerged from the lived experience of Egyptians, yet it simultaneously informs the social and spatial reality of those living and moving within the city.

Throughout this work, I reveal how the dialectic between dance space and professional dancer has served to reify shared perceptions and behaviors toward dance and dancer in Egyptian society, as well as towards the spaces associated with dance and dancers. For centuries, professional entertainers have been a liminal and ambiguous presence in Egyptian social and spatial life. Similarly, spaces of professional entertainment have existed as zones of ambivalence and liminality in the spatial reality of Cairo: heterotopic spaces within which the normal social and spatial boundaries of Egyptian society are blurred, challenged, and upended. The mutually constituting relationship between belly dance space and belly dance practitioner has ensured that each has imparted their ambiguous and liminal qualities on the other.

Additionally, I demonstrate that the meanings inscribed into the Cairo landscape have in many cases persisted despite major changes to the built environment. Dance and dancer have been so deeply written into certain spaces that even the redrawing of the city map could not fully alter this reality. Even the direct action of the state—such as the massive modernization projects of the late nineteenth century—could not erase the meanings that had been embedded in the landscape over the course of centuries.

Chapter One presents a detailed history of belly dance and its professional practitioners in Egypt. Beginning with the female slave entertainers of the ninth century and ending with the belly dancers of the present day, this overview provides a necessary framework for the remainder of the book. Who were Egypt's professional entertainers, and what were they called? What were their roles in Egyptian society, and how did those roles change over the course of Egyptian history? The history outlined in this chapter illustrates that belly dance and its professional practitioners have been a constant presence in Egyptian life for centuries. Although their identities have placed them outside of the mainstream of Egyptian society, these marginal men and women have figured prominently in the social and spatial realities of Egyptians for generations.

Chapter Two illustrates how, with the foundation of al-Qāhirah in 969, spaces of entertainment came to be woven into the geography of the city, establishing a landscape of entertainment that would continue to develop and elaborate in ensuing eras. Over the course of the Fatimid and Ayyubid periods, certain public spaces began to have clear associations in the popular imagination with entertainment and leisure—most notably, the canals and ponds of the city's suburbs, as well as the city's shrines and cemeteries. By the Mamluk era, the suburbs of Cairo, as hubs of recreation and leisure, and the city cemeteries, which played host to a complex mix of sacred and secular activities, had emerged as zones of ambivalence and liminality in the spatial reality of greater Cairo. These were heterotopic spaces, where diverse populations converged and interfaced, and where the normal social order was challenged and occasionally upended. The presence and practice of professional entertainers in these spaces contributed to the re-inscription of heterotopic meanings. Throughout the Mamluk era, the spaces that constituted Cairo's landscape of entertainment continued to be set apart by their ambiguity and liminality, as professional entertainers and other marginal personae lived and worked within them.

Chapter Three traces the evolution and expansion of Cairo's entertainment landscape from the Ottoman conquest until the beginning of the British occupation of Egypt. Under the Ottomans, the area that had come to be known as Azbakīyah, after the pond of the same name, became the focal point of entertainment and leisure in Cairo's western suburbs. Azbakīyah, together with Rumaylah Square, functioned as the main gathering spaces for Cairo's common people, and the city's shrines and cemeteries continued to be important spaces of popular entertainment and recreation, particularly during holidays and festivals. The introduction of coffee houses under the Ottomans, and of formal theaters under the brief Napoleonic occupation, eventually added important new sites to Cairo's entertainment landscape. In the nineteenth century, the modernization projects of Muḥammad ʿAlī Bāshā and his grandson Ismāʿīl drastically transformed the urban geography of Cairo.

Nevertheless, Cairo's "new" downtown carried forward the heterotopic features that had defined the region west of the "old" downtown for hundreds of years, and the association of spaces like Azbakīyah with entertainment and its professional practitioners would persist. Accounts of Egypt's belly dancers become increasingly abundant at this time, due in large measure to the growing European presence in Egypt. Thanks to the Europeans' fixation with these professional entertainers, their accounts paint a vivid picture of how embedded these men and women were in the social and spatial reality of Cairo, and their key role in the ongoing re-inscription of heterotopic meanings in the landscape.

Chapter Four explores the disruptions and the continuities in Cairo's entertainment landscape over the course of the British occupation of Egypt, and how these developments were interwoven with the fortunes of professional belly dancers. Perhaps the most significant development in this era was the proliferation of theaters and music halls—dedicated structures for the performance and consumption of professional entertainment. Though this type of venue was first introduced to Egypt roughly a hundred years earlier, it was at the turn of the nineteenth and twentieth centuries that these establishments would become integral features within the entertainment landscape of Cairo. The majority of these venues were concentrated in Cairo's "new" downtown. Yet, as discussed in Chapter Three, the bustling downtown that was created through the urban design projects of Ismā'īl was situated within what had once been the city's western suburbs, the heart of Cairo's entertainment landscape. Thus the concentration of music halls and theaters here was no coincidence: these venues, ambivalent and liminal sites that enabled experimentation and innovation in traditional Egyptian entertainment, emerged in a space that had been firmly tied to professional entertainment for centuries, and that had long been characterized by its heterotopic qualities.

Belly dancers thrived in these new settings, and they became inextricably associated with the entertainment halls of Cairo. By the end of the 1930s, many dancers had achieved celebrity status, and more than a few owned and managed their own venues, enabling them to play a vital role in shaping the early to mid-twentieth-century Cairo entertainment landscape. Just a stone's throw from downtown Cairo, Muḥammad 'Alī Street blossomed into a commercial and residential center for belly dancers, singers, musicians, and other entertainment professionals. The existence of an entertainers' market in this area as early as the Mamluk era, together with its geographic proximity to both downtown Cairo/Azbakīyah and Rumaylah Square ensured the significance of this space in the entertainment landscape.

Chapter Five examines continuity and change in the Cairo entertainment landscape from the Revolution of 1952 to the present day, and how the circumstances of belly dance and belly dancers in the current moment are directly tied to these developments. The sociocultural, political, and economic upheavals in the wake of the 1950s—in particular, Nasser's experiments with socialism and Sadat's open-door economic policy—have dramatically reshaped the entertainment landscape of Cairo. While the second half of the twentieth century witnessed the emergence and temporary boom of a new space in the entertainment landscape—Haram Street—this period also saw the gradual decline of spaces such as Azbakīyah, 'Imād al-Dīn Street, and Muḥammad 'Alī Street. Downtown Cairo, formerly the western suburb of al-Qāhirah, is no longer at the heart of the entertainment landscape, and Muḥammad 'Alī Street no longer functions as the residential and commercial hub for professional entertainers. Nevertheless, these spaces retain their connections to professional entertainment—and to belly dance and belly dancers—in the popular imagination. Their nostalgic portrayals in recent television and cinema attest to the centuries-long interconnection between these spaces and professional entertainment in the social and spatial reality of Cairo. On the other hand, these portrayals contrast with ambiguous and ambivalent perceptions of the "real life" neighborhoods of downtown Cairo and Muḥammad ʻAlī Street, revealing the persistence of the heterotopic meanings inscribed within them over the course of many centuries.

The scope of this analysis necessitated a careful reconstruction of Cairo's spatial and social realities from the Fatimid era until the present day. Accordingly, I depended on a broad range of primary and secondary source materials in order to conduct this study. Most of these were text sources, although I also relied on period maps, a number of films and audio recordings, and personal interviews. Throughout my research, I attempted to center Egyptian and other Middle Eastern and North African sources as much as possible.

Of vital importance were the works of Egyptian chroniclers such as Abū al-Maḥāsin Yūsuf Ibn Taghrībirdī, ʻAbd al-Raḥmān al-Jabartī, and Taqī al-Dīn al-Maqrīzī, all of which were crucial to my ability to reconstruct the landscape of Cairo in different periods of Egyptian history. The chronicles of al-Maqrīzī, in particular, provided a thorough and detailed accounting of the Cairene landscape from the Fatimid conquest until well into the Mamluk era. William Popper's maps based on Ibn Taghrībird's chronicles were invaluable to my understanding of Mamluk Cairo. And although the *Description de l'Égypte* was an indispensable resource for reconstructing late Ottoman Cairo, al-Jabartī's writings provided the context and the perspective on the city that could never be captured by the French account.

Egyptian and other Middle Eastern and North African authors also provided critical insights into Cairene society at various periods throughout the city's history, and how Cairo's social and spatial realities intersected. Beyond the aforementioned Egyptian chroniclers and other Egyptian authors, the accounts penned by Middle Eastern and North African visitors to Egypt—individuals such as Leo Africanus, Evliya Çelebi, and Nassiri Khosrau—provided some of the most vivid accounts of early Cairo. Occasionally, works of fiction were just as valuable as historical chronicles. The shadow plays of Muḥammad Ibn Dāniyāl, for example, viscerally situated me in Cairo's medieval underworld, while the fictional narratives of Muḥammad al-Muwayliḥī made Cairo's turn-of-the-century night life palpable and real.

Still, certain foreign accounts, such as the *Description de l'Égypte*, were vital to defining the historical landscape of Cairo, as well as in providing interesting details not always present in Egyptian accounts.

Perhaps the greatest value provided by Western sources was their tendency to include painstakingly detailed descriptions of belly dance and its professional practitioners, a feature often strangely absent from Egyptian sources. Yet the value of these sources had to be balanced against their pervasive Orientalist bias. These issues will be discussed further at the outset of Chapter One.

Most of my sources were accessed through libraries and digital archives, though I also depended on my personal collection of books, maps, images, and ephemera. The proliferation of digital archives in recent years has opened up new horizons for independent researchers such as myself. Thanks to archives such as the HathiTrust Digital Library, the Internet Archive, and New York University's Arabic Collections Online, an array of sources is literally at one's fingertips. Through digital archives, I was able to access the chronicles of al-Jabartī and al-Maqrīzī, among others, without which I would not have been able to complete this project.

I hope that this book will be a useful addition to the body of knowledge regarding Egyptian belly dance, and I hope that this work will inspire further research into this dance form, its professional practitioners, and their complicated position in Egyptian society. Thankfully, the past twenty years or so have seen an increasing number of studies focusing on this subject matter. However, conflicted attitudes about this dance in its homeland, as well as popular misconceptions about the dance that persist outside Egypt, continue to stymie efforts to bring more scholarly attention to this dance form and its practitioners. The following chapters make it clear that belly dance, and the men and women who have performed it professionally for generations, are intertwined within the social and spatial reality of Egypt throughout its history: their story is part of Egypt's story, and their story deserves to be told.

ONE

A History of Belly Dance and Its Professional Practitioners in Egypt

In the present day, the most widely recognized professional incarnation of Egyptian belly dance is the dance form known as *raqṣ sharqī*. A relatively young dance form, *raqṣ sharqī* emerged at the turn of the twentieth century from the hybridization of the earlier dance traditions of the female professional entertainers known as the *'awālim* and the *ghawāzī* with elements derived from non–Egyptian dance forms (Ward 2018). The emergence and development of *raqṣ sharqī* is well documented in both Egyptian and foreign primary source materials.

The *'awālim* and the *ghawāzī* can be traced back to the eighteenth century; indeed, these women were somewhat obsessively documented by foreign visitors to Egypt from the eighteenth century onward. From the mid-eighteenth to mid-nineteenth centuries, these two categories of female professional singers/dancers could be distinguished based on the social class of their clientele: the *'awālim* were entertainers for Egypt's ruling elite, while the *ghawāzī* were entertainers for the masses. From the mid-nineteenth century onward, due to a range of social, political, and economic circumstances, the distinction between these groups shifted from one based on class to one based on geography. At the turn of the twentieth century, the *'awālim* were recognized as singers/dancers who provided entertainment for the urban lower and lower-middle classes, while the *ghawāzī* were entertainers for Egyptians dwelling in the towns and villages of the countryside.

The urban *versus* rural connotation of the terms *'awālim* and *ghawāzī* is still generally understood by Egyptians in the present, though the *'awālim* tradition no longer exists, and only a scattering of *ghawāzī* still perform in rural Upper Egypt. The terms *'awālim* and *ghawāzī* are now regarded as somewhat old-fashioned, and a female dancer, whether *ʿālmah*, *ghāziyah*, or practitioner of *raqṣ sharqī*, is generally known as a *rāqiṣah* or *raqqāṣah* (plural *rāqiṣāt* or *raqqāṣāt*, respectively), meaning "dancer," or a *fannānah* (plural *fannānāt*), meaning "artist."

Contemporary with the *ʿawālim* and the *ghawāzī* were the male professional entertainers known as the *khawalāt* (singular *khawal*) and the *jink*.* Like the *ʿawālim* and the *ghawāzī*, these men are well documented by foreign observers. These sources suggest that these men were the male counterparts of the *ghawāzī*—that is, they performed in similar contexts and played a similar role in Egyptian society. Male professional belly dancers continued to practice their trade well into the first half of the twentieth century. After seemingly declining around mid-century, male dancers experienced a resurgence in the late twentieth century and are an important presence in the belly dance industry in the present day. Today, the term *jink* is obsolete, and *khawal* is a negative slang term referring to a male homosexual; a male dancer is now known by the term *rāqiṣ* or *raqqāṣ* (plural *rāqiṣūn* or *raqqāṣūn*, respectively), which simply means "dancer."

At the time of this writing, I have not encountered the terms *ʿālmah*, *ghāziyah*, and *khawal* in reference to professional entertainers in Egypt prior to the eighteenth century (references to *jink* appear somewhat earlier in the Ottoman era). Either these terms were not in common usage, or they were not favored by authors in earlier periods. Nevertheless, there are historical references to professional entertainers who would have played similar roles to the nineteenth-century *ʿawālim*, *ghawāzī*, *khawalāt*, and *jink* in earlier periods of Egyptian history. For example, sources from the Mamluk era include numerous mentions of female performers providing diversion to Egypt's ruling elite, as well as public performers entertaining the masses during special occasions, such as important Coptic and Islamic feast days. References to female professional entertainers in the Tulunid, Fatimid, and Ayyubid periods reveal that the tradition of engaging professional singing and dancing women was established much earlier. Specific mentions of *mukhannathūn*, effeminate male entertainers, in medieval Egyptian sources suggest early historical precedent for the roles of the *khawal* and the *jink*.

The earlier the source, the more difficult it becomes to draw a lineal connection between the song and dance styles of these early entertainers and the well-documented performance styles of Egypt's professional belly dancers in the modern era. Still, it is clear that singers and dancers were a critical part of Egyptian social life long before eighteenth and

* After consulting with multiple native speakers of Egyptian Arabic, I have come to the conclusion that there seems to be no differentiation between the singular and the plural of this term.

nineteenth-century Europeans and Americans made their detailed observations of *'awālim*, *ghawāzī*, *khawalāt*, and *jink*, the first "belly dancers" of modern times. Consequently, the story of professional belly dance in Egypt can best be told by reconstructing the history of professional entertainers.

In building this history, it is important to remember that the practitioners of professional dance in Egypt were rarely exclusively dancers. On the contrary, dance was generally only one of the skills in the repertoire of professional entertainers. As both Shiloah (1962: 469) and Shay (2014: 36–37) have noted, the sort of intense specialization that characterizes art and entertainment in the present day simply did not obtain in earlier eras. Even in the modern day, Van Nieuwkerk has documented how the traditional female entertainers that she met during her research were expected to be *shamla*, well-rounded or "complete"—that is, able to both sing and dance (Van Nieuwkerk 1995: 14, 59, 208). For this reason, it is necessary to examine professional entertainers in general, including those who may be labeled "singers" rather than "dancers" in primary sources.

In this chapter, I will endeavor to trace the history of professional entertainers in Egypt from roughly the ninth century until the present day. Who were these women and men? What were they called? What were their roles in Egyptian society, and how did those roles change over time? What will become clear over the course of this discussion is that Egypt's professional entertainers, though vital to many events and celebrations and deeply woven into the fabric of Egyptian social and cultural life, have existed as marginal figures, individuals who occupy an ambiguous and uncertain position in a society that nevertheless desires them. Despite the vicissitudes of history, the through line connecting these men and women over the course of these many centuries is that their identities place them outside the mainstream of Egyptian society.

Source materials pose a number of challenges to this endeavor—particularly primary sources dating prior to the early twentieth century. With regard to dance, Egyptian sources are often surprisingly lacking in details. I would posit two possible explanations for the lack of attention to dance in Egyptian primary sources. On the one hand, perhaps Egyptian authors felt little need to provide a detailed accounting of a dance which would be largely familiar to their readership. On the other, it seems reasonable to attribute this lack of detail to the authors' conflicted attitudes toward professional dance and dancers. The variability in accounts that do offer in-depth descriptions of dance and dancers manifest this tension.

For example, Muḥammad al-Muwayliḥī's fictional account of a dance performance and its aftermath at a Cairo music hall around the turn of the twentieth century (al-Muwayliḥī 2015, volume 2: 83–117) paints a scathing picture of moral turpitude, both on the part of the dancer and on the part of the men who populate the seedy establishment: the dance performance is associated with a range of vices including drunkenness, adultery, prostitution, and brawling. This contrasts markedly with Tawfīq al-Ḥakīm's warm and affectionate portrayal of the *'ālmah* Labībah (al-Ḥakīm 2019: 83–101), a fictionalized version of a real individual named Ḥamīdah, who was a family friend during al-Ḥakīm's childhood (see Lagrange 2009a). In fact, the entirety of chapter nine of al-Ḥakīm's novel *'Awdat al-Rūḥ* (*Return of the Spirit*) is dedicated to the main character Muhsin's recollections of Labībah, including a lyrical depiction of Labībah's dance during a wedding party (al-Ḥakīm 2019: 99–100).

Non-Egyptian primary sources pose challenges of their own. While Egyptian sources reflect local understandings and perceptions—albeit conflicted—regarding dance and its professional practitioners, European and other Western sources—particularly sources dating prior to the advent of post-colonial scholarship in the late twentieth century—are suffused with Orientalist attitudes toward Egypt and Egyptians. Orientalism, as defined and described by Palestinian-American scholar Edward Said in his seminal work on the subject (Said 1979), is a pattern of thought which creates an essentialist and stereotyped vision of the peoples and cultures of the Middle East, North Africa, and Asia—the so-called "Orient." Orientalism allows the "West" to define itself by constructing and controlling an opposing "East." Within the Orientalist paradigm, the Orient is characterized by its timelessness, irrationality, disorder, and depravity, while the Occident is regarded as progressive, rational, orderly, and virtuous. Orientalism does not merely define the Orient: it also provides the framework within which the Occident engages with the Orient. Edward Said writes:

> Taking the late eighteenth century as a very roughly defined starting point Orientalism can be discussed and analyzed as the corporate institution for dealing with the Orient—dealing with it by making statements about it, authorizing views of it, describing it, by teaching it, settling it, ruling over it: in short, Orientalism as a Western style for dominating, restructuring, and having authority over the Orient [Said 1979: 3].

While Western primary sources often include detailed and meticulous descriptions of Egypt's professional entertainers and their dance, these descriptions are generally pervaded by Orientalist value judgements of the subject matter. Particularly in sources from the eighteenth and nineteenth centuries, the inferiority of the Oriental to the Occidental is presumed; Egyptian dance is presented, at best, as a curiosity and at worst, as a primitive vulgarity. In light of this, though Western primary sources are replete with information about dance and dancers, they must be treated with caution. The unique circumstances and motivations behind each source must be carefully considered, and the information provided by foreign sources must be weighed in light of evidence from local sources.

Before the Mamluk Period

Female professional entertainers, particularly slave entertainers, are widely documented in the medieval Islamicate world, beginning in earnest with the rise of the Abbasid caliphate in the eighth century (Caswell 2011, Meyers Sawa 1987, Nielson 2017, Richardson 2009). Female slave entertainers were particularly prized among the Abbasid rulers and the nobility; the trade in slave women was booming and lucrative. This trade was not exclusively the domain of men: Myrne (2017: 63–64) notes that women owned, trained, and traded in slaves as well, and the ownership of female slaves was a mark of prestige for elite women.

In the literature of the time, the term *jāriyah* (plural *jawārī*) was used broadly to refer to a slave girl or concubine, as well as specifically to designate a female slave entertainer (see Myrne 2017: 66*n*, Nielson 2017: 79). A female slave singer might also be known as a *mughannīyah* (female singer, plural *mughannīyāt*) (Nielson 2017: 79), though this term could also refer to a free woman singer. Among the female slave entertainers was an elite class of slave courtesans known as the *qiyān* (sometimes *qaynāt*, singular *qaynah*) (Nielson 2017: 78–81, Richardson 2009).

Women entered into slavery through one of two means: they were either captured in warfare, or they were born to slave parents (Tolmacheva 2017: 163). As a result, slave women hailed from a broad range of ethnicities, including Armenians, Ethiopians, Greeks, Indians, Persians, and many others. Female slaves were destined for domestic service, which could also encompass entertainment functions. While many female slaves received some degree of musical training, those who displayed aptitude or talent went on to much more extensive and intensive musical education, since female slaves with musical ability were particularly prized as concubines. Female slaves with potential were sent by slave traders to train under famous musicians and singers, though sometimes training was provided by the slave traders themselves (Nielson 2017: 83).

Nielson (2017: 78–81) argues that although the terms *jāriyah*, *mughannīyah*, and *qaynah* are often used interchangeably in medieval Arabic sources to denote a "musical concubine" or woman musician, the term *qaynah* connotes a higher degree of musicianship, and by implication, courtesanship. The *qiyān* were set apart from other female slave entertainers by their extensive training, their exceptional skill set, and the extraordinary prices that they commanded on the slave market. Though frequently referred to as "singing girls" or "songstresses" in the English language, it is important to note that *qiyān* received training not only in music, but in a variety of other subjects, ranging from poetry recitation to courtly etiquette (Nielson 2017: 81–84, Richardson 2009: 110–111). The training of *qiyān* was a profitable enterprise: the famous Abbasid-era musician and singer Ibrāhīm al-Mawṣilī made a lucrative business of training and selling them (Caswell 2011: 17, Nielson 2017: 83).

Importantly for the current discussion, it is evident that some of these women were also trained in dance and included it in their performance repertoires (Richardson 2009: 114, Reynolds 2017: 117). Richardson (2009: 114) writes: "The qiyan could sing and play an instrument as a solo act, perform in ensemble recitals that combined instrumentalism, song, and dance, or even participate in competitions between highly rated singers." Shiloah (1962) makes a strong case that dance was an important and valued art form that was inextricably linked to music performance in the Islamicate courts. Nevertheless, as both Sawa (2018: 312–321) and Shiloah (1962) have noted, detailed accounts of dance are few and far between in medieval Arabic sources. Shiloah (1962: 463) attributes this absence to moralistic attitudes regarding dance: "Hostile in a certain sense to music, the Muslim religion was to be all the more hostile to dance, which could undermine morality." Yet, as Sawa points out, although music was also viewed as morally questionable by many, this certainly did not prevent medieval authors from writing extensively about it (Sawa 2018: 312). This puzzling lack of attention to dance (in comparison to music and song) in the Arabic-language primary sources is a phenomenon that persists into later periods.

The primary performance context of Abbasid-era female slave entertainers was the *majlis* (plural *majālis*), a musical event held in the court or in an elite household (Caswell 2011: 236–237, Nielson 2017: 86).* A *majlis* could be planned or impromptu, and it could involve considerable expense. Nielson (2017: 86) writes:

> The format of a *majlis* was highly ritualized and organized, with standing conventions of behavior, appearance, and subject matter. In addition, the visual element was an important aspect of the performance, and a great amount of effort and expense was made to set the proper environment for the musical event.

Beyond the *majlis*, performances of female slave entertainers could be enjoyed in certain public houses (Caswell 2011: 25–31, Nielson 2017: 84).

* The term *majlis* also refers to the salon in which such gatherings took place (see Shiloah 1995: 12).

Nielson notes that it is unclear whether these establishments were houses for the musical training of slaves, actual brothels, or some combination thereof (Nielson 2017: 84). Caswell indicates that these public houses were widespread in Abbasid Baghdad and Kufa (Caswell 2011: 25).

Female slave entertainers occupied a complex and ambiguous social and moral position relative to other slave and free women of the time. Unlike free women of the nobility, who were bound by rules regarding veiling and seclusion, slave entertainers were generally unveiled and mingled freely with their male patrons (Richardson 2009: 112–113).

Moreover, the *qiyān*, due to the unique skill set that made them highly desired in the royal court and in noble households, possessed a degree of social mobility that most other women—slave or free—did not (Gordon 2017, Myrne 2017, Nielson 2017, Richardson 2009). Myrne (2017: 66) notes: "The investment that owners made in the education of some slave women provided them with the intellectual and cultural capital that made it easier for them to control their life course to some extent." A *qaynah* leveraged all the tools at her disposal—beauty, intelligence, wit, musical prowess—to maneuver the intricacies of Abbasid courtly life and to improve her station.

Like other female slaves, female slave entertainers were sexually available to their male owners. Should a slave give birth to the master's child, she became *umm walad* (mother of a child), a status that granted her a number of legal protections (Richardson 2009: 106–108). She could never be sold, she would be manumitted upon her master's death, and her child would not inherit her slave status. These benefits hinged on the master's acknowledgment of paternity. Moreover, male slave owners, aware of the financial and legal consequences of slave pregnancy, were cautious about impregnating their female slaves. Nevertheless, such pregnancies did occur, and the sons of slave women often rose to considerable rank: as Richardson notes, several Abbasid caliphs were the sons of slave mothers (Richardson 2009: 115).

The training of and commerce in female slave entertainers appears to have declined in the eastern Islamicate lands in the latter half of the ninth century, due in large measure to political upheavals in the heart of the Abbasid empire (Caswell 2011: 258–266). Notably, this political instability enabled the governor of Egypt, Aḥmad ibn Ṭūlūn (r. 868–884), to break away from the empire and establish independent control; his son, Khumārawayh (r. 884–896), retained female entertainers in the royal palace, near the future site of the Cairo Citadel (Raymond 2000: 27, al-Maqrīzī 1906: 216–219).

Despite the decline in the east, the institution of the *qiyān* continued: beginning in the ninth century, the cities of al-Andalus became important centers for the training and trading of female slave entertainers (Reynolds 2017). The scope of training for *qiyān* appears to have been considerably broader in al-Andalus. Reynolds cites several accounts of Andalusian *qiyān* being trained in fields as diverse as the physical sciences, Quranic recitation, and fencing (Reynolds 2017:113–116). Of particular interest for the current discussion is the following account dating to the thirteenth century:

> She might also be skilled on all of the different instruments, as well as all forms of dance and shadow-puppetry, and possess her own instrument and her own servant-girls who accompany her with percussion and wind instruments, in which case she is known as "complete" and is sold for several thousand Maghribi dinars [Aḥmad al-Tīfāshī, cited in Reynolds 2017: 117].

This text reinforces that some *qiyān* were indeed trained in dance. It is also noteworthy that it was possible to purchase not only a single *qaynah*, but her entire entourage of accompanists.

In addition to the female slave entertainers, two additional categories of professional entertainers are important to describe here: the *ghulāmīyāt* and the *mukhannathūn* (Rowson 1991, 2003). Both groups were characterized by their inversion of mainstream contemporary gender roles. The *ghulāmīyāt* (singular *ghulāmīyah*) were female professional entertainers, generally slave women, who adopted the dress and mannerisms of pubescent boys. The *mukhannathūn* (singular *mukhannath*), on the other hand, were male professional entertainers who assumed effeminate dress and behaviors.

The *mukhannathūn* are documented from as early as the time of the Prophet Muḥammad (Rowson 1991). Later, in the Umayyad period, a group of these singers and musicians flourished in the city of Medina. Their music appears to have been distinguished by a characteristic "lightness," and they accompanied themselves with the frame drum known as the *duff*, at the time perceived as a women's instrument. These early *mukhannathūn* had access to the women's quarters of elite homes and often functioned as marriage brokers and go-betweens. Notably, the Umayyad-era *mukhannathūn* were not presumed to engage in homosexual behavior, though the general view was that they lacked sexual interest in women.

The *mukhannathūn* were periodically persecuted, culminating in the castration of the Medina *mukhannathūn* under the caliph Sulaymān in 717 (Rowson 1991: 687–693, 2003: 57). The Umayyad persecution of these men was prompted not by their inversion of gender norms, but by broader concerns about policing activities viewed as frivolous and leading toward immorality, such as music and drinking. In fact, Sulaymān's extreme action was rooted in the caliph's concerns that the *mukhannathūn* were endangering *women's* morality with their music and song.

The *mukhannathūn* survived this event, but in the Abbasid period, their situation was significantly different. They continued to be associated with light musical entertainment, shifting from the *duff* to the long-necked lute known as the *ṭunbūr* as their favored instrument, but they appear to have been valued more for their wit and humor than for their musicianship. In contrast to their predecessors, the Abbasid-era *mukhannathūn* were assumed to be passive homosexuals. Rowson (2003: 59) notes: "*Takhannuth* [effeminacy] went from being a category conceptually distinct from, but overlapping with, *bighā'* [passive homosexuality], to being a subset of it." The role of the *mukhannath* would persist for centuries in the Islamicate world.

In contrast to the *mukhannathūn*, the institution of the *ghulāmīyāt* appears to have been a phenomenon unique to the Abbasid era (Rowson 2003). As Rowson notes, although there are mentions of women dressing as men in earlier periods, the specific institution and associated terminology have no precedent prior to the Abbasids. The term *ghulāmīyah* is a female adjective derived from the word *ghulām*, meaning "boy" but also used to refer to a male slave. The *ghulāmīyāt* wore the tunic, sash, and turban favored by teenage boys of the time, and they adopted the latter's fashionable hairstyles, either by growing long side curls on the cheeks, or else by painting them on.

The institution of the *ghulāmīyah* was a function of male sexual proclivities of the era. Unlike the *mukhannath*, whose role as a potential sexual partner was secondary to his role as a professional entertainer, the *ghulāmīyah*'s *raison d'être* was to satisfy the sexual desires of aristocratic men. Rowson (2003: 66) writes: "The point of the [*ghulāmīyah*] was to charm the ordinary man through a combination of female and boyish sexual attractions; the [*mukhannath*] offered entertainment to ordinary society that had nothing to do with sexual attraction, but depended on the freedom offered by gender inversion and the consequent abandonment of dignity." Importantly, the identity of *ghulāmīyah* was generally one that was imposed on a woman, whereas the role of *mukhannath* was voluntarily adopted.

Turning now to ninth-century Egypt, it is clear that Egypt's rulers followed the established Abbasid practice of retaining female slave entertainers in their courts. According to al-Maqrīzī's history of the Tulunid dynasty, Khumārawayh, son of the dynasty's founder Aḥmad ibn Ṭūlūn, created a special *majlis*, or salon for entertaining guests,* within the royal palace at al-Qaṭā'i' (al-Maqrīzī 1906: 216–217; 1906–1908, volume 2:

* As noted earlier, the term *majlis* can refer to a musical gathering as well as to the salon in which musical entertainments took place (see Caswell 2011: 236–237, Nielson 2017: 86, Shiloah 1995: 12).

108–109). This *majlis* was known as *bayt al-dhahab* (house of gold) because of the opulence of its décor. Upon the walls were affixed elaborate wooden sculptures of Khumārawayh, his wives, and his female slave singers; the sculptures were painted and ornamented with gold and precious stones.

The practice of retaining female slave entertainers would continue under Egypt's Fatimid-era rulers and nobility. As was the case elsewhere in the Islamicate world of the time, the ownership of female slaves, including female slave entertainers, remained commonplace and would persist long after the end of the Fatimid dynasty. Fatimid elites acquired their female slaves through conquest, through purchase, or as gifts; slave women given as gifts proved to be an important means of diplomatic exchange (Cortese and Calderini 2006: 78).

Though enslaved, these women were sometimes able to transcend their origins and achieve high status: Cortese and Calderini recount the story of Raṣad, the slave who became consort to the caliph al-Ẓāhir li-I'zāz Dīn Allāh (r. 1021–1036) and mother to the caliph al-Mustanṣir bi-llāh (r. 1036–1094) (Cortese and Calderini 2006: 110–114). When al-Mustanṣir was a minor, Raṣad acted as regent and exercised considerable political power. Decades later, Shajar al-Durr (r. 1250) would ascend even higher (Fairchild Ruggles 2015). Wife to the last reigning Ayyubid sultan of Egypt, she briefly assumed the throne after her husband's death and the assassination of his heir; she also became wife to the first Mamluk sultan and conspired with other Mamluks to arrange his murder, a turn of events that would lead to her own demise.

The Fatimid elites, like their predecessors, appear to have had a particular fondness for worldly pleasures like music, song, dance, and drink, and female slave entertainers were central to their luxurious lifestyle. According to al-Maqrīzī, al-Ẓāhir was notoriously fond of music and drink (al-Maqrīzī 1920: 22) and spent a great deal in his pursuit of female entertainers:

> He was passionate about pleasure, a great fan of singing. It was during his reign that they began to seek out singers [*mughannīyāt*] and dancers [*raqqāṣāt*] in Egypt, and this passion came at a considerable expense [al-Maqrīzī 1920: 26; 1906–1908, volume 2: 169].

Thanks to a brief fluorescence of figural representation in the early Fatimid era, the opulent lifestyle of the Fatimid rulers and nobility is recorded in Fatimid artwork, with its lively portrayals of singers, dancers, and revelers (Figure 1) (see Bloom 2007: 89–115).

Undoubtedly, Fatimid-era female professional entertainers included both free and slave women. Unfortunately, there appears to be very little documentation of free female entertainers from this era, particularly

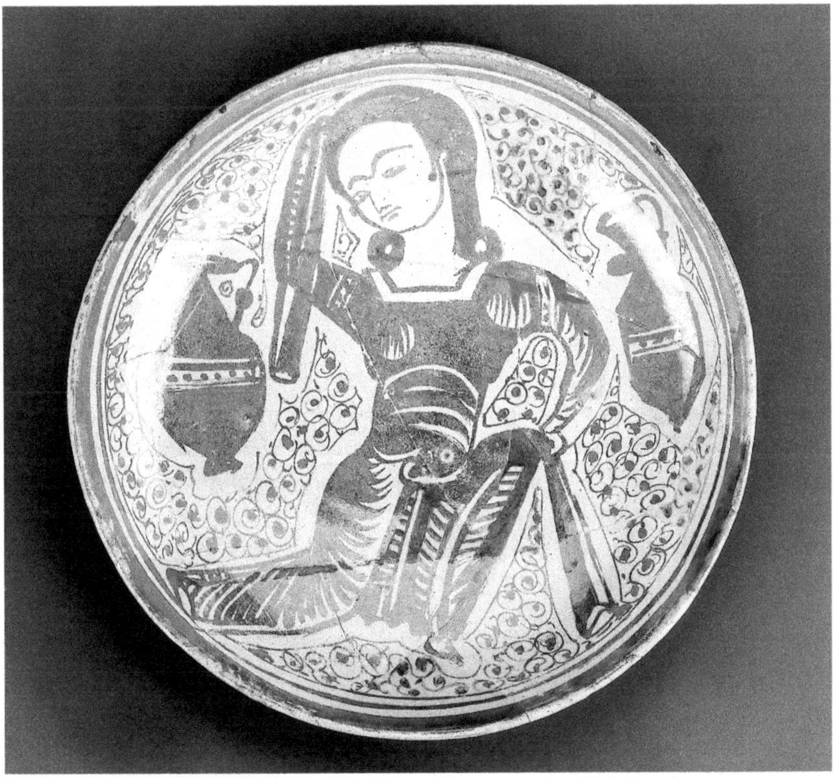

Figure 1: Fatimid-era female entertainer (Fatimid-era ceramic bowl, National Museum of Asian Art, Smithsonian Institution, Freer Collection, Purchase—Charles Lang Freer Endowment, F1946.30).

the popular entertainers who provided entertainment to the Egyptian masses; al-Maqrīzī shares an interesting account of a prominent singer named Nasab (al-Maqrīzī 1906–1908, volume 3: 203–205). According to al-Maqrīzī, Nasab so pleased the caliph al-Mustanṣir with a song in his honor that he gifted her with an expanse of land to the northwest of Fatimid Cairo. This account implies that Nasab was a free woman. Notably, al-Maqrīzī indicates that Nasab performed her song outside al-Mustanṣir's palace: this suggests that she may have been a popular entertainer who performed in public settings (rather than a slave entertainer who performed within the palaces and households of the elite). However, it is impossible to determine this for certain based on the currently available evidence.

What of male professional singers and dancers in Egypt before the Mamluk period? Rowson (2003: 65) cites two examples of eleventh-century *mukhannathūn* as recorded by the Fatimid historian al-Musabbiḥī. In one of these cases, a *mukhannath* was punished for acting as a procurer of several women. In the other, a wealthy *mukhannath* was murdered: "We are told that he was a rich man and a musician, who maintained singing slave girls in his home but was himself enamored of beardless boys, on whom he spent much money" (Rowson 2003: 65).

Shoshan cites examples of government action against *mukhannathūn* around 865, during the first period of Abbasid rule in Egypt, and 913, during the second Abbasid period (Shoshan 1993: 49, 112*n*). In fact, al-Maqrīzī mentions several crackdowns on the *mukhannathūn* by Abbasid governors (al-Maqrīzī 1906: 201–203; 1906–1908, volume 2: 102, 125). In one instance, the *mukhannathūn* were chased from Fusṭāṭ; though the exact date is unclear, this action took place sometime between 856 and 867. In another, occurring in 867, the *mukhannathūn* were imprisoned. In a third instance, taking place around 907, the *mukhannathūn* were suppressed. These frequent mentions of government intervention suggest that the *mukhannathūn* were fairly commonplace in Egyptian popular entertainment from at least the Abbasid period onward through the Fatimid era.

Mamluk Period

Female professional entertainers are frequently mentioned in sources from the Mamluk period, including the chroniclers al-Maqrīzī and Ibn Taghrībirdī. What is particularly noteworthy is that Mamluk-era sources provide documentation of two distinct classes of female professional entertainers in Egypt ('Abd ar-Rāziq 1973: 66–69). The first class consisted of the female slave entertainers who provided entertainment to the ruling elite, as they had in prior centuries. The second class was comprised of popular entertainers, presumably free women, who entertained the Egyptian population at large. A female professional entertainer, whether slave or free, was generally known as a *mughannīyah* or a *qaynah*, and apparently sometimes as a *raqqāṣah* (see al-Maqrīzī 1906–1908, volume 2: 169). 'Abd ar-Rāziq also mentions the term *rayyisah* (1973: 66), meaning chief or leader (of a troupe of entertainers).

Egypt's Mamluk aristocracy adhered to the established and centuries-old tradition of retaining female slave entertainers. At the height of the Mamluk era, every prominent *amīr* retained a band (*jūqah*) of female slave entertainers ('Abd ar-Rāziq 1973: 66, Rapoport 2007: 9). The Mamluk sultan Ṣalāḥ al-Dīn Ḥajjī (r. 1381–1382, 1389–1390), for example, maintained a band of 15 slave singers (Popper 1954: 104; Ibn Taghrībirdī 1929–1972, volume 11: 380).

The names of some of the most famous of these female slave entertainers, as well as a few tantalizing clues about their lives, were recorded by Mamluk-era historians. Khūbi was known as an excellent player of the *ʿūd* (Arabic lute); she was purchased for the price of 10,000 dinars and housed at her owner's mansion on the banks of the Birkat al-Fīl (ʿAbd ar-Rāziq 1973: 68, Rapoport 2007: 10). Ittifāq began her career as a slave to the *ḍāminat al-maghānī*, the female tax farmer of singers and prostitutes (see below), in the Delta town of Bilbays (Rapoport 2007: 10–11). She was then sold to the *ḍāminat al-maghānī* of Cairo, who then gifted her to the household of the sultan al-Nāṣir Muḥammad ibn Qalāwūn (r. 1293–1294, 1299–1309, 1310–1341). Ittifāq went on to become concubine and wife of three consecutive Mamluk sultans (ʿAbd ar-Rāziq 1973: 68, Rapoport 2007: 10–11).

Nevertheless, there are indications that the elite practice of retaining female slave entertainers may have peaked in the Mamluk era. Rapoport (2007: 13–16) describes historical evidence for important changes in the female slave trade in fifteenth-century Egypt, changes which would have implications for the role of the female slave entertainer. As Rapoport notes, there appears to have been a substantial decline in female slavery throughout the fifteenth century. This decline may have been tied to the advent of the Black Death in Egypt in the fourteenth century. Slaves, who were generally of foreign ethnicities, appear to have been more vulnerable to the plague than native Egyptians, and contemporary sources indicate that female slaves were hit particularly hard during plague outbreaks (see Rapoport 2007: 13).

Alongside this decline was a change in social attitudes toward female slaves. Rapoport notes that in the fifteenth century, slave concubines were valued much more for their domestic skills and piety than for their good looks and musical abilities. In some instances, a concubine served as a substitute for a wife. In her discussion of Ibn Baṭṭūṭah, Tolmacheva (2017) illustrates how the famed Maghrebi traveler depended on concubines to fulfill his needs—both domestic and sexual—during his extensive journeys, noting that "he found concubines a suitable alternative, and sometimes a replacement, for his wealthier and well-connected wives" (Tolmacheva 2017: 167).

While the female slave trade continued for many more centuries, the role of the female slave entertainer in elite society appears to have declined steadily from the fifteenth century onward, eventually disappearing in the Khedivial era. Nevertheless, entertainments like music, song, and dance would continue to be integral to the lifestyle of Egypt's elite. As will become apparent in the later discussion of the Ottoman period, entertainers for hire, including the female professional entertainers known as the *'awālim*, would take over the roles previously fulfilled by slave entertainers.

The popular class of female professional entertainers is fairly well-documented in the Mamluk period. Popular entertainers performed at important social occasions such as weddings and births, as well as at the periodic public festivals that punctuated the Egyptian year. Al-Maqrīzī notes the presence of female singers (he uses the term *mughannīyah*), along with an array of other public entertainers, as well as prostitutes, at a now-obsolete Coptic festival called the Feast of the Martyrs (al-Maqrīzī 1895: 194–197; 1906–1908, volume 1: 110–112). This feast took place during the Coptic month of Bashans (roughly May in the Gregorian calendar), and revolved around a ritual designed to ensure an adequate Nile flood: the Copts immersed into the river a reliquary containing the severed finger of one of their deceased saints. Public debauchery provided the pretense for authorities to crack down on the festival, and the Feast of the Martyrs was banned temporarily from 1302 to 1338, and permanently from 1355 onward; al-Maqrīzī's description of the festival suggests female professional entertainers analogous to the *ghawāzī* of later centuries.

Popular entertainers also performed at public celebrations and processions related to the political and military successes of the ruling elite. For example, Ibn Taghrībirdī describes the following scene in Cairo upon the return of the sultan al-Mu'ayyad Shaykh (r. 1412–1421) from one of his Syrian campaigns:

> Thus the Sultan passed on until he alighted at his mosque which he had built near Zuwaila Gate. Cairo had been decorated in honor of his arrival; the shops had been illuminated with candles and lamps; and the singing girls sat in rows above the shops, beating their tambourines [Popper 1957: 52].

Ibn Taghrībirdī describes similar celebrations in the streets of Cairo after the sultan al-Ashraf Barsbāy's (r. 1422–1438) conquest of Cyprus in 1426 (Popper 1958: 43–44).

Apparently, female entertainers of the popular class were so prevalent and integral to Egyptian life at this time that the government found it worthwhile to tax them; al-Maqrīzī reveals that these women were subject to taxation throughout much of the Mamluk era. Interestingly, he refers to this as a tax on *qiyān*, with an implication that these women were prostitutes (al-Maqrīzī 1895: 255; 1906–1908, volume 1: 144). His choice of this term indicates that in the Mamluk era, the word *qiyān* could be used not only for female slave entertainers, but for free female professional entertainers as well as prostitutes.

The tax on female entertainers was collected by means of a tax farm (*ḍamān*), a system in which a government contracts with a private individual to collect tax on its behalf. The tax farmer is given the right to collect tax in the name of the state, as well as to keep any amount beyond what is owed to the state, often resulting in the extortion of the local population by the tax farmer. In the case of female entertainers, both the entertainers themselves and the clients who hired them were responsible for remitting taxes to their tax farmer. More information is supplied by al-Maqrīzī:

> The tax farming of singers [*ḍamān al-aghānī*] was an abominable institution which consisted of extracting money from prostitutes. If one of the most respected women went out in Egypt to indulge in debauchery and have her name registered with the tax farmer, the latter provided her with everything she needed, and it was impossible for the greatest man in Egypt to prevent her from engaging in debauchery. If this woman gave birth, or became betrothed, or rubbed her hands with henna, or if someone proposed to her in marriage, she had to pay the duty imposed by the tax farmer. Anyone who hired a singer for a wedding or for a birth without the permission of the tax farmer was subjected to unheard-of annoyance [al-Maqrīzī 1895: 306–307; 1906–1908, volume 1: 171–172].

According to al-Maqrīzī, the sultan al-Nāṣir Muḥammad ibn Qalāwūn called for the abolition of the tax on female entertainers, though it appears that the abolition was not formally implemented until the reign of sultan al-Ashraf Sha'bān (r. 1363–1377), during al-Maqrīzī's lifetime (al-Maqrīzī 1895: 306; 1906–1908, volume 1: 171). This state of affairs was apparently short-lived, as just a few years later, under sultan al-Ẓāhir Barqūq (r. 1382–1389, 1390–1399), the tax was abolished *again* in a number of small towns in the Egyptian countryside (Popper 1954: 42; Ibn Taghrībirdī 1929–1972, volume 11: 291). The taxation of female professional entertainers would be reinstated and abolished multiple times over the course of Egyptian history, though systematic government regulation of the entertainment trades would not be introduced until the late nineteenth century.

It should also be noted that there appears to have been some overlap between the trade in female slave entertainers and the business of popular entertainment. As noted earlier, there are examples of *ḍāmināt al-maghānī* (the female tax farmers of female professional entertainers and prostitutes) owning and trafficking in female slave entertainers. It seems quite likely that some of the female professional entertainers of the popular class may have begun their careers in slavery.

What of male professional entertainers in this period? In his description of the Coptic Feast of the Martyrs noted above, al-Maqrīzī mentions the presence of *mukhannathūn* among the array of entertainers and merry-makers (al-Maqrīzī 1895: 194–197; 1906–1908, volume 1: 110–112). *Mukhannathūn* also figure prominently in one of the surviving shadow plays of Muḥammad Ibn Dāniyāl (see Kahle 2015). A pair of *mukhannathūn* appear in the play *al-Mutayyam*: one sings a raunchy song, then the other, after reciting some scatological prose, dances and drinks until passing out (Rowson 1997: 180). Robert Irwin (2004: 165) refers to the Mamluk-era *mukhannathūn* as "transvestite prostitutes." However, the earlier precedent of *mukhannathūn* as entertainers, and the persistent popularity of effeminate male entertainers in the ensuing Ottoman era (see below), suggests that the role of Mamluk-era *mukhannathūn* was more nuanced. Nevertheless, in the eyes of much of the Egyptian public, who generally assumed the immorality of singers and dancers, the distinction between professional entertainer and prostitute was fuzzy at best.

It is likely that many, perhaps even most, of Egypt's Mamluk-era popular entertainers were members of a loose confederation known until the late thirteenth century as the Banū Sāsān (Sons of Sāsān), and later as the Ghurabā' (Strangers). Though traditional historiography has cast the Banū Sāsān simply as criminals and tricksters, denizens of the medieval Islamic underworld, recent scholarship by Kristina Richardson (2022) demonstrates that the Banū Sāsān is better understood as a tribal entity: "The Banū Sāsān was a multiethnic, multiconfessional group that consciously styled itself as a tribal nation, with an eponymous founder, subtribes organized by profession, local shaykhs, and a mixed language called Sīn" (Richardson 2022: 15).

Over the course of medieval Islamic history, the Banū Sāsān/Ghurabā' encompassed a broad range of ethnic and linguistic groups. These diverse groups were unified by their conscious estrangement from mainstream society and their use of Sīn or Sīm, a mixed language consisting of a substitutive vocabulary inserted into the grammatical structure of other languages. The Banū Sāsān/Ghurabā' defies traditional ethnic and linguistic typologies, rather being defined by "otherness" relative to majority societies. The people of the Banū Sāsān/Ghurabā' were characterized by their work in socially marginal occupations: they were entertainers, beggars, astrologers, fortune tellers, animal trainers, etc.

Ottoman and Khedivial Periods

Over the course of the Ottoman era, Egypt's professional entertainers came to be known by a variety of new terms, including *'awālim* and *ghawāzī* (used to describe various female professional entertainers), *khawal* (used to describe certain male professional entertainers), and *jink* (used to describe male *and* female entertainers at various times). Western interest in these professional singers and dancers began in earnest, and the accounts of foreign visitors to Egypt from the eighteenth century onward offer detailed descriptions of these men and women, their performances, their costuming, and other aspects of their profession. Notably, in Ottoman-era sources, there is a much more explicit association of the *'awālim*, *ghawāzī*, *khawalāt*, and *jink* with dance than was evident in their predecessors in earlier periods. The persistence of terms like *'awālim* and *ghawāzī* as colloquial designations for professional belly dancers, even into the present day, indicates that these entertainers are a meaningful bridge between the professional entertainers of earlier periods and the professional belly dancers of today.

Here it is important to discuss an apparent disconnect between Western sources and Egyptian reality. Western accounts of the *'awālim*, *ghawāzī*, *khawalāt*, and *jink* generally lead to the conclusion that each represents a discrete and well-defined category of professional entertainers. The *'awālim* and the *ghawāzī*, in particular, are described by foreign observers as distinct and more or less mutually exclusive groups: the *'awālim* were private entertainers catering to Egypt's elite, while the *ghawāzī* were public entertainers performing for the masses. However, an examination of contemporary Egyptian sources, particularly the detailed chronicle of 'Abd al-Raḥmān al-Jabartī (al-Jabartī 1904), suggests that these categories were not entirely clear-cut. Moreover, the infrequency and inconsistency in how these terms were used in Egyptian chronicles such as al-Jabartī's suggest that these were somewhat flexible colloquial designations.

In 1801, during Napoleon's occupation of Egypt, the French military compiled a list of trade guilds in Cairo (Raymond 1957). On this list were three guilds of female entertainers: corporation 137 ("*chanteuses du Caire*"—female singers of Cairo), corporation 200 ("*danseuses qui sont au Caire dites Rakassin*"—female dancers who are in Cairo, called Rakassin), and corporation 192 ("*danseuses et musiciens qui les accompagnent qui sont au Caire*"—female dancers and male musicians who accompany them, who are in Cairo). The terms *'awālim* and *ghawāzī* are not mentioned in this list. In addition, the list included two guilds of male entertainers: corporation 126 ("musiciens du pays et chanteurs qui sont au Caire"—local male musicians and male singers who are in Cairo) and corporation 139 ("*danseurs qui sont au Caire*"—male dancers who are in Cairo). The terms *khawal* and *jink* are not mentioned. It is not clear whether the French list is complete, but it hints at the scope and complexity of the Egyptian entertainment business at the turn of the eighteenth and nineteenth centuries.

For comparison, consider al-Jabartī's description of the inappropriate behavior of a group of Egyptian soldiers during Ramadan in 1814 (al-Jabartī 1888–1896, volume 9: 102–103; 1904, volume 4: 227–228). In this account, Al-Jabartī laments that the soldiers, who were encamped just outside Bāb al-Futūḥ, not only brazenly broke the Ramadan fast by eating, drinking, and smoking, but engaged in a range of morally reprehensible activities, including carousing with prostitutes and smoking hashish. According to al-Jabartī, many women of "ill-repute" gathered around the soldiers' encampment; among those specifically listed were *baghāyā* (prostitutes), *ghawāzī*, and *raqqāṣūn* (al-Jabartī 1904, volume 4: 228).

The mention of *raqqāṣūn** suggests a direct correspondence with corporation 200 from the French guild list, and the fact that al-Jabartī distinguishes the *raqqāṣūn* from the *ghawāzī* raises the possibility that the latter correspond to corporation 192. Are the *raqqāṣūn* the women elsewhere referred to as *'awālim*? While some Western accounts assert that the *'awālim* were exclusively singers, it is quite clear that at least some of the *'awālim* danced as well. Edward Lane (2005 [1836]: 355) inadvertently confirms this in his attempt to distinguish the *'awālim* from the *ghawāzī*: "There are many of an inferior class, who sometimes dance in the hareem; hence travellers have often misapplied the name of 'almé,' meaning 'ál'meh, to the common dancing-girls." Yet it would seem that not all of the dancing *'awālim* were "of an inferior class." Lane's sister, Sophia Lane-Poole (1846: 96), offers this firsthand account from the royal wedding of Zaynab Hānim, the youngest daughter of Muḥammad 'Alī:

> These girls were succeeded by two 'A'lmehs, the first Arab singers of Egypt; and the band struck up some beautiful Arab airs; but on that evening the 'A'lmehs did not sing; they only danced in the Arab manner, for which performance they are also celebrated as the first of their day.

Lane-Poole's account is particularly valuable, since she had access to female-only entertainments that her brother did not (see Fraser 2002). Her description makes it clear that these *awālim* were esteemed and prestigious enough to be hired for a lavish event hosted by Egypt's ruling family. Leaving aside the issue of prestige, however, consider how the *'awālim* and *ghawāzī* are defined in the French-Arabic dictionary compiled by Ellious Bocthor, a Coptic Egyptian and contemporary of al-Jabartī who eventually became a professor of colloquial Egyptian Arabic in Paris. In Bocthor's dictionary, both *'ālmah* and *ghāziyah* are listed under the entry for *danseuse* (*femme publique*)—female dancer (public woman) (Bocthor 1828: 231).

---

* *Raqqāṣīn/ raqqāṣūn* are the plural forms of the word *raqqāṣ*, which signifies a male dancer. The plural form can be used to refer to a group of male dancers, or to any collective of dancers, regardless of gender. The -īn and -ūn suffixes represent accusative/genitive and nominative cases, respectively. See also Wehr (1976: 354).

On the other hand, the existence of at least *three* guilds of female professional entertainers in late eighteenth-century Cairo suggests that the reality of female singers and dancers was more complex than the binary categorization of *'awālim versus ghawāzī* that is so often described by Western sources (a point noted by Fraser 2015: 38–42). Indeed, if some *'awālim* were exclusively singers, and some were both singers and dancers, then it is quite feasible that women from both corporations 137 and 200 were known colloquially as *'awālim*. All of these factors suggest that it is necessary to take a somewhat flexible approach to the terminology for these entertainers moving forward.

Generally speaking, an *'ālmah* was a female entertainer skilled in poetry, music, and dance, and frequently hired to entertain in upper-class Egyptian households on important social occasions (Figure 2). Though favored by the Egyptian elite, the *'awālim* belonged to the lower strata of Egyptian society (Chabrol 1826: 41–42). The *'awālim* were gifted singers with the ability to improvise both verse and melody (Chabrol 1826: 41–42, Savary 1785: 149–150). Though some of the *'awālim* of the eighteenth and nineteenth centuries were exclusively singers, as noted above, it is clear from contemporary sources that many *'awālim* excelled at the native Egyptian dance (Lane-Poole 1846: 96, Savary 1785: 150–153, Villoteau 1826: 169–170).

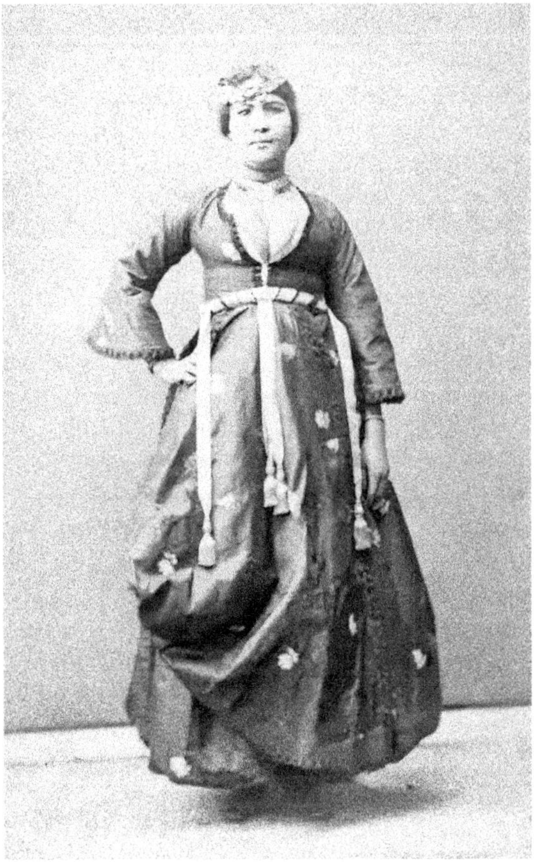

Figure 2: An *'ālmah* or *ghāziyah* of the mid-nineteenth century (Délié et Cie. *carte de visite, circa* 1860s).

The *'awālim* generally performed within the *ḥarīm*, or women's quarters, of elite homes, where men could hear them, but not see them (Clot-Bey 1840: 86, Villoteau 1826: 169–170). Edward Lane (2005 [1836]: 354–355) offers this detailed description:

> The 'Awâlim are often hired on the occasion of a *fête* in the hareem of a person of wealth. There is generally a small, elevated apartment, called a "tukeyseh," or "mughanna,"adjoining the principal salon of the hareem, from which it is separated only by a screen of wooden lattice-work, or there is some other convenient place in which the female singers may be concealed from the sight of the master of the house, should he be present with his women. But when there is a party of male guests, they generally sit in the court, or in a lower apartment, to hear the songs of the 'Awâlim, who, in this case, usually sit at a window of the hareem, concealed by the lattice-work.

Such accounts should not lead to the conclusion that the *ʿawālim* were never seen or heard by people outside of elite households, however. For example, Lane-Poole notes that during festive occasions, the elite *ḥarīm* was accessible to women of all social classes, a phenomenon that she observed during the wedding of Zaynab Hānim in 1845 (Lane-Poole 1846: 126). Nor should accounts like Edward Lane's lead to the conclusion that the *ʿawālim* never appeared in front of men. Accepting that *raqqāṣūn/raqqāṣīn* refers to at least some of the *ʿawālim*, al-Jabartī indicates that they marched along with the members of at least 70 different Cairo guilds in a public procession for the new bride of ʿAlī Āghā, *khazindār* of the *amīr* Muḥammad Āghā al-Barūdī, near the end of the eighteenth century (al-Jabartī 1888–1896, volume 5: 152–153; 1904, volume 2: 238). Moreover, as noted earlier in al-Jabartī's account of the events of Ramadan 1814, some of these women performed for male clients.

The role of the *ʿawālim* as the favored female professional entertainers of Egypt's wealthy elites evokes that of the *qiyān* of earlier centuries, suggesting that the *ʿawālim* were the inheritors of their legacy. It is interesting that the term *ʿālmah* literally means learned/knowledgeable-woman (see Lane 2005 [1836]: 354), much as the term *qaynah* originally meant something akin to "trained technician" (see Beeston 1980: 2). Yet, the *ʿawālim* differed from their predecessors in being free entertainers for hire, rather than slave women.

As discussed earlier, changes in the female slave trade beginning in the fifteenth century appear to have initiated a decline in the practice of retaining female slave entertainers. Most notably, female slaves were increasingly valued for domestic services rather than entertainment functions. It seems probable that this change contributed to the rise of the *ʿawālim*, since the elite demand for musical entertainment continued even as the institution of female slave entertainers declined. Still, the role of the female slave entertainer did not entirely disappear until the mid- to late nineteenth century. Clot-Bey (1840: 90), who resided in Egypt in the first half of the nineteenth century, observed the retention of slave entertainers by the nobility: "As dance is an amusement which is very popular with ladies, there are dancing slaves among the great lords."

Contemporary with the *'awālim* were the female professional entertainers known as the *ghawāzī* (Chabrol 1826: 119–120, Jomard 1829: 441, Savary 1785: 155–156, Villoteau 1826: 170–171). The most significant difference between the *ghawāzī* and the *'awālim* was their typical clientele. While the *'awālim* generally performed for the elite, the *ghawāzī* provided entertainment to the Egyptian lower classes. They also differed in where they performed. Whereas the *'awālim* usually performed in the privacy of the *ḥarīm* of the homes in which they were hired, the *ghawāzī* frequently danced and sang in public spaces for mixed-gender or male audiences. Nevertheless, it is important to bear in mind that the boundary between the *'awālim* and the *ghawāzī* was likely more porous than presented in many Western sources of the time. For example, Isabella Romer (1846: 127) observed with dismay that the Turkish daughter of the last Dey of Algiers, a member of Cairene high society, had accepted a *ghāziyah* into her household: "She was formerly one of the public ghawazee of Cairo, but her performance possessed so many charms for the Dey's daughter that she took her into her household, and has loaded her with jewels, and pays no visits without being accompanied by her."

There has been a great deal of speculation on the origin of the term *ghawāzī*. *Ghāziyah* is the feminine form of the noun *ghāzī*, meaning "raider" or "invader." The latter term was used to refer to a warrior who engaged in military campaigns in the name of Islam, and it became a common honorific in the Ottoman era. In the documentary *The Romany Trail* (1992), Su'ād Māzin, the eldest sister of the famous Banāt Māzin *ghawāzī* of Luxor, suggests a poetic interpretation of the term *ghāziyah*: "They call us by the name *ghāziyah*. To them, it's a dirty word. But to us, it means that we invade their hearts with our dance and in any other way they want."

Nearing (2004b) points to the possibility of a more mundane origin: the term *ghawāzī* may actually derive from a specific type of coin nicknamed a *ghāzī*. These coins, minted in the Ottoman era, were imprinted with the names and titles of Ottoman Sultans, many of whom assumed the honorific *ghāzī*, perhaps explaining the origin of the nickname. These coins were used to tip a dancer by licking the coin and sticking it to the dancer's forehead or body. This usage of the *ghāzī* coin is mentioned by the French author Gérard de Nerval (1884: 88–89). This tipping practice is also noted by both Clot-Bey and Lane, though neither offers a specific name for the coins (Clot-Bey 1840: 94, Lane 2005 [1836]: 495). To date, I have not encountered the term *ghawāzī* in reference to female professional entertainers prior to the Ottoman period. Since it seems that *ghāzī* coins were not minted prior to the Ottoman era, the idea that the term *ghawāzī* emerged due to the practice of tipping dancers with these coins is rather compelling.

It has been suggested that the *ghawāzī* were of a distinct "race" or "tribe" (Lane 1860: 379–381, Lane 2005 [1836]: 373–376). Indeed, some modern-day *ghawāzī* self-identify with the various Dom ethnolinguistic groups that reside in North Africa and the Middle East, suggesting that at least some of the *ghawāzī* are ethnically distinct from other Egyptians (Nearing 1993). Among the various groups of Dom in Egypt are the Ghajar, the Ḥalab, and the Nawar (Marsh 2000, Thomas 2000).* These groups are well-documented by several nineteenth-century sources, including Lane (1860: 386–387, 2005 [1836]: 382–383), Newbold (1856), and Von Kremer (1864).

In more recent times, the researcher Nabil Sobhi Hanna conducted fieldwork among a group of Ghajar in a rural community near Cairo (Hanna 1982), and Alexandra Parrs researched Dom groups in Cairo and Alexandria (Parrs 2017). Lane makes no specific connection between the *ghawāzī* and Egyptian Dom, though he notes with interest that both groups occasionally claim descent from the Barāmikah (Lane 1860: 379–381, 387; Lane 2005 [1836]: 373–376, 382). By contrast, Von Kremer treats the *ghawāzī* as a Dom group (Von Kremer 1864: 264). Newbold makes no mention of the *ghawāzī* in his quite detailed overview of the Ghajar, the Ḥalab, and the Nawar, though he notes that many Ghajar women worked as rope dancers and musicians (Newbold 1856: 292).

Present-day sources make it clear that while some *ghawāzī* are Dom, others are not. The Banāt Māzin *ghawāzī* of Luxor identify as Nawar (Nearing 1993, 2004a, 2004b). On the other hand, Umm Hāshim, a popular *ghāziyah* from the Upper Egyptian village of Abū Shūshah, adamantly denies being a part of any of these groups (personal communication, November 17, 2022). Hanna, based on firsthand experience with the Ghajar, indicates that some families of Ghajar work as professional entertainers, with the women singing and dancing, and the men providing musical accompaniment (Hanna 1982: 31–33). However, Hanna states:

* In the English language, the Dom, along with the Rom, and similar groups, are often collectively referred to as "Gypsies." Due to the stereotypical and derogatory connotations of that term, I am avoiding its usage as much as possible. It is also important to note that the terms Ghajar, Ḥalab, and Nawar carry derogatory connotations in the Arabic language, though their meanings vary from region to region within the Middle East and North Africa, and individuals belonging to these groups still refer to themselves by these appellations.

> Although financially well off, the people who practice this profession are despised by Ghagar and non-Ghagar alike. Some even pretend to have given up entertaining or say that they have forbidden their daughters and wives to sing and dance [Hanna 1982: 31–33].
>
> For the Ghagar who work as singers and dancers, there is a high frequency of marriages where both spouses have the same profession. The Ghagari girls who are dancers marry early because their work is considered an important source of income. Other Ghagar men who are not in this profession would not want a dancer for a wife [Hanna 1982: 41].

Hanna's findings indicate that even among Egyptian Dom, the entertainment trades were undesirable occupations.

The overlap, but lack of clear equivalence, between the Dom and the *ghawāzī* suggests that these groups are united not by a shared ethnic identity, but by a shared marginality relative to mainstream Egyptian society. Accordingly, it may be more fruitful to view these groups as descendants of the medieval Banū Sāsān/Ghurabā'. This is supported by the research of Parrs (2017), which demonstrates that modern-day Dom identity creation is a process of constant re-negotiation of insider-outsider boundaries between the Dom and the majority society, much as Banū Sāsān/Ghurabā' identity was defined by the group's collective "otherness" and marginality.

More tellingly, Sīn/Sīm has survived in the dialects of both Dom and popular entertainers in the modern era (Newbold 1856, Richardson 2022: 42–46, Van Nieuwkerk 1995: 96–102, Von Kremer 1864). Viewing these groups as modern-day incarnations of the Banū Sāsān/Ghurabā' collective helps to explain the *ghawāzī*'s connectedness to the Dom while allowing space for the ambiguity and multiplicity of ethnic identities among the *ghawāzī*.

In the early nineteenth century, the primary performance contexts of the *ghawāzī* were public markets and festivals, particularly *mawālid*, and celebrations of birth or marriage among lower-class Egyptians. In addition to these settings, the *ghawāzī* could be found performing within or in front of Egyptian coffee houses (Fraser 2015: 76–78). These were not formal performances; rather, the *ghawāzī* seem to have lingered in or around coffee houses, occasionally providing spontaneous performances either as a way to earn a few piasters or as a means to advertise their availability for more lucrative engagements such as weddings (see, for example, Jollois 1826: 533). Egyptian musicians and storytellers similarly frequented the coffee houses, providing impromptu entertainment (Lane 1860: 333, 391; Lane 2005 [1836]: 335, 386).

Unlike the *'awālim*, the *ghawāzī* were rarely invited to perform in the homes of the well-to-do. Further, Muslim families were far less likely to invite the *ghawāzī* into their homes than Europeans and non-Muslim

Egyptians (Clot-Bey 1840: 90–91). If the *ghawāzī* were engaged to entertain in the private home of a Muslim family, the performance took place in the *mandarah*, the sitting room in which the male members of the household received guests. The women of the home and the female guests observed the event from a window or balcony overlooking the *mandarah*. The *ghawāzī* might provide a separate performance for the women in the interior of the *ḥarīm*.

Alongside the female professional entertainers just described were the male professional entertainers generally known as the *khawalāt* and the *jink* (Figure 3) (Clot-Bey 1840: 94–95, Lane 1860: 381–382, Lane 2005 [1836]: 376–377).* The primary distinction between the two was their ethnic origin: the *khawal* was native Egyptian, while the *jink* was foreign (usually Armenian, Greek, Jewish, or Turkish). The Egyptian Arabic term *jink* derives from the Turkish *çengi*, which can refer to a male or a female dancer (And 1963: 26). Male *çengis* were extremely popular in Ottoman Turkey, and the appearance of the term *jink* in Egyptian Arabic seems to coincide with Ottoman control of Egypt. However, as has already been noted, a tradition of male professional entertainers existed in Egypt prior to the Ottoman conquest.

The *khawalāt* and the *jink* appear to have inherited the legacy of the *mukhannathūn* of earlier periods. They are described as male performers who assumed effeminate dress and behaviors, and like their predecessors, they were recognized as men in spite of their attire and mannerisms. Lane (2005 [1836]: 376–377) writes:

> As they personate women, their dances are exactly of the same description as those of the Ghawázee, and are, in like manner, accompanied by the sounds of castanets; but, as if to prevent their being thought to be really females, their dress is suited to their unnatural profession, being partly male and partly female. It chiefly consists of a tight vest, a girdle, and a kind of petticoat. Their general appearance, however, is more feminine than masculine. They suffer the hair of the head to grow long, and generally braid it, in the manner of the women. The hair on the face, when it begins to grow, they pluck out; and they imitate the women also in applying kohl and henna to their eyes and hands. In the streets, when not engaged in dancing, they often even veil their faces; not from shame, but merely to affect the manners of women.

In other words, like the *mukhannathūn*, they were not meant to "pass" as women.

These male performers are noted in Egyptian sources long before Western authors became fascinated with them. Over a century before Lane, the chronicler Aḥmad al-Damurdāshī describes how Ismā'īl Bāshā, Ottoman

* Raymond (1974: 151), citing al-Jabartī, mentions a third term, *ghāyish* (plural *ghiyāsh*).

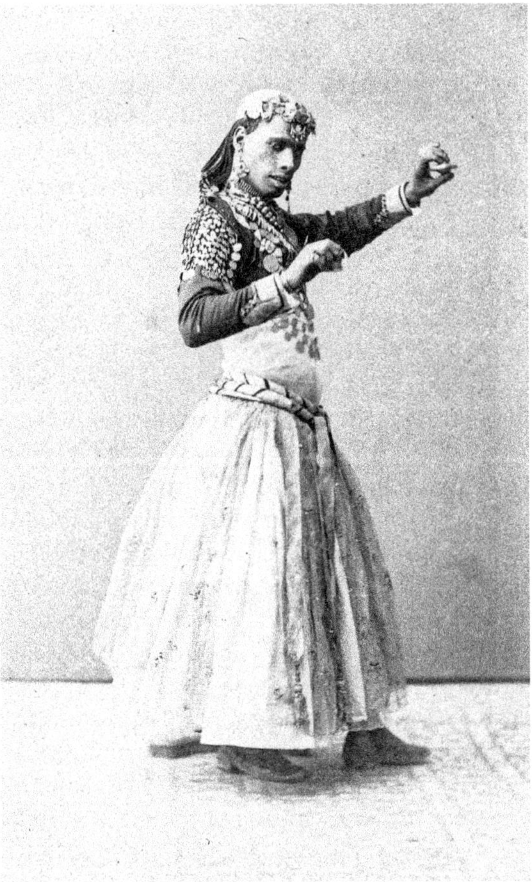

Figure 3: A *khawal* or *jink* of the mid-to-late nineteenth century (Délié and Béchard *carte de visite*, *circa* 1870s, Getty Research Institute, Los Angeles [2008.R.3]).

governor of Egypt from 1695 to 1697, hired male dancers to perform at the celebration for the circumcision of his two sons (al-Damurdāshī 1991: 64–67). Two separate troupes are mentioned, and one of the troupe leaders was prominent enough to be mentioned by name (*ibid.*, 65): "Abu al-Yusr al-Cenki (*cengi*) [the public dancer] came to the Diwan al-Ghawri with his slaves (*mamalik*); the public dancer of the Jews performed in the diwan of Qa'itbay."

The *khawalāt* and the *jink* performed in many of the same settings as the *ghawāzī*. In fact, these men were often preferred over the *ghawāzī*, since they posed less of a threat to the moral order than female performers (a preference that most contemporary Western observers found incomprehensible). Clot-Bey (1840: 94) writes: "As Muslims are not supposed to be allowed to see women dancing, they have historically had young male dancers (*khowals*) dressed in female costume." He goes on to note that the number of these male performers increased when the Egyptian government banned public performance by female entertainers (an event which occurred in the 1830s, and which will be discussed below). Similar observations are offered by Lane (2005 [1836]: 376–377) and Nerval (1884: 89).

As noted above, the Turkish term *çengi* can refer to a male or a female dancer, and until around the turn of the nineteenth century, this was the case with the Egyptian Arabic term *jink* as well. Sources indicate the existence of a separate category of female *jink*, sometimes rendered *jinkiyah* (plural *jinkiyāt*) (see al-Sayyid Marsot 1995: 119 for two examples). Villoteau (1826: 182) describes the female *jink* as "Jewish women who teach dancing, and who sometimes, mounted on donkeys, follow the wedding procession, playing the *rebâb* or the *târ*." The *jink* is mentioned by al-Jabartī several times in his chronicle, but it is not always clear whether he is referring to male or female entertainers. However, his mention of a *jink*, along with a group of singers, leading a wedding procession for an elite family whose women were pious and sequestered suggests the female *jink* as described by Villoteau (al-Jabartī 1904, volume 1: 209).

Another curious note by al-Jabartī seems to reference the female *jink*. In 1818, Egyptian troops under Muḥammad 'Alī's son Ibrāhīm won a commanding victory over the Wahhabis in Arabia, thus bringing the Islamic holy sites of Mecca and Medina under Ottoman control. In describing the massive citywide celebrations in Cairo, al-Jabartī mentions that there were music and dance performances in some quarters (al-Jabartī 1904, volume 4: 318). Specifically, he uses the term *jink raqqāṣāt*, perhaps indicating that the *jink* was the leader of a troupe of dancers. Interestingly, alongside *jink raqqāṣāt*, al-Jabartī mentions *qiyān*, indicating that the latter term was still in use, seemingly to refer to female singers.

As in the earlier Mamluk period, Ottoman-era professional entertainers were taxed by the Egyptian government. However, in contrast to the Mamluk period, wherein taxes were extracted by tax farmers, Ottoman-era taxation was accomplished by means of the guild system (Baer 1964; Raymond 1957, 1974). Each guild was headed by a *shaykh* who was responsible for ensuring that the guild's taxes were remitted to the appropriate government official. Guilds of professional entertainers paid their taxes to an official called the *amīn al-khurdah*. Ottoman sources mention a woman called the *shaykhat al-maghānī*, the head of the guild of female singers. However, it is currently unclear if and how this individual relates to the specific guilds of female professional entertainers noted by the French in 1801. As discussed earlier, the French guild list includes a variety of guilds of professional entertainers, both male and female (Raymond 1957).

It is unclear whether this list reflects a complete accounting of all the professional entertainer guilds of Cairo in 1801, let alone the number and nature of such guilds earlier in the Ottoman era. As Raymond notes, the available lists of Ottoman Cairo guilds are generally incomplete and do not perfectly overlap (Raymond 1974: 90–93).

The taxation of professional entertainers was not accompanied by systematic regulation of their trades. In fact, the taxation of entertainers was not particularly systematic either: these taxes were alternately passed and abolished throughout the Ottoman era. Raymond (1974: 172) notes that a tax on female singers (*maghānī*) and dancers (*jinkiyāt*) that was instituted under the Ottoman governor Muḥammad Bāshā (in office from 1637 to 1640) was abolished just a few years later under Maqsūd Bāshā (governor from 1642 to 1644), then reinstated shortly thereafter.

Yet, entertainers were frequently subject to government crackdowns. Until the late nineteenth century, these actions generally corresponded to periods of repeal or abolition of the entertainment taxes. The chronicler al-Damurdāshī offers this detailed account from 1703. From 1703 to 1705, 'Alī Āghā, the head of the Janissaries, was given broad authority in fiscal matters, a post he accepted only on condition of being able to shut down taverns, brothels, and the like. Individuals working in "immoral" trades such as entertainment and prostitution were the targets of 'Alī Āghā's wrath. Al-Damurdāshī (1991: 122) writes:

> In the Husayniya quarter, he demolished the *buza* [an alcoholic beverage made from fermented grain] cafe of al-Zulaqa and drove the prostitutes from it. He raided the house of al-'Anza, who was the head of the female singers' guild (*shaykhat al-maghani*) in Egypt, but didn't find her there. The merchants, the inhabitants of the city and the members of the guilds (*ahl al-sina'i*) wouldn't give wedding parties for their daughters without including the female singers, but ['Ali Agha] abolished all these [immoral] practices. [Because of these measures] the merchants destroyed the silver ornaments [used in the wedding parties]. The public singers and their leader took refuge in the house of 'Ali Hasan Katkhuda which was part of the house of Shahrab Efendi and dared not leave for fear of 'Ali Agha until she ['Anza] married her daughter to a public weigher and then died.

One of the most substantial government actions against professional entertainers occurred in the early 1830s, when Muḥammad 'Alī Bāshā took the drastic action of banning all public dance performances by female professional entertainers in Cairo and Alexandria (Clot-Bey 1840: 90, Lane 1860: 377, Lane 2005 [1836]: 566). The same decree also banned prostitution in Egypt's urban centers. It appears that Muḥammad 'Alī was responding to public agitation stemming from three sources. First was the moral indignation, particularly among the *'ulamā'* (an elite class of Islamic scholars) and other pious Egyptians, regarding the government's receipt of revenue from the taxation of morally reprehensible occupations, a factor which certainly contributed to the repeal of such taxes in the past.

Second, corruption and abuses in the application of the taxes on female entertainers and prostitutes generated significant public outrage. For example, St. John (1834: 115) notes that the official responsible for the taxation of prostitutes was convicted of adding "several respectable ladies" to his rolls "apparently through revenge" (but probably also to extort money for himself) (see also Tucker 1985: 151–152). Finally, as female entertainers and prostitutes increasingly plied their trades among foreigners, public indignation and resentment grew over this overt expression of foreign dominance in Egypt.

Punishments for violating the law were severe. According to Lane (2005 [1836]: 566): "Women detected infringing this new law are to be punished with fifty stripes for the first offence, and for repeated offences are to be also condemned to hard labor for one or more years." Many female professional entertainers fled the cities, while some were actually deported after they were found in violation of the law (see, for example, Didier 1860: 341).

The *ghawāzī* were the hardest hit by this action, since they primarily performed in public settings. The *'awālim*, who were favored by the elites, and who mostly entertained within elite households, were in many cases able to continue working. Recall that Sophia Lane-Poole witnessed several *'awālim* singing and dancing during Zaynab Hānim's wedding festivities in 1845. Nevertheless, it is probable that some *'awālim* and female *jink* faced repercussions as well. There was overlap among these categories, and some *'awālim* and female *jink* performed in the same public settings as *ghawāzī*. As discussed earlier, al-Jabartī's account of the incident in Ramadan 1814 describes *raqqāṣūn*—again, probably *'awālim*—performing alongside *ghawāzī* (al-Jabartī 1888–1896, volume 9: 102–103; 1904, volume 4: 227–228).

The ban forced many female professional entertainers to migrate to the smaller towns and villages of the Delta and Upper Egypt, where life was more uncertain. The *fallāḥīn*, the poor farmers who formed the majority of the rural population, could not afford to hire entertainers for their weddings, leaving the rural *mawālid* and performances for foreigners as the primary sources of income (Van Nieuwkerk 1995: 34). Further, security risks outside of the metropolitan centers of Alexandria and Cairo, combined with economic uncertainty, made some entertainers vulnerable to extortion by pimps, protectors, money lenders, and sometimes even the local police (Van Nieuwkerk 1995: 35–36). Thus, cross-purposes with the intent of the ban, the move to rural towns such as Isnā, Qinā, and Luxor actually propelled female entertainers further into performing for foreigners, as well as into prostitution.

Ultimately, the 1830s ban further blurred the boundaries between the various categories of female professional entertainer, and over the course of the next century, the terms *'awālim* and *ghawāzī* gradually shifted in meaning, while the term *jink/jinkiyah* for a female entertainer faded from common usage.* Though the term *ʿālmah* continued to be used for female singers even into the early twentieth century, by the 1930s, *muṭribah* became the preferred term for esteemed singers, as *ʿālmah* came to designate a common singer/dancer who performed for the lower and middle classes of urban Cairo and Alexandria (Lagrange 2009b: 227–228). The term *ghāziyah* increasingly referred strictly to singer/dancers working in the rural villages and the *mawālid*. In essence, the terms *ʿawālim* and *ghawāzī* began to convey a distinction between urban and rural singer/dancers, and neither group was highly esteemed in Egyptian society.

Male professional entertainers enjoyed a brief surge in popularity after the institution of the ban. According to Clot-Bey (1840: 95): "What is immoral in the dance of the almées becomes infamous in that of the *khowals*; and yet, since the ban on public female dancers, the number of these foolish men has increased, to the shame of morality, to which their existence bears the most degrading outrage." In fact, male dancers would continue to be popular in Egypt for decades to come. However, the designations *khawal* and *jink* would eventually be replaced by the more general term *rāqiṣ* or *raqqāṣ*, "dancer." The term *jink* faded into obsolescence, and the term *khawal*, though still used for a male dancer at the turn of the nineteenth and twentieth centuries, eventually came to refer to a male homosexual.

While it has been suggested that the 1830s ban on public performance by female professional entertainers was lifted during the reign of ʿAbbās Bāshā (r. 1848–1854) (for example, Van Nieuwkerk 1995: 36), Fraser points out that the ban continued to be vigorously enforced throughout his reign (Fraser 2015: 161–165). Taxation of both prostitutes and female entertainers resumed as early as 1866 (Duff Gordon 1875: 94–95), perhaps a manifestation of the substantial increase in taxation that took place under the administration of Khedive Ismāʿīl (Chalcraft 2005: 40–44). Yet, counter to earlier periods, when restrictions on entertainers generally coincided with the repeal of entertainment taxes, governmental restrictions on prostitution and public dance by female entertainers persisted even as taxation resumed.

Both Leland (1873: 130–131) and Warner (1900: 160) indicate that restrictions were in effect in Cairo in the 1870s. At the same time, female professional entertainers could be seen at private events hosted by the wealthy (Leland 1873: 130–131) and within at least one *café chantant* near the Azbakīyah Gardens (Linden 1884: 52, Warner 1900: 101–102). Adding to the confusion, Charmes indicates that female dancers performed

* The term is still understood, however, in both Egypt and the Levant. A Palestinian informant (male, aged mid-sixties) relayed to me that he remembered "*zay jinkiyah*" ("like a dancer") being used to criticize someone behaving ostentatiously.

publicly at the celebration of the Mūlid al-Nabī (the *mūlid* of the Prophet Muḥammad) in Cairo in the late 1870s (Charmes 1883: 179–181). These discrepancies suggest that governmental regulation of female professional entertainers in the latter half of the nineteenth century was somewhat arbitrary and inconsistent. In contrast to the situation in the urban centers, public performances by both male and female dancers at rural weddings and *mawālid* continued to be commonplace (see, for example, Ebers 1887: 82, Klunzinger 1878: 187–191, and Warner 1900: 46).

The situation would change dramatically with the advent of the British occupation in 1882. Under the occupation, the Egyptian government's bureaucratic and administrative functions became increasingly systematized, and governmental regulation of entertainment and entertainment venues became intrusive and methodical. These changes had profound implications for professional entertainers.

British Occupation

At the outset of the British occupation, the female professional entertainers known as *'awālim* and *ghawāzī* continued to ply their trades (Figure 4). However, in contrast to the *'awālim* of the late eighteenth century, who were entertainers to Egypt's elites, the *'awālim* of the late nineteenth century were largely popular entertainers who performed for Egypt's urban lower and (growing) middle classes. The tastes of Egypt's elites had shifted to European style entertainments such as opera, though they continued to occasionally patronize talented *'awālim*. The rural counterparts to the urban *'awālim* were the *ghawāzī*, who performed in the towns and villages of the Delta and Upper Egypt. Alongside the *'awālim* and *ghawāzī* were the male professional dancers, less numerous, but still common. The *mawālid* were largely the domain of male dancers and *ghawāzī*.

By the 1890s, some of Egypt's female professional entertainers had begun to perform in the newly-established music halls and theaters of Cairo and Alexandria. Though the first European-style theater was created in Cairo during Napoleon's brief occupation (see Sadgrove 1996: 27–31), it was in the second half of the nineteenth century that venues dedicated to the performance of comedy, drama, song, and dance would become commonplace in both Cairo and Alexandria. The first such venues were targeted at European consumers, offering European-style music, operettas, and the like. However, by the end of the century, there were a variety of venues offering Egyptian-style entertainment for the enjoyment of Egyptian audiences.

For Egypt's female dancers, in particular, these venues offered an

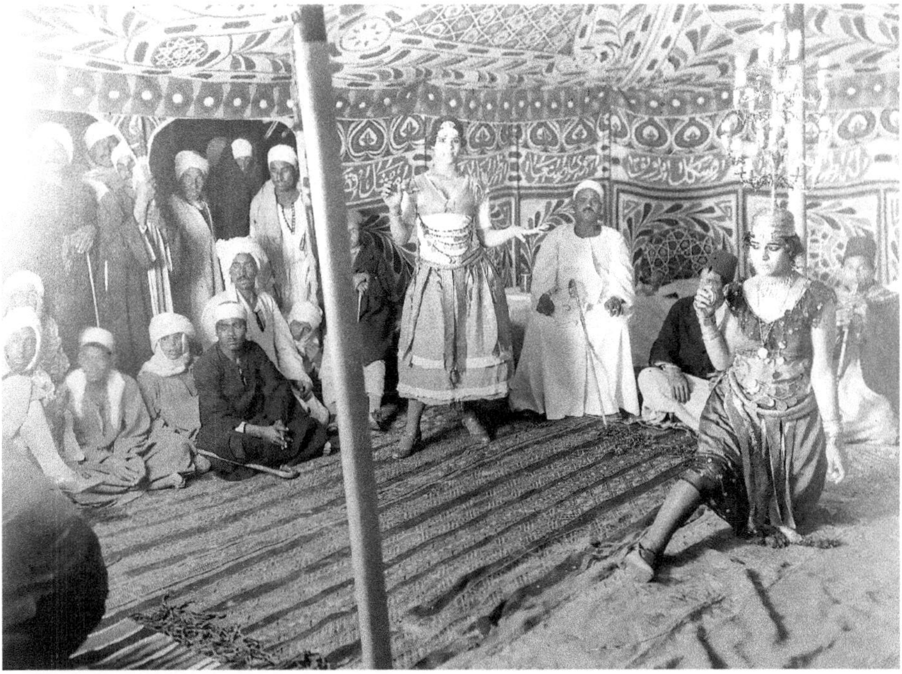

Figure 4: *Ghawāzī* of the early twentieth century (photo by Publishers Photo Service, *circa* 1920s).

opportunity to continue working in spite of the ongoing regulation of their trade. As noted above, restrictions on public dance in Egypt's urban centers continued long after Muḥammad 'Alī's ban. Such restrictions persisted—and even intensified—during the British occupation. In contrast to Charmes' observations in the 1870s, Leeder indicates that female dancers were completely absent from Cairo's Mūlid al-Nabī in the 1910s (Leeder 1913: 253). Even more telling, a brief 1894 article in the Arabic-language arts and literature magazine *al-Hilāl* commends the Egyptian government for implementing a ban on dance by female performers in public cafés (*al-Hilāl* 1 August 1894: 729). It is quite possible that this move was a direct response to popular outcries about public dance: just a few years earlier, *al-Ahrām* newspaper had published a complaint about female dancers gathering and performing at cafés in Cairo's Muḥarram Bik neighborhood (*al-Ahrām* 10 April 1891: 3). Notably, the 1890s ban applied only to public performances by *native* dancers, a point of frustration for the author of the *al-Hilāl* article (*al-Hilāl* 1 August 1894: 729).

Yet, multiple sources indicate that native female dancers were performing in Egyptian cafés, music halls, and theaters after the ban was put into effect. Guide books for travelers mention the "native dancing girls" of the El Dorado entertainment hall beginning in the 1890s (see, for example, Baedeker 1898: 24, Reynolds-Ball 1898b: 12). Frederic Penfield (Penfield 1899: 30), an American diplomat stationed in Cairo in the 1890s, describes the widespread presence of female dancers in Cairo's entertainment venues by the end of the century: "Another widely described institution, satisfying most spectators with a single view, is the dancing of the Ghawâzi girls, to be witnessed at a dozen Cairo theaters and cafes." A closer examination of the Egyptian government's approach toward entertainment and entertainment venues at the turn of the century is necessary to resolve this contradiction.

Legal restrictions on public dance at the turn of the century coincided with broader and more systematic government regulation of a wide array of public establishments, including bars, cafés, hotels, and theaters. In 1889, 1891, and 1904, a series of ordinances were passed to regulate such establishments, including those presenting entertainment (Brunyate 1906: 64–65, Fonder 2013: 61–72, Scott 1908: 278). The 1889 legislation enabled the policing of public establishments, while the legislation of 1891 created licensing requirements. Laws Number One and Thirteen of 1904 amended and supplemented the earlier laws, further detailing the licensing requirements for public establishments, including those presenting music, song, and dance (Brunyate 1906: 64–65).

Journalist Sydney Moseley describes the legislation that was in effect during his time in Egypt in the 1910s. Though not explicitly stated in his text, it is likely that he is referencing Laws Number One and Thirteen of 1904:

> One result of public agitation was the enactment of a drastic law curtailing the privileges of these night cafés, cabarets, music halls, and such places of rendezvous.... The new law divides public establishments into two categories. The first includes cafés, restaurants, cabarets, concert halls, sporting establishments, places of entertainment, clubs, and other similar places open to the public. The second comprises hotels, pensions, furnished apartment houses, and other similar establishments offering lodging to the public. In addition to the new law, theatres, etc., will be subject to the Theatre Law of 1912 [Moseley 1917: 207–208].*

Moseley goes on to detail how the "new law" established zoning regulations, licensing requirements for the sale of alcoholic beverages, and restrictions on hours of operation. Importantly, the new law also stipulated the following:

* Van Nieuwkerk (1995: 42–43) dates the Theatre Law to 1904 and states that amendments to the law were passed in 1911.

> No immoral entertainment or meeting can be held in these establishments, and no music, dances, or songs can be performed without a special permit, renewable yearly. No game of hazard can be played nor hashish be permitted on the premises [Moseley 1917: 209].

By the end of the 1920s, regulation of entertainment in public establishments had extended beyond the urban centers of Cairo and Alexandria to the towns and villages of the Egyptian countryside (Ward 2018: 56–57).

In its efforts to regulate entertainment and entertainment venues, the Egyptian government repeatedly found its hands tied by the Capitulations. Established under the Ottoman Empire, the Capitulations granted extraterritorial rights to certain European powers (Abu-Lughod 1971: 127). In essence, European nationals residing and doing business in Egypt were largely subject to the jurisdiction of their nation's consulate, rather than Egyptian law. Thus, though the Egyptian government passed numerous regulations pertaining to entertainment and entertainment venues, it sometimes found itself challenged to enforce them in cases involving foreign nationals. Brunyate (1906: 65), describing the legislation pertaining to public establishments that was passed in 1904, states:

> It is of a somewhat rudimentary character, owing to the fact that effective legislation as to such establishments would inevitably come into conflict with rights consecrated by the Capitulations, but it represents some advance towards effective control.

Given the previous discussion, it is noteworthy that many (if not most) of the venues that presented Egyptian dance in the 1890s and 1900s, including El Dorado, were owned and/or managed by foreigners—particularly Greeks and Italians. One need only glance through the various commercial directories published at the time to find listings for the many foreign-owned brasseries, cafés, cafés-concerts, and theaters (see, for example, The Egyptian Directory and Advertising Company, Limited 1907; Poffandi 1896, 1901, 1904; Société Anonyme Égyptienne de Publicité 1912). A 1913 article in the Arabic-language magazine *al-Zuhūr* notes that in the latter years of the nineteenth century, numerous cafés and theaters focused on Egyptian dance were opened by Greek entrepreneurs in Cairo and Alexandria (*al-Zuhūr* November 1913: 359–360). The article goes on to state that the Egyptian government closed several of these venues (*al-Zuhūr* November 1913: 361). Although the author does not provide a specific date, the text suggests that the government took this action sometime between 1887 and 1897.

It is possible that the government was enforcing the 1890s dance ban mentioned in *al-Hilāl* (*al-Hilāl* 1 August 1894: 729). In fact, I would posit that the 1890s action described in *al-Hilāl* may have been a crackdown on venues that were in violation of the licensing requirements established in 1891. Notably, the *al-Zuhūr* article states that the café and theater owners took their case to the courts and were able to re-open. It is probable that these Greek entertainment hall owners were able to overcome governmental restrictions on public dance due to the privileges afforded to them under the Capitulations.

The implication here is that at the turn of the century, foreign-owned entertainment venues likely held a particular attraction for Egyptian dancers, because they provided a means to evade contemporary restrictions on public dance. This is further corroborated by way of an anecdote from Muḥammad al-Muwayliḥī's fictional narrative *Ḥadīth 'Īsā Ibn Hishām* (*What 'Īsā Ibn Hishām Told Us*) (al-Muwayliḥī 2015, volume 2: 83–117). Originally published in serial form between 1898 and 1902, *Ḥadīth 'Īsā Ibn Hishām* is a sharp and satirical look at the uneasy juxtapositions of tradition and modernity in turn-of-the-century Egypt, and the struggle of Egyptians to navigate life under foreign occupation. Al-Muwayliḥī, the son of a businessman and newspaper publisher with connections to the aristocracy, paints a vivid picture of the (in his view) vice and profligacy at the heart of urban Cairo, when three of his main characters—a provincial *'umdah* (village mayor), a Westernized "playboy," and an urban merchant—watch a dance show in an Azbakīyah music hall. In this particular anecdote, al-Muwayliḥī inadvertently supplies some very useful information regarding the strategies employed by Egypt's female professional dancers to dodge restrictions on their trade:

> The [dancer's] husband is one of the Maghribi riffraff attached to a foreign government, a status that makes him immune to the authority of Egyptian laws. Prostitutes like this woman have habitually chosen to rely on men like him; they marry such a man and pay him a fixed amount on which to live. So while he's her husband in name, in fact she can be everyone's girlfriend. In return he serves and protects her. The woman sticks with her so-to-say husband so as to get foreign protection. Thus, whenever she happens to get in a situation in which Egyptian law will seek to punish her, the fact that she's married to this man will serve to protect her from the law. Whenever, in the name of modesty and decency, the government attempts to stop her dancing, behaving in a lewd fashion, and blatantly promoting sex, she can't be stopped. If the government forces her, the crafty woman can go to the Mixed Courts because of her relationship with her husband and claim damages for being forced out of work [al-Muwayliḥī 2015, volume 2: 113].

Al-Muwayliḥī's anecdote, though fictional, illustrates how the loopholes provided by the Capitulations enabled Egyptian dancers to keep working in spite of heavy government regulation.

By the end of the nineteenth century, Egypt's female professional dancers were a fixture in urban music halls and theaters. These venues represented a fundamental departure from traditional modes of entertainment in Egypt. Prior to the establishment of these venues, professional entertainment occurred in the context of traditional social occasions—weddings, circumcisions, public markets, and saint's day festivals—or at one of Egypt's many coffee houses. With the creation of dedicated spaces for performance, professional entertainment was no longer embedded in the traditional occasions and settings that had previously justified its performance. As Danielson states, it was "cut loose from the moorings of religious or celebratory occasions and removed from familial environments" (Danielson 1999: 118). Professional entertainment could now be sought after and enjoyed for its own sake, by anyone willing to pay the cost of admission. In these settings, the traditional dances of the *'awālim* and the *ghawāzī* gradually transformed into the concert dance form that would come to be known as *raqṣ sharqī* (Ward 2018).

A female dancer who performed *raqṣ sharqī* in one of these many urban entertainment venues was described as a *rāqiṣah* or *raqqāṣah*, rather than an *'ālmah* or a *ghāziyah*. The terms *'ālmah* and *ghāziyah* continued to be in common usage: *'ālmah* continued to be associated with the common singer/dancers who performed at the weddings and other celebrations of the lower and middle classes of urban Cairo and Alexandria, while *ghāziyah* remained tied to singer/dancers working in the rural villages and the *mawālid*. In Joseph Habeiche's French-Arabic dictionary, the entry for *danseuse* (female dancer) lists both *raqqāṣah* and *ghāziyah* (Habeiche 1890: 136), and the entry for *cantatrice* (female singer) lists *'ālmah* and *mughannīyah* (Habeiche 1890: 79).

Similarly, Socrates Spiro's English-Arabic dictionary from 1897 lists *ghāziyah* for female dancer (Spiro 1897: 134) and *'ālmah* for female singer (Spiro 1897: 441). Also, it is worth noting that female singers who appeared in music halls and theaters were occasionally referred to as *'awālim*. For example, an 1895 advertisement in *al-Ahrām* announces a musical performance by "*al-'ālmah, al-muṭribah* [the singer], *al-sayyidah* [the lady]" al-Lāwandīyah (*al-Ahrām* 26 March 1895: 3). However, neither *'ālmah* nor *ghāziyah* appears to have been used with any regularity to refer to a dancer performing in an urban entertainment hall.

In spite of this terminological distinction, many of these dancers were *'awālim* and *ghawāzī* who found work in the theaters and music halls of Cairo and Alexandria—at least initially. Further, the use of the term *rāqiṣah/raqqāṣah* should not lead to the conclusion that these early performers of *raqṣ sharqī* specialized exclusively in dance. Many of these women, like their predecessors throughout Egyptian history, were well-rounded entertainers who not only danced, but sang. Shafīqah al-Qibṭīyah was a turn-of-the-century entertainment hall performer who has often been linked to a specific dance act known as *raqṣat al-sham'adān* (i.e., the candelabrum dance, in which a candelabrum is balanced on the dancer's head) (Ward 2013). Photographs of Shafīqah and a number of other contemporary dancers are included in Maḥmūd Ḥamdī al-Būlāqī's 1904 book, *Mufriḥ al-Jins al-Laṭīf wa-Ṣuwwar Mashāhīr al-Raqqāṣīn* (*Joy of the Fair Sex and Pictures of Famous Dancers*). The popularity of Shafīqah and her dance hall is recorded in the notes of Muḥammad Sa'īd Shīmī Bik, an Interior Ministry spy of Khedive 'Abbās Ḥilmī (r. 1892–1914) (see, for example, HIL/15/21–22 in *Abbas Hilmi II Papers*). Nevertheless, it is clear that Shafīqah was also known to be a singer. S.H. Leeder notes:

> For years the most scandalous of the public singing women in Cairo bears a name which she has made so famous that I have never met an intelligent person anywhere in Lower Egypt who was not most familiar with it—*Shafika el Coptieh*, or Shafika the Copt [Leeder 1918: 107].

One of Shafīqah's singing and dancing performances is spoofed in a *circa* 1908 Odéon recording by the singer Bahiyah al-Maḥallāwīyah (*Raqṣ Shafīqah* 1908). Singing continued to be part of a *rāqiṣah/raqqāṣah*'s repertoire well into the twentieth century.

However, by the 1930s, the entertainment circuit of theaters, music halls, and the like had begun to diverge from the traditional entertainment circuits of the *'awālim* and the *ghawāzī*, with the result that there was less and less overlap between the dancers who performed in these different settings. The music halls of the 1910s and 1920s evolved into the nightclubs of the 1930s and 1940s. In this environment, female dancers thrived. Many were able to achieve celebrity status, and some went on to own or manage entertainment venues of their own. However, this success often came at great cost and with substantial risk. Government regulation of professional entertainment persisted, though its intensity waxed and waned throughout the first half of the twentieth century (Van Nieuwkerk 1995: 46–48). The abolition of the Capitulations was initiated in 1937 (Vatikiotis 1991: 293), removing one mechanism for evading regulation. Some entertainers fell victim to protection rackets: such was the case of the dancer Imtithāl Fawzī, who was murdered inside her own nightclub for refusing to accede to the demands of a local gang (Cormack 2021: 284–287).

Beginning in the 1920s and 1930s, the female professional dancers of Egypt's urban entertainment venues ventured into a new and growing entertainment medium: the cinema. Over the course of the 1930s and 1940s, the nightclub and cinema circuit became increasingly distinct from the traditional circuit. As the cinema became available to a wider Egyptian public, cinema portrayals of Egyptian belly dance began to shape public perceptions and expectations regarding style, technique, and costuming. Over the course of the twentieth century, the *raqṣ sharqī* performers of the cinema would become the standard against which all Egyptian belly dancers were judged, and *raqṣ sharqī* would eclipse the dances of the *'awālim* and the *ghawāzī* as the normative style of Egyptian belly dance.

Egypt's first film screening took place in 1896, in a café in Alexandria (el-Charkawi 1963: 3). According to el-Charkawi, by 1908, there were five cinemas in Cairo, three in Alexandria, and one each in Port Sa'īd, Manṣūra, and Asyūṭ (el-Charkawi 1963: 3). Initially, audiences consisted of Europeans and the Egyptian elite. However, film gradually became more accessible to a wider cross-section of the Egyptian public, not only due to the addition of additional cinemas, but also because film screenings were added to the variety programs presented in Egyptian entertainment halls.

Although the earliest films screened in Egypt were produced by foreigners, Egyptians soon began to establish their own production companies and to create films that were targeted towards the interests and aesthetics of the native population. The silent film *Layla*, considered by many to be the first Egyptian feature-length film (el-Charkawi 1963: 5), premiered at Cairo's Metropole Cinema in 1927. A few years later, in 1935, Egyptian businessman Ṭal'at Ḥarb established Studio Miṣr, which would remain an influential force in the Egyptian cinema for years to come (el-Charkawi 1963: 11–13).

Egyptian films from the 1930s onward often contained scenes that provided pretexts for music and dance numbers. Scenes set in nightclubs were particularly common and ensured the frequent appearance of female professional dancers in film. As Shafik has noted, the Egyptian cinema became "frantically obsessed" with these venues and the belly dancers who performed within them (Shafik 2006: 163–165). Cinematic portrayals of the nightclubs varied widely. While they were sometimes depicted as dens of vice, in other cases, they provided a path to wealth, fame, and success for an aspiring protagonist. Similarly, film portrayals of female professional dancers were decidedly mixed. As Dougherty states:

> Female dance stars from the 1930s to the present day have certainly played dancers who were home wreckers, gold-diggers, unreconstructed girlfriends of gangsters, and enslaved, drug-addicted creatures of pimps. But they have also portrayed dancers as loving daughters, faithful wives and partners, good mothers, and successful artists making a contribution to the cultural development of Egyptian society [Dougherty 2005: 153].

These variable depictions reflect Egyptians' complex and conflicted opinions regarding professional belly dancers, as well as their ambivalent attitudes towards dance in professional entertainment venues, where it was being performed without the social justification provided by a festive occasion such as a wedding.

The belly dancers who appeared in Egyptian films from the 1930s through the 1960s were generally *raqṣ sharqī* performers who got their start in the very venues depicted in such complex and conflicted ways on the silver screen. For example, one of the most prolific dance stars of the twentieth-century Egyptian cinema, Taḥīyah Carioca, started her career working in the entertainment halls of Su'ād Maḥāssan and Badī'ah Maṣābnī (Adum n.d., *Badia Masabni in 1966 Television Interview* n.d.). Similarly, the beloved dancer Sāmiyah Jamāl got her start at Badī'ah Maṣābnī's Casino Opera (Adum n.d., *Badia Masabni in 1966 Television Interview* n.d.).

The *'awālim* and the *ghawāzī* were periodically depicted in Egyptian film; however, they were rarely portrayed by actual *'awālim* and *ghawāzī*. A few notable exceptions exist. For example, the legendary *'ālmah* Zūbah al-Klūbātīyah can be seen executing impressive balancing acts in a number of Egyptian films, including *al-Khamsah Jinīh* (1946), *Fatāt al-Sīrk* (1951), and *Wa'd* (1954). The famous *'ālmah* Nazlah al-'Ādil can be seen performing her signature splits to the accompaniment of her finger cymbals in *Qaṣr al-Shūq* (1966). Additionally, the Banāt Māzin *ghawāzī* appear in at least two films from the 1960s: *al-Zawjah al-Thāniyah* (1967) and *Anā al-Duktūr* (1968). These are the exceptions that prove the rule, however. More often than not, *'awālim* and *ghawāzī* were played by *raqṣ sharqī* performers.

Still, it is important to note that many *raqṣ sharqī* performers of the early-to-mid twentieth century did have connections to urban *'awālim* culture. As noted earlier, many of the first dancers to appear in Egypt's entertainment halls were *'awālim* and *ghawāzī*. As the century progressed, various performers emerged from Cairo's Muḥammad 'Alī Street neighborhood, the area where many *'awālim* continued to be based. For example, Na'amat Mukhtār, a popular dancer who frequently appeared on film in the 1950s and 1960s, resided with her mother in a Muḥammad 'Alī Street flat that they rented from Zūbah al-Klūbātīyah (*About Naemet Mokhtar* n.d.). Though she denied any associations with the *'awālim*, the gymnastic backbends that she frequently performed were atypical of *raqṣ sharqī* in her day and suggestive of the *'awālim* style. Another dancer with explicit *'awālim* connections was Nabawīyah Muṣṭafa, who appeared in many films throughout the 1940s and 1950s. Like Na'amat Mukhtār, she performed flamboyant, gymnastic movements more similar to the *'awālim* style than to contemporary *raqṣ sharqī*. Importantly, Nabawīyah's mother was an *'ālmah* from Muḥammad 'Alī Street (*al-Muṣawwa*r 1958). While these examples argue for a continuing connection between the *ʿawālim* and the performers of *raqṣ sharqī*, the profound stylistic differences between Naʿamat Mukhtār and Nabawīyah Muṣṭafa and the vast majority of their contemporaries indicate that the ongoing stylistic influence of *ʿawālim* dance on *raqṣ sharqī* was minimal. Indeed, the growing stylistic disconnect between *raqṣ sharqī* performers and the *ʿawālim* and *ghawāzī* highlights the divergence of their respective entertainment circuits.

Important implications emerge from *raqṣ sharqī* performers playing varied Egyptian dance roles. A *raqṣ sharqī* dancer, whether playing a Cairo nightclub entertainer, an *ʿālmah* dancing at a lower-class Cairo wedding, or a *ghāziyah* performing at a village *mūlid*, danced in a fairly similar manner. The resulting homogeneity of technique and style would begin to shape public perceptions and expectations with regards to professional belly dance. In essence, Egyptian cinema established a unified vision of what constituted good technique, proper costuming, and an interesting and engaging style. Cinema stars such as Taḥīyah Carioca and Sāmiyah Jamāl became the benchmarks against whom other dancers would be measured. In this manner, *raqṣ sharqī* would eventually be able to overshadow the dances of the *ʿawālim* and the *ghawāzī* to become the *de facto* representation of professional belly dance to the Egyptian public.

Still, because the audiences for the cinema were (and still are) primarily urban (see Shafik 2006: 282–285), the portrayal of *raqṣ sharqī* in Egyptian film had limited impact beyond Egypt's urban centers until the advent of television in the 1960s. Roushdy states:

> What is unquestionably a crucial contribution of Egyptian cinema to the dance culture, not only in Egypt but in the entire Middle East, is the diffusion of the style developed in the nightclubs of Cairo to the public, a style that continues to characterize the structure of the *baladi* dance observed today. Moreover, when television was introduced, these movies entered the Egyptian household and familiarized the wider public with the cabaret style, which was originally limited to a small segment of the population. It played a crucial role in the socialization of young Egyptians into the local dance culture and continues to influence the performance style of professional and non-professional dancers [Roushdy 2009: 38].

As Roushdy and others have noted, the films of the 1930s through the 1960s are still regularly broadcast on Egyptian television, ensuring the continued influence of this cinematic vision of *raqṣ sharqī* on the public imagination. Indeed, many of the *raqṣ sharqī* performers of those early films are still viewed as beloved national icons.

Even as female professional belly dancers made their way onto stage and screen, *ʿawālim* and *ghawāzī* continued to perform at the popular celebrations of ordinary Egyptians. The early decades of the twentieth century were a golden age for the *'awālim*, who were a necessary feature of urban lower and middle class weddings. The *'awālim* occasionally worked in the *mawālid* of Cairo and the Nile Delta as well (Van Nieuwkerk 1995: 53–54). The majority of Cairo's *'awālim* resided on Muḥammad 'Alī Street, as well as in the smaller streets and alleys near the main boulevard (Van Nieuwkerk 1995: 50). Famous *'awālim* hung signs outside of their homes to announce their availability for weddings and parties; many also advertised their services in local newspapers and magazines. Literary depictions of the *'awālim* in the early twentieth century, such as al-Hakim's *Return of the Spirit* and Naguib Mahfouz's *Cairo Trilogy*, attest to the importance of the *'awālim* in Egyptian popular culture at the time.

The *ghawāzī* were a fixture at the *mawālid*, with the exception of a period of government repression of these festivals during the 1930s (see McPherson 1941). McPherson, who documented a broad array of Egyptian *mawālid* in the early twentieth century, makes frequent note of the "dancing girls" that performed there. At the larger *mawālid*, there were tent theaters that featured variety entertainment, including male and female belly dancers. At the 1934 *mūlid* of Ḥusayn, centered on the saint's mosque and mausoleum in Fatimid Cairo, the *ghawāzī* could be seen in a mile-long line of tent theaters that extended from the end of the Sikkat al-Jadīdah (the eastern extension of al-Mūskī Street), skirting the wasteland to the east of the city (McPherson 1941: 220).

Alongside the *'awālim* and the *ghawāzī* were the male dancers, who remained popular well into the twentieth century. Male dancers appear to have been fairly commonplace at *mawālid* throughout the early decades of the twentieth century, excepting the government repression of the 1930s. McPherson (1941: 84–85) documented a popular performer named Ḥusayn Fu'ād:

> A very well known character, a star unique in his way, has not been *en evidence* very recently. He danced always in the dress, ornaments, hair, lipstick, and manners of a woman, and people who watched for the umteenth time could hardly be made to believe that he was not what he appeared. He generally made a simpering round of the audience, and with a smirk presented his photo under which was printed, [in Arabic] "The celebrated Egyptian dancer, Husein Foad" and his address for private appointments to weddings, &c. Whether of his own free will, he "walked sober off," or whether he attracted the attention of the "city fathers" and was shoved off, I cannot say [McPherson 1941: 84].

There is also anecdotal evidence of male dancers performing in theaters and music halls. In an interview with journalist Yūsuf al-Sharīf, Zūbah al-Klūbātīyah indicated that she learned *raqṣat al-sham'adān* by imitating a male performer whom she witnessed at a venue called Ṣalāḥ

'Izz al-Dīn in Cairo (Yiḥyā 2017)—most likely sometime during the 1930s. Male actors sometimes performed in drag in the entertainment halls, even portraying female belly dancers (for example, Dinning 1920: 275–276). This phenomenon would continue to be commonplace in Egyptian cinema. The actor Ismā'il Yāsīn was particularly famous for his drag roles (see Shafik 2006: 160–162). However, performances by actual male professional belly dancers were uncommon in film.

At the turn of the century, both *rāqiṣ* or *raqqāṣ* and *khawal* were in use to refer to male dancers; the term *jink* appears to have already faded away. Habeiche's dictionary lists *raqqāṣ* (Habeiche 1890: 136), while Spiro's dictionary lists two terms: *khawal* and *ghāyish* (Spiro 1897: 134). Apparently, the term *khawal* had assumed its present-day connotation of male homosexual by the time Spiro published his second edition in 1923. The 1923 edition offers two definitions for *khawal*: "dancing-man" or "effeminate, catamite" (Spiro 1923: 165). Spiro's second edition includes both *rāqiṣ* and *raqqāṣ*, as well as *ghāyish* (Spiro 1923: 186, 196, 313). Notably, Ḥusayn Fu'ād used the term *rāqiṣ* on his professional photos (as described by McPherson1941: 84).

The Nasser Era and Beyond

On July 23, 1952, Egypt witnessed its second revolution of the twentieth century, when a group of young military officers overthrew the Egyptian monarchy. While the 1952 revolution shared the anti–British orientation of the earlier 1919 revolution, the class divisions brought to the fore in 1952 presented a stark contrast to the cross-class unity that characterized the revolution of 1919. Under the presidency of Gamal Abdel Nasser (1954–1970), the wealth and influence of foreigners and of Egypt's landed aristocracy were effectively dissolved through the institution of state socialism, and Egyptian nationalism was linked to a broader vision of pan–Arab unity. In the entertainment industry, the state found an important mechanism for propagating its ideology of Egyptian nationhood. The cinema was nationalized in 1963, and from the 1960s onward, the state encouraged the institutionalization and professionalization of the entertainment industry by supporting institutional forms of training in the arts (Shafik 2006: 108, 282–283; Van Nieuwkerk 1995: 62–63).

Nasser's regime espoused an ideology of popular unity that celebrated the important role of the ordinary folk—the lower class and the peasantry—in Egyptian society, and in the newly-established genre of theatrical folk dance, the state found a powerful and effective mechanism for propagating this ideology. Two folk dance companies were founded in short succession. First came the Firqat Riḍā (the Riḍā Troupe), created by Maḥmūd Riḍā in 1959 and nationalized in 1961. It was followed almost immediately by the Firqat al-Qawmīyah lil-Funūn al-Sha'bīyah (the National Troupe of Folk Arts), when the Egyptian government hired Boris Ramazin, a former Moiseyev Dance Company member, to create an Egyptian folk dance company in the mold of the Riḍā Troupe.

In reality, the vision of the "folk" embodied by these troupes was very much informed by urban elite sensibilities, and their romantic portrayals of the Egyptian "everyman" and "everywoman" deliberately avoided aspects of traditional folk dance that the upper classes deemed "unseemly." Shay (2002: 136) writes:

> As has been the case in many nations with a large peasantry, while despising the peasant as unlettered, poor, and dirty, urban upper-class individuals also romanticize the peasants and their supposed bucolic lives.... Both of these elements—the romantic and the avoidance of actual peasant movements, music, and costume—are woven into the choreographies of Mahmoud Reda. Like Igor Moisiyev and Amalia Hernandez, Reda clearly manifests the need to "improve" the original materials through the use of fantasy stories, urban-designed costumes, large theater orchestras, and sanitized movements.

Most noticeable was the removal or alteration of movements associated with belly dance. Shay (2002: 148) notes:

> Among the many specific choreographic strategies that [Maḥmūd Riḍā] utilized, in my opinion his most striking modifications, alterations, and inventions relate to his treatment of solo-improvised dance, the general term that I employ to cover the most widespread Egyptian dance genre, of which the best known example is belly dancing.

Urban elite discomfort with this widely practiced traditional dance demanded the "sanitization" of the movement vocabulary.

A particularly troubling aspect of belly dance was its blurring of masculine and feminine roles. In social settings, belly dance is practiced by both men and women, and the movements are entirely the same, regardless of the dancer's gender. Further, as noted throughout this chapter, there is a long history of male professional belly dancers in Egypt, and in most cases these men have adopted feminine attire and mannerisms. In keeping with contemporary elite attitudes regarding masculinity and femininity, the theatrical folk dance troupes strictly differentiated masculine and feminine roles, leaving no space for belly dance's gender ambiguity:

> Mahmoud Reda did not permit males on his stage to perform any [belly dance] movements, thus following the colonial gaze, now shared by elite decision makers in the Egyptian government, of what constitutes proper and

> improper movements for the male (English, and now Egyptian body). Mahmoud Reda's new theatrical genre thus attempts to erase the actual performance practices of the people, both urban and rural [Shay 2002: 148].

The strict gender binary represented by the theatrical folk dance troupes did not reflect on-the-ground realities: both men and women continued to practice belly dance in social settings, and male professional belly dancers continued to exist, though they may have been less common than in prior decades. For example, a young male dancer is described (and pictured) in a 1955 article in the Egyptian entertainment magazine *Ahl al-Fann*. Like his predecessors in earlier periods, this dancer wore female attire (in this case, a skirt and blouse) and make-up.

The government's actions with respect to arts and entertainment had dire implications for professional belly dancers. The professionalization of the entertainment industry—in particular, the institutionalization of training—created a split between "high" and "low" art. The theatrical folk dance troupes, which embraced a formalized mode of classroom training based on the Western ballet model (see, for example, Fahmy 1987: 25–27), fit well within an institutional structure. Artists and entertainers with institutional training found themselves with more and better employment opportunities than those without formal training.

> For [belly] dancers, professionalization has generally had an unfavorable effect. From the 1960s, the Ministry of Culture has patronized ballet and folk-dance groups, such as the Reḍa Troupe and the National Troupe of Folk Arts. Belly dancing has been left without any form of schooling or recognition [Van Nieuwkerk 1995: 63].

The various forms of professional belly dance, which generally followed a more traditional mode of learning centered on individual training and mentoring by an experienced performer, would be effectively sidelined by an entertainment industry that favored institutionally-trained, credentialed theatrical folk dancers representing a state-supported vision of wholesome Egyptianness. There would be no academies or institutes for belly dance, and there would certainly be no state sponsorship. Belly dance and its professional practitioners—male and female—did not fit within the state's vision of the "folk."

The establishment of provincial troupes in the mold of the Cairo-based folk dance groups at the various "Palaces of Culture" throughout Egypt ensured widespread dissemination of the state's vision. To this day, these institutions propagate the cultural policies of the Ministry of Culture at the local level. Saleh, writing in 1979, describes how the theatrical folk dance genre became so pervasive that it even began to impact the source dances upon which it was based:

> As concerns the status of dance, it is worthy of note that for the past twenty years they have been subjected to a concentrated campaign bent on "improving" them, to make them more befitting to the new image of Egypt. The result to date has been a proliferation of theatricalized versions of a number of dances. These have, in their transition to stage and night-club, almost lost any resemblance to the authentic material, whether in regard to pattern, gesture, costume, music, or custom. The regrettable tendency of these innovations is then, by means of the vast media network and Palaces of Culture, to revert to their home base, there affecting the source of original inspiration [Saleh 1979: 462].

Around the same time that the government was throwing its support behind theatrical folk dance, film portrayals of belly dancers were beginning to change. According to Dougherty:

> Through my viewing and research I found that in the first three decades of Egyptian cinema, dancers in cinema are portrayed by women who are themselves professional dancers; after about 1960 and ever since, dancers tend to be portrayed by women who are originally actresses and not dancers.... When dancers are portrayed in film by non-dancers, the tendency to present a negative image of the profession is much greater [Dougherty 2005: 167].

Compounding the ideologically-driven impacts initiated under the Nasser regime were the profound effects of the economic policies of Nasser's successor, Anwar Sadat (1970–1981). Sadat, in a dramatic retreat from the socialist policies of Nasser, relaxed government controls over the Egyptian economy and encouraged private investment. The *nouveau riche* who benefited from Sadat's policy of *infitāḥ* (openness) were profligate spenders on leisure and entertainment, as were the wealthy Persian Gulf tourists who eventually became a common sight in Cairo's popular nightclubs.

For professional belly dancers in Egypt's urban centers, this was initially a booming period with abundant work and high pay, and these benefits attracted many individuals from outside the belly dance profession to enter the trade. Unfortunately, the boom rapidly turned to bust, leaving dancers struggling to survive in an oversaturated market with declining demand. The mass influx of outsiders disrupted the traditional networks that existed among singers and dancers in places like Cairo's Muḥammad 'Alī Street; these networks were the means by which professional entertainers maintained standards of artistry and enforced unwritten rules of behavior. Van Nieuwkerk notes:

> *Khushnî* (plural: *khashânâ*) is the word the older generation uses to denote the "intruders," the people without roots in the trade who have recently entered it. It is derived from the Standard Arabic *khishin*, "coarse" or "rough," and means that the newcomers are still ignorant of the subtleties and rules of the trade [Van Nieuwkerk 1995: 100].

Outside of the traditional networks, individual entertainers were left to fend for themselves, and to minimize risk, female dancers increasingly aligned themselves with male impresarios. Male managers and agents certainly existed prior to this period. For example, in a 1958 interview in the popular Egyptian magazine *al-Muṣawwar*, Muḥammad ʿAlī Street *ʿālmah* Anūs laments the incursion of males into the business, revealing that male impresarios were already an important and influential part of the trade as early as the 1950s (*al-Muṣaww*ar 1958: 26). However, with the boom and bust of the 1970s and the flood of outsiders into the trade, male impresarios rapidly ascended to dominate the business of belly dance. As Van Nieuwkerk notes, the market had become "impersonal and hazardous," and for individual female dancers in this unstable environment, there was security and stability in aligning with a male impresario (Van Nieuwkerk 1995: 57–58). As a consequence of these developments, from the 1970s onward, female dancers have largely lost control over their trade, and male impresarios have assumed control of booking parties, setting fees, and most other aspects of the business.

By the end of the twentieth century, the *ʿawālim* tradition had largely ceased to exist. Today, most of the final generation of *ʿawālim* have passed away. I have been unable to find any of the surviving *ʿawālim* who are willing to discuss their prior involvement with the trade. In fact, even family members are often unwilling to speak on these matters, as I discovered in several futile attempts to secure an interview with the daughter of the *ʿālmah* Nazlah al-ʿĀdil in 2014.

In the present day, female professional belly dancers (*rāqiṣāt/raqqāṣāt* or *fannānāt*) in Egypt's urban centers are divided into tiers depending on their work setting (Figures 5 and 6). At the top of the pyramid are the elite dancers who perform in discos, five-star hotel nightclubs, and upper-class weddings (and who occasionally cross over into film and television roles). Next are the dancers who perform in the myriad Nile cruise boats that cater primarily to tourists and some well-heeled Egyptians, as well as some higher-end cabarets. Below these are the dancers of the lower-class cabarets and nightclubs, and the dancers who perform at the urban weddings of the lower classes. Echoes of the old *ʿawālim* dance style can still be glimpsed in the dancing of the lower-class cabaret and wedding performers, though none of these dancers can be properly termed *ʿawālim*.

The state-sponsored theatrical folk dance troupes that emerged in the middle of the twentieth century have had a direct impact on the technique and aesthetic of present-day *raqṣ sharqī*. In the latter decades of the twentieth century, former members of the Riḍā Troupe and the National Troupe of Folk Arts entered the world of belly dance as solo performers and trainers/choreographers of *raqṣ sharqī*. Rāqīah Ḥassan, a former company

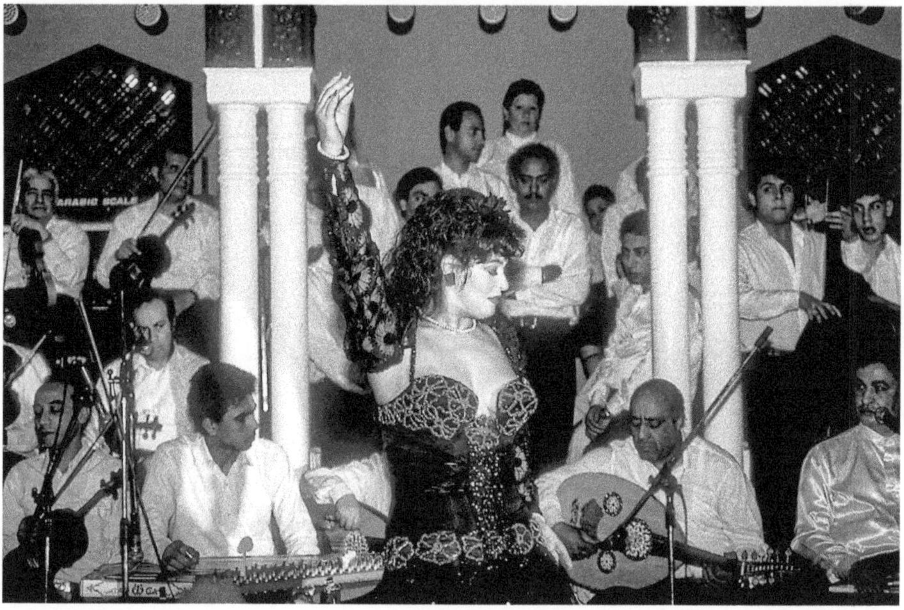

Figure 5: Fifi ‘Abduh, one of the most famous Egyptian dancers of the late twentieth century, and today a popular film and television star, here performing at the Cairo Sheraton in 1992 (Christine Osborne Pictures / Alamy).

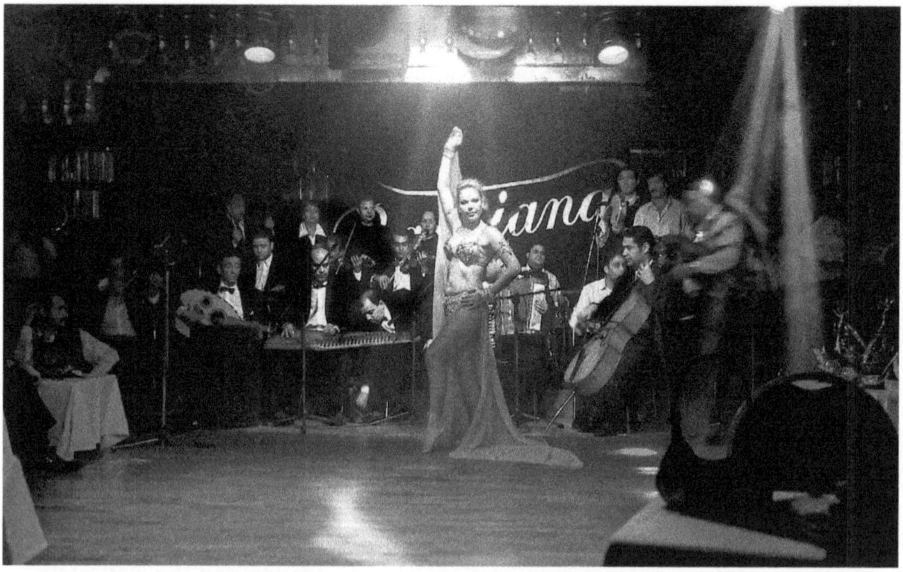

Figure 6: The popular dancer Lucy performing at her Parisiana nightclub (Horizons WWP / Alamy Stock Photo).

dancer of the Riḍā Troupe, is a trainer and choreographer to some of the most celebrated *raqṣ sharqī* performers of the present day. Former members of the theatrical folk dance troupes, like Ḥassan, as well as their protégés, tour and train dancers around the world; they also organize dance festivals targeted at non-Egyptian practitioners. As a result, their vision of *raqṣ sharqī*, one that is heavily informed by the stylization of the theatrical folk dance troupes, has come to dominate the international market.

As noted earlier, the theatrical folk dance genre firmly differentiated masculine and feminine roles, and the genre could not accommodate the gender ambiguity that is characteristic of belly dance. Nevertheless, many male dancers from the theatrical folk dance troupes have worked as belly dance trainers and choreographers. A few have worked as professional belly dancers themselves. However, their performances within Egypt have generally been limited to the tourist-oriented Red Sea resorts or to the dance festivals targeted at foreign practitioners. Indeed, in the current era, Egypt's male belly dancers find their most lucrative opportunities on the international workshop and festival circuit rather than in the weddings and nightclubs of their home country.

Outside of Egypt's urban centers, the rural *ghawāzī* have persisted. Today, they primarily perform at weddings, circumcisions, and other family celebrations. The *mawālid*, once the backbone of the *ghawāzī* livelihood, are now largely devoid of professional belly dancers. Government suppression is the likely culprit: Schielke (2006: 196) notes that in the 1990s the Egyptian government issued bans on female dancers at "most mawlids" and a "tent with transvestite shows" at the *mūlid* of Ḥusayn. Nevertheless, Parrs (2017: 205) indicates that when she was conducting her research in the 2010s: "I was provided with a few examples of 'secret tents' where Ghawazi were still, almost clandestinely, dancing or 'showing part of their bodies' to enthusiastic crowds."

Most of the remaining *ghawāzī* are located in Upper Egypt, in the vicinity of Luxor, Qinā, and Sūhāj. The *ghawāzī* who still actively perform are based out of these towns and out of nearby villages, particularly the villages of Abū Shūshah and Naj' Ḥammādī. In personal interviews with dancers and musicians in Luxor and Abū Shūshah in January 2022, I was told that a great deal of the current demand for the traditional *ghawāzī* dance style is located in the vicinity of Naj' Ḥammādī, and further south in Kom Ombo, Edfu, and Aswan.

The *ghawāzī* of Lower Egypt appear largely to have vanished, having been replaced by urban *rāqiṣāt/raqqāṣāt*.* Indeed, the proximity of Cairo

* Interestingly, one of my informants, Riḍā Ḥankish, a well-known and well-respected musician from a famous Muḥammad 'Alī Street family, used the term *raqqāṣīn* for these women (personal communication, January 23, 2022).

and Alexandria and their ready supply of belly dancers, combined with the decline of belly dance at *mawālid*, likely spelled the doom of the Delta *ghawāzī* tradition. While the current dancers fulfill the same social functions as their *ghawāzī* predecessors—providing entertainment at weddings and other celebrations—they have no familial or social ties to the *ghawāzī* who once performed in the region (Riḍā Ḥankish, personal communication, January 23, 2022).

I would posit that, in much the same way that outsiders disrupted the traditional networks of Muḥammad ʻAlī Street, urban *rāqiṣāt/raqqāṣāt* have contributed to the disruption and decline of the traditional networks that maintained the integrity of the *ghawāzī* tradition in Lower Egypt. Until now, the *ghawāzī* of Upper Egypt have avoided a similar fate, probably due to their geographic distance from Cairo and Alexandria. However, it is important to note that belly dancers from Cairo and Alexandria are frequently imported to perform in Upper Egyptian hotels and Nile cruise boats, and even at local weddings. Under pressure of competition from urban *rāqiṣāt/raqqāṣāt*, local *ghawāzī* perform urban *raqṣ sharqī* when their audiences request it. Nevertheless, the persistence of local demand for the traditional *ghawāzī* style of dance has ensured the survival of the Upper Egyptian *ghawāzī* tradition.

Conclusion

The history outlined here demonstrates the deep roots of belly dance and its professional practitioners in Egypt. For centuries, professional entertainers have been woven into the fabric of Egyptian social and cultural life, even as their identities have positioned them outside of the mainstream of Egyptian society. In spite of their marginality, these men and women have figured prominently in the social and spatial realities of Egyptians for generations. From the female slave entertainers and *mukhannathūn* of the ninth century, to the *raqqāṣāt* and *raqqāṣīn* of today, the professional entertainers of Egypt have been a constant presence in Egyptian life.

The following chapters explore the dialectical interplay between Egypt's professional entertainers and the spaces that they have occupied within the Cairo landscape. The presence and practice of entertainers have contributed to the production and reproduction of meaningful spaces constituting Cairo's landscape of entertainment. At the same time, these meaningful spaces have informed the perceptions and actions of the individuals moving within them. In essence, the dialectical relationship between entertainers and entertainment spaces has embedded belly dance and its professional practitioners in the lived experience of Cairenes, both socially and spatially. From the emergence of a landscape of entertainment in the Fatimid era, through the elaboration of this landscape over the ensuing centuries, until its restructuring in the twentieth century, the remaining chapters of this book reveal the mutually constituting relationship between Cairo's landscape of entertainment and Egypt's professional entertainers.

Two

Fatimid Beginnings

The nucleus of the modern city of Cairo was established in 969, when the Fatimids conquered Egypt and created the city of al-Qāhirah ("The Victorious") as their capital. However, the story of Cairo began over three hundred years earlier, with the Arab conquest of Egypt in the year 640. The conquering general, 'Amr ibn al-'Āṣ, would establish a capital called Fusṭāṭ (later Miṣr) in 642.

Fusṭāṭ was founded on the east bank of the Nile, at the location of the Roman and Byzantine fortress of Babylon, far to the south of the modern-day city center of Cairo (Raymond 2000: 11–16). The site was a sensible strategic choice for the invading Arab army: Babylon was situated at the interface of Upper and Lower Egypt, with easy access to the Nile, as well as to the land route to Arabia. The city began as a military encampment organized into distinct quarters or cantonments based on the various ethnic units that composed the invading Arab army. Over the next several decades, this army camp town would transform into a permanent city that would function as the administrative and commercial capital of Egypt for several more centuries, until this role was overtaken by al-Qāhirah.

Over the next 350 years, three satellite cities would be founded to the northeast of Fusṭāṭ, in succession: al-'Askar, al-Qaṭā'i', and al-Qāhirah (Abu-Lughod 1971: 13–25, Alsayyad 2011: 39–54, Raymond 2000: 23–30). In contrast to Fusṭāṭ, each was founded as a dynastic city, marking the accession of a new caliphate. While camp towns like Fusṭāṭ developed organically and with little attention to aesthetics, dynastic cities, as symbols of the power and authority of the ruling class, were carefully planned and replete with monumental construction. Al-'Askar ("The Cantonment") was established by the Abbasids in 750, al-Qaṭā'i' ("The Wards") was founded by Aḥmad ibn Ṭūlūn—of the short-lived Tulunid dynasty—in 868, and al-Qāhirah was established by Egypt's Fatimid conquerors in 969.

Of these three cities, only al-Qāhirah would transcend its beginnings as a dynastic city and supplant Fusṭāṭ as Egypt's capital. Over the course of roughly one century, al-'Askar was gradually absorbed into Fusṭāṭ. Al-Qaṭā'i' was sacked in 905, when the Abbasids retook control of Egypt from the Tulunids. The imposing mosque of ibn Ṭūlūn remains as one of the only vestiges of this once impressive royal city. Al-Qāhirah would live on for centuries, absorbing neighboring Fusṭāṭ into a conurbation that has become one of the most populous cities in the world.

The Fatimid City

The plan for al-Qāhirah was laid out almost immediately after the Fatimid conquest (Figure 7). The early city, sited to the northeast of Fusṭāṭ, was planned as a rectangular walled enclosure with eight gates, bordered on the west by the Khalīj (see below) and on the east by the Muqaṭṭam hills. The rectangle was bisected by a main thoroughfare (*qaṣabah*)

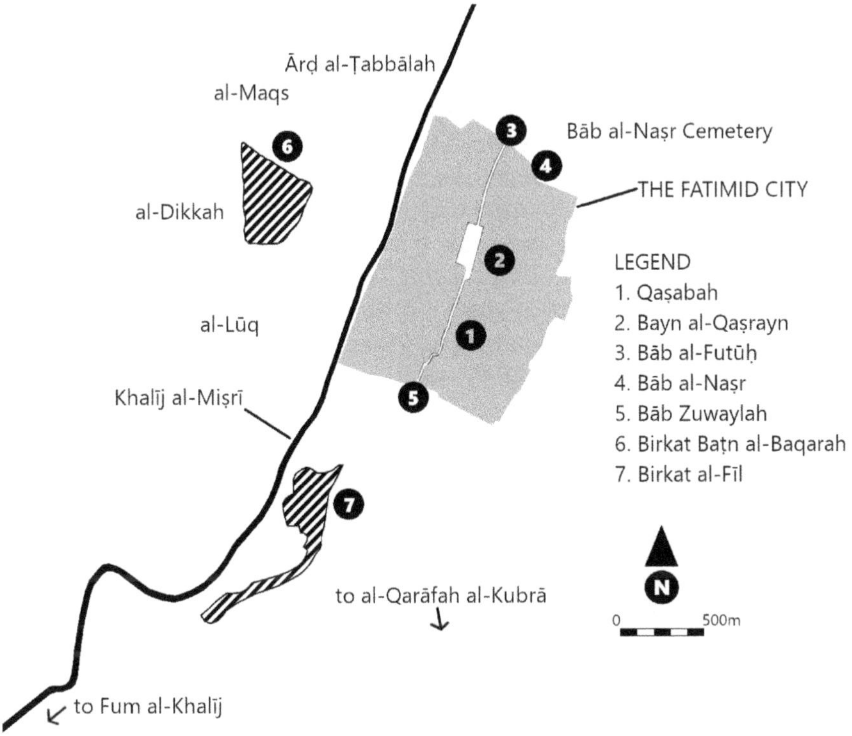

Figure 7: Fatimid Cairo (map by the author).

running from Bāb al-Futūḥ (Gate of the Conquest) in the north to Bāb Zuwaylah (Zuwaylah Gate) in the south. Between the Eastern Palace and the Western Palace of the Fatimids, the *qaṣabah* widened, creating a public square known as Bayn al-Qaṣrayn ("between the two palaces").

Abu-Lughod (1971: 23) writes: "The city of the Fāṭimids had a social system and a physical shell—partly imposed but partly the inevitable counterpart of its system of social organization—that influenced the form the medieval city was to take." Importantly, the internal structure of al-Qāhirah was organized on ethnic and occupational lines, and this mode of organization would persist as the city developed. Initially, several cantonments (*khiṭaṭ*) were set aside in a portion of the city for the various ethnic contingents of the Fatimid army and their families; these would eventually evolve into quarters, known as *ḥārāt* or *ḥawārī* (singular *ḥārah*). The *ḥārāt* emerged as a central organizing feature of Cairo, both socially and administratively, and would continue in this role for centuries (Al-Messiri Nadim 1979). Each *ḥārah* was occupied by a relatively homogeneous group—either ethnically or occupationally. The *ḥārah* was a fairly closed community, both socially and spatially: it was protected by a gate that was closed at night and during times of crisis.

Yet, although al-Qāhirah was conceived as a city reserved for the caliph, his family, his court, and his army, a large population soon began to occupy the areas between the military quarters, and commercial activity in the city steadily increased. As Raymond (2000: 79) notes, the distance between al-Qāhirah and Fusṭāṭ made it difficult for the latter to adequately support the former, effectively ensuring the development of the city's commercial aspect. New *ḥārāt* developed alongside the original *ḥārāt*, and specialized markets appeared. The number of *ḥārāt* in al-Qāhirah expanded from some 10 to 15 at its founding to 37 at the height of the Mamluk era (Abu-Luhgod 1971: 42–43).

Expansion of the city outside its original boundaries was slow but inexorable. Under the Ayyubids, the city grew southward, pulled in that direction by the construction of the Citadel and the subsequent relocation of political and military power there. Concerns about security prompted Ṣalāḥ al-Dīn's (r. 1174–1193) plan for fortifying the city with a massive new wall, with the Citadel as its lynchpin (Abu-Luhgod 1971: 27–30, Raymond 2000: 83–92). However, as Raymond notes, the Sunni Ṣalāḥ al-Dīn's distaste for settling in the palaces of his Shi'ite predecessors likely also played a role in his decision to build the new fortress (Raymond 2000: 83).

Under the Mamluks, the city would begin a westward expansion, made possible as the Nile's course shifted to the west and opened up a broad expanse of fertile land. Development west of the Khalīj was likely also encouraged by the security afforded by Ṣalāḥ al-Dīn's northern wall, which extended from the Khalīj to the Nile port of al-Maqs (Abu-Luhgod 1971: 30). The western suburbs extended from the western boundary of the city to the Nile, and included the areas known as al-Dikkah and al-Lūq. Yet, settlement in the area proceeded very slowly, and the area retained a suburban quality until the nineteenth century. Notably, al-Maqs was home to a large Coptic Christian community, and the western suburbs would eventually encompass the largest Christian quarter in Cairo (Behrens-Abouseif 1985: 26).

Among the most important landmarks in the geography of early Cairo were the various canals and ponds that shaped the suburban landscape to the west and south of the urban center. Most significant of these was a canal originating far to the southwest of the urban center of al-Qāhirah and terminating northeast of the city at a pond called Birkat al-Ḥājj (so called because it provided a resting place for pilgrims traveling to and from Mecca). Variously referred to as the Khalīj al-Ḥākimī (Canal of Ḥākim), after the Fatimid caliph Ḥākim bi-Amr Allāh (r. 996–1021) who restored it, Khalīj al-Miṣrī (Cairo Canal), or simply the Khalīj (Behrens-Abouseif 1985: 1), this canal formed the western border of Cairo during pre-Mamluk times and would remain a boundary between Cairo and its western suburbs from the Mamluk era until the nineteenth century.

In addition to the Khalīj, the landscape between Cairo and the Nile was dotted by a number of ponds or small lakes. The ponds, some of which were natural depressions, others of which were intentionally dug at the behest of the ruling elite, were filled by canals, or else by the infiltration of rising water from the Nile flood (Behrens-Abouseif 1985: 20). Two of the ponds are worth noting here. One was a pond dug by Fatimid caliph al-Ẓāhir in the area of al-Dikkah to the west of the Khalīj: later known as Baṭn al-Baqarah (Cow's Belly), this pond would form the basis of the Birkat al-Azbakīyah in the Mamluk period (Behrens-Abouseif 1985: 6). The other was a pond called Birkat al-Fīl (Elephant Pond), located to the south of the urban center of al-Qāhirah. Both of these ponds would become focal points for ongoing suburban development in the Mamluk era.

Also important to the geography of Fatimid Cairo were its shrines and cemeteries. To the southeast of al-Qāhirah was a massive necropolis, today known as al-Qarāfah al-Kubrā (The Great Cemetery), or simply al-Qarāfah (the Cemetery). The cemetery predates the existence of al-Qāhirah: its origins can be traced back to the establishment of Fusṭāṭ (El Kadi and Bonnamy 2007: 28). At the core of this early development was the cemetery of members of the tribe of Quraysh, the tribe of the Prophet Muḥammad; under the Ayyubids, this cemetery would become the site of an impressive mausoleum and *madrasah* (religious school) dedicated to the Sunni scholar Imām al-Shāfi'ī (d. 820). Over the next several hundred years, with the successive foundations of al-'Askar, al-Qaṭā'i', and al-Qāhirah, al-Qarāfah gradually expanded northward. By the arrival of the Fatimids, the cemetery stretched from Birkat al-Ḥabash in the south to the mosque of ibn Ṭūlūn in the north.

Under the Fatimids, another cemetery was established outside of Bāb al-Naṣr, one of al-Qāhirah's northern gates (El Kadi and Bonnamy 2007: 129). Prior to the creation of the cemetery, this area was the site of a *muṣallā*, or open prayer ground, established by the Fatimid general Jawhar for the celebration of the 'Īd al-Fiṭr, the festival marking the end of the month of Ramaḍān, in 969 (Sanders 1994: 45). This *muṣallā* figured prominently in the ceremonials of the Fatimid court, and the first tombs of the cemetery were built in its vicinity. The emergence and development of the cemetery were roughly contemporaneous with the neighboring suburb of Ḥusaynīyah, and as El Kadi and Bonnamy note, the residential district and the burial ground regularly encroached upon one another (2007: 129–131). Geographic constraints would ensure that the Bāb al-Naṣr cemetery would remain modest in comparison to al-Qarāfah.

The Spaces of Entertainment in the Fatimid City

As detailed in the previous chapter, professional entertainers have been a steadfast presence in Egyptian social and cultural life. Historical documentation demonstrates that even before the Fatimid conquest, Egypt's ruling class followed the Abbasid practice of retaining female slave entertainers in their courts. Similarly, multiple allusions to *mukhannathūn* in historical sources make it clear that these male entertainers were commonplace throughout the Abbasid era. Female popular entertainers, though less well-documented, were undoubtedly present long before the Fatimids built their new capital, a point supported by al-Maqrīzī's anecdote about Nasab (see below).

With the establishment of al-Qāhirah, Egypt's professional entertainers were integrated into the social and spatial geography of the new city. The foundation of al-Qāhirah established a landscape within which entertainment spaces were interwoven. These entertainment spaces included both private settings, such as the interiors of the royal palaces, as well as public settings, particularly within the bucolic landscape located to the west and south of the city core. Importantly, over the course of the Fatimid and Ayyubid periods, certain public spaces began to have clear associations in the popular imagination with entertainment and leisure, and the ongoing presence of professional entertainers in these spaces would ensure that the interconnection between these spaces and entertainment would persist into later centuries. These public spaces included the canals and ponds of the suburbs, as well as the city's shrines and cemeteries.

Canals and Ponds

The canals and ponds of Cairo were strongly associated with entertainment, leisure, and vice from the Fatimid period onward. As Behrens-Abouseif (1985: 10) notes: "There is not a single description in Maqrīzī's *Ḫhiṭaṭ* of a site located beside the Ḫhalīğ or the ponds of Cairo that does not refer to the amusements and frivolities which took place there." Particularly during the annual flood season, the pleasant vistas and cool breezes afforded by these sites proved attractive to both the elites and the masses. The general population could enjoy picnics on the banks, while the ruling elites plied the ponds and canals with their pleasure boats. Professional entertainers were drawn to these sites, where they found ready audiences, particularly during popular festivals.

The reputation of the Khalīj and its environs as sites of leisure and entertainment—as well as debauchery—continued from the Fatimid period into the ensuing Ayyubid and Mamluk eras. The Andalusian scholar Ibn Sa'īd al-Maghribī, who spent time in Cairo in both the late Ayyubid and early Mamluk periods (Raymond 2000: 95), says of the Khalīj: "It is constricted on both sides by numerous pavilions greatly populated by people given over to merriment, to banter, and to bawdiness, so that people of respectable morals and the great do not allow themselves to cross it in a boat" (quoted in al-Maqrīzī 1920: 58–59).

Pavilions or belvederes, known as *manāẓir* (singular *manẓarah*), were constructed by the Fatimid-era nobility along the Khalīj, as well as in the vicinity of the ponds located outside the city proper, and these became focal points for amusement and entertainment (Behrens-Abouseif 1985: 2–4, 103; al-Maqrīzī 1906–1908, volume 2: 183–184; al-Maqrīzī 1920: 48–49). These were elevated structures that provided panoramic views of the local landscape, and they allowed the elites to observe social and military activities taking place in the vicinity. Behrens-Abouseif notes that a typical *manẓarah* was likely a substantial structure, since *manāẓir* were sometimes used as residences by the caliph and members of his court (Behrens-Abouseif 1985: 103).

According to Pradines and Khan (2016: 24): "Socially, a belvedere symbolizes hierarchy and status.... It is a manifestation of the Caliph's position that he can see more than ordinary people can. Observing from this vantage point is a sign of privileged status because the luxury of having a broader view was not available to everyone." Certainly, the pavilions themselves were indisputably the property and the domain of the ruling elite, and they reinforced the status and wealth of the ruling class. Yet, the spaces around these structures were in many cases accessible to the common people, with the result that the *manāẓir* actually became points of confluence between the elites and the masses—a phenomenon alluded to in the statement by Ibn Sa'īd al-Maghribī quoted above.

The scene near the al-Lū'lū'ah (Pearl) and Dār al-Dhahab (House of Gold) pavilions, located between the western city wall and the Khalīj; is described by al-Maqrīzī:

> Between Bāb Sa'ādah, Bāb al-Khūkhah, and Bāb al-Faraj [on the one hand] and the Khalīj [on the other hand] there was a plain without construction, and the pavilions overlooked the gardens to the west of the Khalīj, behind which was the Nile. The population went between the pavilions and the Khalīj to indulge in the amusements. There gathered an innumerable crowd of idlers and onlookers, and to tell all that was offered to them of amusements and entertainment, there would not be enough paper. It was especially at the time [of the flood] of the Nile when the caliph went to al-Lū'lū'ah, and his favorites went to Dār al-Dhahab and the surroundings; then the pleasures multiplied, thanks to the abundance of resources and the extent of wealth at that time [al-Maqrīzī 1906–1908, volume 2: 183–184; 1920: 48].

The al-Lū'lū'ah *manẓarah* was located near Bāb al-Qanṭarah; it overlooked the Khalīj to the west, and the Kāfūr gardens to the east. Constructed by the caliph al-'Azīz bi-llāh (r. 975–996), it would be destroyed by Ḥākim and subsequently rebuilt by al-Ẓāhir (Behrens-Abouseif 1985: 2). It continued to be a popular retreat for the nobility, as well as a gathering place for the common people, in the subsequent Ayyubid period; al-Maqrīzī also offers an account of the revelries that took place near al-Lū'lū'ah on the occasion of the annual Nayrūz festival in 1188. Nayrūz, the Coptic New Year celebration (celebrated by Muslims and Christians alike), was characterized by its wild revelry, leading to its occasional regulation and eventual suppression by the authorities in Cairo (al-Maqrīzī 1906: 48–54; 1906–1908, volume 2: 30–33; Shoshan 1993: 40–51). Citing a contemporary source, al-Maqrīzī writes: "Rich and debauched gathered under Qaṣr al-Lū'lū'ah, where the Caliph could see them; they had musical instruments with them; the songs were rising; they openly drank wine and *mazr*" (al-Maqrīzī 1906: 53; 1906–1908, volume 2: 32).

Manāẓir were also erected to the north of the city, in the vicinity of an area known as the Ārḍ al-Ṭabbālah (The Drummer's Land) (al-Maqrīzī 1906–1908, volume 2: 184; 1920: 48–49). Here, the connection between space and professional entertainers is explicit: it is embedded in the very name of the place (Figure 8); al-Maqrīzī provides a detailed history of the Ārḍ al-Ṭabbālah and how it acquired its name (al-Maqrīzī 1906–1908, volume 3: 203–205; see also Ibn Taghrībirdī 1929–1972, volume 5: 12). In 1058, the Shi'a Fatimids celebrated a temporary victory over the Sunni Abbasids, when the Shi'a *khuṭbah* (sermon) was recited in Baghdad in the name of the Fatimid caliph al-Mustanṣir bi-llāh. Outside al-Mustanṣir's palace in Cairo, a famous singer played her drum and recited a poem in honor of the occasion; al-Maqrīzī states that her name was Nasab, or possibly Ṭarab (neither of which is a proper Arabic name, suggesting a nickname), and he refers to her variously as a *mughannīyah* (singer) and as a *ṭabbālah* (drummer).*

Apparently, the caliph was so pleased with Nasab's performance that he gifted her the stretch of land that would come to be known as Ārḍ al-Ṭabbālah.† The Drummer's Land and the lake that would eventually be created nearby—Birkat al-Raṭlī—carried associations with entertainment

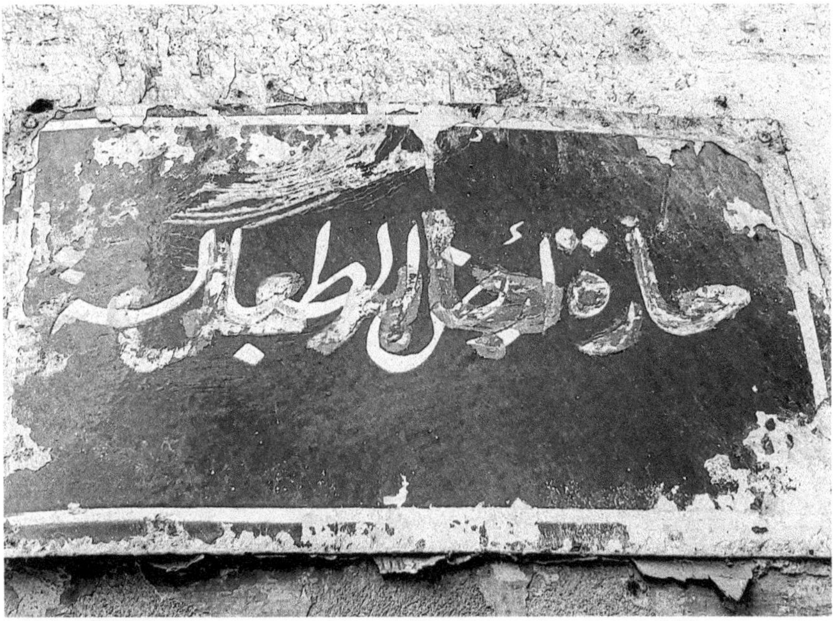

Figure 8: Street sign that reads "Ḥārat Ārḍ al-Ṭabbālah" (photo taken by the author in 2022).

* Behrens-Abouseif (2012) speculates that a Fatimid-era bronze figurine of a woman with a tambourine may be a representation of the *ṭabbālah*.

† Ibn Taghrībirdī's account is similar (see Ibn Taghrībirdī 1929–1972, volume 5: 12). By contrast, the chronicler ʿAbd al-Raḥmān al-Jabartī, writing at the time of the Napoleonic conquest of Egypt, set the story of the *ṭabbālah* several decades earlier, during the reign of al-Muʿizz li-Dīn Allāh. According to al-Jabartī's telling, the *ṭabbālah* pleased the caliph with singing and drumming upon his triumphal entry into Cairo (al-Jabartī 1888–1896, volume 6: 200–201; 1904, volume 3: 109–110).

and leisure (and, periodically, with debauchery and vice) from the Fatimid period until the dawn of the Khedivial era.

Cairo's ponds and canals were integral to the most significant festival of the Egyptian year: the celebration of the annual Nile flood with the opening of the Khalīj (Figure 9). As Sanders points out, Egypt's dependence on the Nile was expressed in a variety of Nile cults (Sanders 1994: 99). Celebrations of the Nile flood had existed for centuries, and some sort of canal cutting celebration likely existed before the Fatimid era. Under the Fatimids, this festival evolved into an elaborate royal ceremony accompanied by widespread popular festivities (Sanders 1994: 100–104, Shoshan 1993: 72–73).

The Persian scholar Nassiri Khosrau, describing this event in the eleventh century, writes: "The whole population of Misr and Kaire flock to enjoy this spectacle, and they indulge in all kinds of entertainment" (Khosrau 1881: 136–143). When the Nile began its annual rise (in early July), dams were constructed across the Khalīj and the smaller canals.

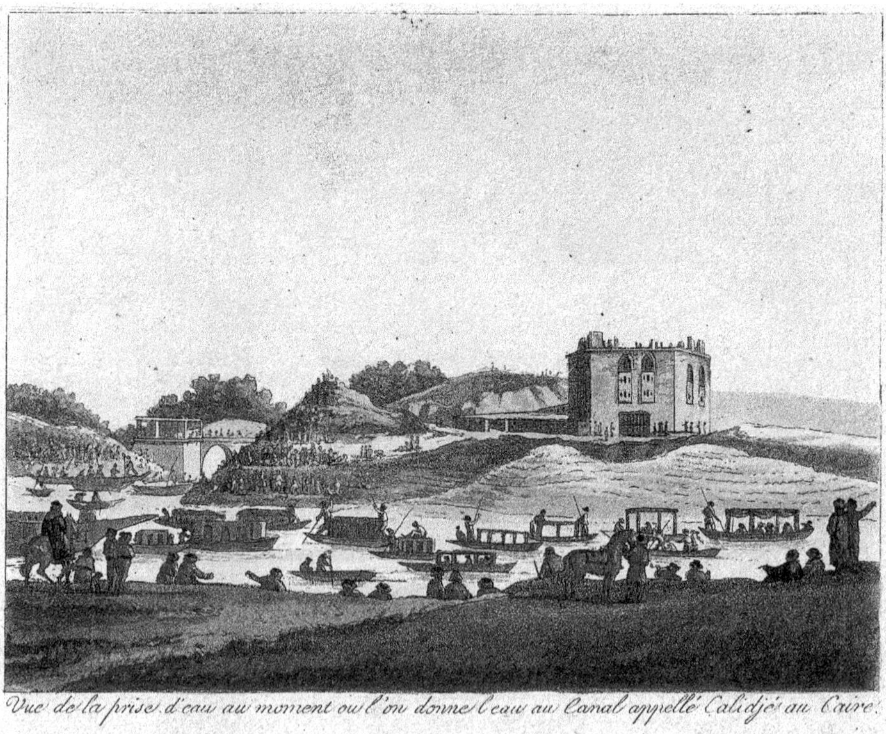
Vue de la prise d'eau au moment ou l'on donne l'eau au Canal appellé Calidjé au Caire.

Figure 9: The cutting of the Khalīj (engraving of an earlier work by Luigi Mayer, from Jean-Baptiste Joseph Breton's *L'Égypte et la Syrie*, 1814).

Once the Nile reached a sufficient height as determined by the Nilometer, the ruler and his entourage assembled at Fum al-Khalīj (the Mouth of the Canal, located just north of Fusṭāṭ and across the river from al-Rawḍah Island) to supervise the cutting of the dam. The dams of the smaller canals were also cut, allowing the floodwaters to inundate the lowlands. Upon the opening of the dam, the pleasure boats of the wealthy sailed into the canals and ponds of suburban Cairo, and popular celebrations took place upon the banks.

The canals and ponds, already zones of confluence between the elites and the masses, hosted multitudes from all levels of Egyptian society for the various ceremonies and celebrations associated with this important festival. Sanders (1994: 103), citing the Fatimid historian al-Musabbiḥī, writes:

> al-Musabbiḥī also reported the popular gathering of Christians and Muslims in Muḥarram 415/1024, on the third day following the opening, at the Church of al-Maqs, where they set up tents next to the bridge (*qanṭara*) for eating, drinking, and merriment. The festivities continued until the caliph al-Ẓāhir sailed in a boat (*markab*) to al-Maqs. He spent some time there and then returned to his palace.

In the late Fatimid period, the caliph and his entourage gathered at the pavilion known as al-Sukkarah (Sugar Pavilion), as well as in lavish tents erected nearby, while the elites of Cairo erected tents all along the canal from the gardens near al-Sukkarah to the gardens of al-Dikkah far to the north (Pradines and Khan 2016: 9–11, Sanders 1994: 104–112). Simultaneously, the ordinary citizens of Cairo gathered nearby in the vicinity of the canals and ponds, as well as in specially-constructed observatories for watching the cutting of the dam (Pradines and Khan 2016: 10–11, Shoshan 1993: 73).

Shrines and Cemeteries as Sites of Recreation

Cairo's shrines and cemeteries were never merely repositories for the dead. On the contrary, the living have engaged with and even inhabited these spaces for centuries (Taylor 1999: 16–18, 22). Abu-Lughod (1971: 63) writes:

> From early times, among the shrines were found monasteries and schools for various religious and mystic orders. Some of these served as free hostels for itinerant scholars or travelers. In addition, guarding each family tomb was a resident retainer and his dependents. To this population must be added a few temporary and permanent squatters who found the rent-free stone and wooden structures of the "tomb city" more spacious and substantial than the mudbrick huts available to them within the city proper. With such a resident

> population, it was perhaps inevitable that some artisans and shopkeepers should gravitate to the area to fulfill the demand for daily goods and services.
>
> Nor were these the only functions of this unique land use. Just as the marshlands provided open recreational space for the militaristic sports pursued by the Mamluks, the Cities of the Dead provided recreational facilities for the bulk of the population who repaired there weekly and, in even greater numbers, on the major festival occasions. While this custom originated as a means of paying respect to the tombs of saints and relatives, it attained a momentum of its own, with festivities rather than solemnity usually accompanying the exodus.

In short, Cairo's cemeteries and shrines have served as sites of religious devotion and education, as residential sites, as workplaces, and even as places of leisure and recreation, and all of these functions have overlapped throughout the city's history.

The Fatimids contributed to the development of Cairo's cemeteries with monumental constructions that expressed their devotion to Shi'a Islam while asserting the legitimacy of their rule over the Sunni majority. Egypt's Fatimid rulers were adherents to the Ismā'īlī branch of Shi'ism, central to which is the cult of the *ahl al-bayt*, the family of the Prophet Muḥammad.

Accordingly, the Fatimids constructed or renovated numerous tombs and shrines to honor the saints and martyrs descended from Muḥammad's son-in-law 'Alī (Williams 1983, 1985). According to Williams (1983: 40), the renovation of the mausoleum of Sayyidah Nafīsah (d. 824) in al-Qarāfah was the first such project officially undertaken by the Fatimid state (Figure 10). A direct descendent of the Prophet through his grandson Ḥassan, Sayyidah Nafīsah spent her last years in Egypt, where she was renowned for her piety and reputed to perform miracles. The location of the shrine near the main road connecting al-Qāhirah—the capital of the Shi'a Fatimids—and Fusṭāṭ—with its predominantly Sunni population—offered an opportunity for symbolic unity between the two, which may have prompted the Fatimid efforts at refurbishing the mausoleum (Williams 1983: 40–41).

The Fatimid elites also constructed lavish tombs and mausolea for themselves, along with congregational mosques and associated structures. Though the Fatimid caliphs were interred within the Eastern Palace (Sanders 1994: 42, Williams 1985: 39), in many cases, wives, children, other family members, and Fatimid notables were buried in al-Qarāfah or in the Bāb al-Naṣr cemetery (Cortese and Calderini 2006: 93, El Kadi and Bonnamy 2007: 31). Within the cemeteries, the Fatimids constructed palatial residences, places where they could live comfortably while visiting the mausolea of their deceased family members, as well as the tombs

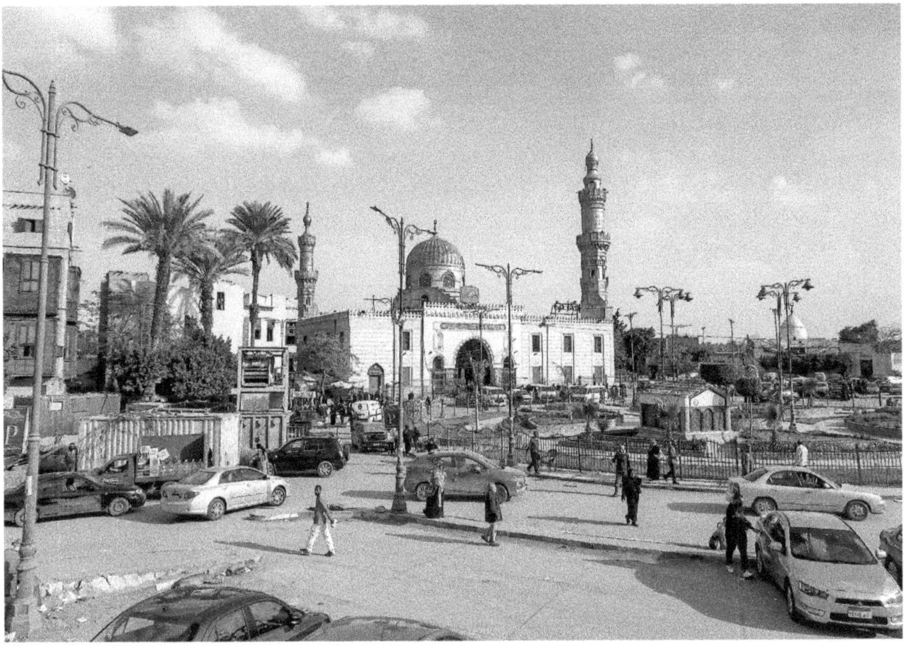

Figure 10: The shrine of Sayyidah Nafīsah (photo taken by the author in 2022).

and shrines of the *ahl al-bayt*. The construction of residential structures as well as places of worship necessitated the construction of supportive infrastructure (El Kadi and Bonnamy 2007: 31). The al-Qarāfah constructions commissioned by Durzān, mother of the caliph al-ʿAzīz, illustrate the scale and scope of these Fatimid building projects (Cortese and Calderini 2006: 167–169, Taylor 1999: 23–24). Her constructions included a palace, a public bath, a mausoleum, and an immense mosque, the Jāmiʿ al-Qarāfah.

The monumental constructions undertaken by the Fatimids became focal points for a wide range of religious observances. Among these were the observances sacred to all Muslims, whether Shiʿa or Sunni, including Friday prayers, ʿĪd al-Fiṭr, and ʿĪd al-'Aḍḥā (Festival of the Sacrifice, commemorating Abraham's willingness to sacrifice his son as an act of obedience to God). These sites also became central to observances instituted by the Fatimids, many of which were focused on devotion to the *ahl al-bayt*. Among these celebrations were *mawālid* in honor of Muḥammad, his daughter Fāṭimah, her husband ʿAlī, and their sons Ḥassan and Ḥusayn. Other Fatimid-era religious celebrations include the festivals of ʿĀshūrā' and Ghadīr, and the four Layālī al-Wuqūd (Nights of Lighting Fires).

Some of the observances instituted by the Fatimids, though distinctly Shiʿa in flavor, appealed to Shiʿa and Sunni Egyptians alike, particularly those focused on the *ahl al-bayt*. As Williams (1985: 56) notes, the tradition of commemorating the *ahl al-bayt* predated the Fatimid presence in Egypt. Thus, the *mawālid*, with their focus on honoring the Prophet and his immediate family, inevitably appealed to both Shi'a and Sunni Egyptians (though some religious scholars considered *mawālid*, even the *mūlid* of the Prophet, to be unacceptable innovations). Nevertheless, the *mawālid* of the Fatimid era were primarily courtly celebrations, unlike the popular festivals that they would become in later periods (Schielke 2006: 164–165). The festivities generally involved state banquets, Qur'ān recitation, and the distribution of food to the common people. Still, by instituting these celebrations, the Fatimids established a festive tradition of honoring the Prophet and other Muslim saints, a tradition that would persist and thrive in later centuries.

Like the *mawālid*, the festival of 'Āshūrā', celebrated on the tenth day of the Islamic month of Muḥarram, attracted Shi'a and Sunni alike. This day is sacred for a variety of reasons, including the commemoration of the martyrdom of Ḥusayn, making it relevant to both Shi'a and Sunni Muslims. The recovery of the head of Ḥusayn by the Fatimid vizier Badr al-Jamālī (see Williams 1983), the relocation of this relic to Cairo, and the subsequent establishment of a major shrine in Ḥusayn's honor ensured the continuing significance of this festival in Egypt.

Besides the *mawālid* and 'Āshūrā', one of the four Layālī al-Wuqūd, though not specifically tied to the *ahl al-bayt*, was also attractive to both Shi'a and Sunni Egyptians. This was the fourteenth night of the month of Sha'bān, on which, according to popular belief, the fate of every living person was decided for the following year. The night of mid-Sha'bān continued to be observed for centuries, often with visits to Cairo's cemeteries.

In short, some of the observances instituted under the Fatimids took hold among the general populace, both Shi'a and Sunni, and persisted long after the end of the Fatimid state. On the other hand, some Fatimid-era celebrations were destined to disappear with the return of Sunni control of Egypt, such as the 'Īd al-Ghadīr (Sanders 1994: 121–134). This festival takes its name from the pond of Ghadīr Khumm, the site at which, according to Shi'a belief, Muḥammad named 'Alī as his successor. The 'Īd al-Ghadīr, with its focus on the legitimacy of the Shi'a caliphate of the Fatimids, would not stand under the Sunni Ayyubids.

The Fatimid construction projects within al-Qarāfah and Bāb al-Naṣr, together with their centrality to the cult of the *ahl al-bayt* and other Islamic religious observances, contributed to the urbanization of the cemeteries. As noted above, the construction of residential structures and congregational mosques required infrastructural developments within the cemeteries. Additionally, these constructions necessitated a population dedicated to related service and support functions.

However, monumental construction and state-sanctioned religious observances were not the only driving force in the development of Cairo's cemeteries. The popular practice of *ziyārah*—the visitation of tombs and shrines—ensured that the cemeteries were cities for the living as well as resting places for the dead. This practice, which remains popular even into the present day, was a favorite outing for Cairo's lower classes, especially lower class women. Visiting the tombs of family members offered an opportunity both to remember and to commune with the deceased, while visits to the tombs and shrines of saints and martyrs provided a means to seek blessings and intercessions.

Sources from later periods offer more detail regarding these cemetery outings (Early 1993: 122–130; Lane 1860: 479–480, 2005 [1836]: 474–475; Lutfi 1991: 114–115). Tomb and shrine visits were festive occasions, and for women in particular, they provided an opportunity for socialization with friends and family. Although they could occur on any day of the week, Thursday evenings and Fridays were particularly popular, as were the various festivals that punctuate the Egyptian calendar year. Visitors would pack food for the occasion, and would sometimes camp out overnight at the cemetery. There was a joyful and party-like atmosphere to these visits, especially on the occasion of a festival. Notably, sources from later periods reveal that professional entertainers sometimes plied their trades in the cemeteries (see, for example, al-Jabartī 1888–1896, volume 2: 178–179; 1904, volume 1: 225).

The origins of *ziyārah* are unclear, though it certainly existed even before the establishment of al-Qāhirah. That it existed under the Abbasids is demonstrated by their attempts to ban its practice by women in 867 (al-Maqrīzī 1906: 202; 1906–1908, volume 2: 102). Attempts to regulate or to prohibit *ziyārah* persisted in the Fatimid period, particularly under caliph Ḥākim, who enacted a number of restrictions on women in public spaces (Cortese and Calderini 2006: 192–199, Shoshan 1993: 69).

Why did the Egyptian government take issue with *ziyārah*? It seems that the drive to regulate this popular practice could be attributed to the view among some Islamic scholars that *ziyārah* was a deviation from orthodox interpretations of Islamic doctrine. While cemetery visitation is certainly permissible, even encouraged, in Islam, many aspects of *ziyārah* push against the boundaries of orthodoxy. First and foremost is the act of seeking intercessions and blessings from saints and martyrs, rather than directly from God, which some viewed as bordering on *shirk* (idolatry or polytheism). Second is *ziyārah*'s disruption of gender roles and gender segregation. The practice of tomb and shrine visitation was particularly popular among women, and their participation meant that women were a common sight at Cairo's cemeteries. For some Islamic scholars, the increased visibility of women in public spaces, and the unchecked intermingling of men and women, were evidence of social disorder. In addition to these issues, *ziyārah* was associated with a range of secular activities that some believed had no place among the tombs and shrines of the dead.

As Shoshan (1993: 69) notes, the concerns of the ruling elites were twofold. First, viewing themselves as defenders of the faith, Egypt's rulers were compelled to take action against practices that endangered public morality. Second, however, Egypt's ruling class was concerned with the maintenance of public order and was quick to attack practices that could threaten it. Thus, "While the learned provided the ideological weaponry, it was mainly rulers who took practical measures to combat and repress those cultural phenomena that could be characterized as popular" (*ibid.*).

It is important to note that *ziyārah* was not an exclusively Muslim phenomenon: Egypt's Christian and Jewish populations also engaged in pilgrimages to shrines and tombs. Given the discussion above, it is noteworthy that there is evidence for the regulation and repression of these activities *within* these minority communities as well. In the eleventh century, local rabbis compiled a list of regulations for pilgrims visiting the Synagogue of Moses in Dammūh; among the rules and regulations were an admonition against brewing beer, a ban on marionette shows and other popular entertainments, and prohibitions against singing and dancing (Schielke 2006: 162). It seems that the religious authorities in these communities shared Islamic scholars' concerns regarding the intermingling of the sacred and the secular.

The Heterotopic Nature of Cairo's Public Entertainment Spaces

The public entertainment spaces just described—the canals and ponds of the suburbs, the shrines and cemeteries—were both socially and spatially distinct from the rest of the city. As noted earlier, the internal structure of the Fatimid city was organized along ethnic and occupational lines. The *ḥārāt* of al-Qāhirah were relatively homogeneous communities, each distinguished from the others according to ethnic identity, religious affiliation, and common craft or trade. As the caliphal city transformed into a thriving residential and commercial center, specialized markets began to emerge. Many of these were situated along the *qaṣabah*, foreshadowing the future importance of Cairo's main thoroughfare as a hub of commercial activity.

Recall also that al-Qāhirah was founded as the dynastic capital for the Fatimids, and as such, it included public spaces that were controlled by the ruling elite and used for political and ritual purposes. Bayn al-Qaṣrayn, the public square created by the widening of the *qaṣabah* between Eastern and Western Palaces, functioned as a parade ground for the Fatimid rulers (see Sanders 1994: 42). This square was an important site for state ceremonies and rituals, particularly during the major Islamic and Ismāʿīlī Shiʿa religious holidays. Similarly, the *muṣallā*, or open prayer ground, to the northeast figured prominently in court ceremonials. As Sanders (1994) details, elaborate processions from the Fatimid palaces to the *muṣallā* during Ramadan and at major feast days underscored the authority of the Fatimid rulers and their Ismāʿīlī Shiʿa brand of Islam. Through these public spaces and the processions, ceremonies, and rituals orchestrated within them, the Fatimid elite asserted both secular and sacred hegemony over a local population that did not share their theology.

Cairo's public entertainment spaces defied the typical social and spatial organization that characterized the rest of the city. These were heterogeneous spaces, contrastingly markedly with the city's fairly homogeneous residential neighborhoods, and while the elites were certainly present in these spaces, they did not control or direct the social and spatial narrative here as they did in public spaces like Bayn al-Qaṣrayn. Indeed, by the time the Mamluks assumed control of Egypt, the suburbs of Cairo, as hubs of recreation and leisure, and the city cemeteries, as host to a complex mix of sacred and secular activities, had emerged as zones of ambivalence and liminality in the spatial reality of greater Cairo. These spaces played host to the sort of carnivalistic mésalliances described by Bakhtin. Within them, the normal social and spatial boundaries of Egyptian society were blurred, challenged, or even upended. Socially distant individuals were no longer spatially distant: Egyptians from radically different social contexts converged in the same spaces. These were ambiguous spaces where the "rules" of society were bent or sometimes broken. Here, Egyptians engaged in activities and behaviors that were elsewhere frowned upon, pushing and pulling at social norms, and playing in the space between.

The canals and ponds of the suburbs were zones of confluence among a variety of disparate social groups: rich, poor, Muslim, Christian, male, female. The ruling elites were in a social world apart from indigenous Egyptians: ethnically distinct, possessing massive wealth and power, and living a lifestyle far removed from the daily experience of the masses. Yet, both classes were brought together on the banks of the canals and ponds. At festive occasions, ordinary Egyptians gathered and amused themselves around the suburban *manāẓir* of the elites, who observed the revelries—as during the celebrations of Nayrūz in 1188, when the public congregated at al-Lūʾlūʾah.

Muslims and Christians enjoyed these spaces together, even though these groups tended to reside in separate neighborhoods, and in spite of periodic tensions between them. Annual festivals like the celebration of the Nile flood and the opening of the Khalīj were celebrated *en masse* by all Egyptians, regardless of religious affiliation. Yet, this ecumenical spirit was not limited to secular festivals like the flood celebration. On the contrary, it is quite clear that Muslims sometimes participated in Christian festivities. Such was the case with the Coptic Feast of the Martyrs: al-Maqrīzī indicates that most of the inhabitants of al-Qāhirah and Fusṭāṭ attended this Coptic Christian festival, centered on the banks of the Nile at Shubrā (al-Maqrīzī 1895: 194–197; 1906–1908, volume 1: 110–112).

Men and women intermingled around the ponds and canals. However, not only did ordinary men and women interact within these spaces: they mingled together with professional entertainers, individuals who routinely violated normative gender roles. At the Feast of the Martyrs, for example, were female singers, prostitutes, and *mukhannathūn* (al-Maqrīzī 1895: 194–197; 1906–1908, volume 1: 110–112).

Many of the activities and behaviors that took place in these spaces were outside of social norms. Contemporary observers decried what they perceived to be debauchery in the suburban zone of canals and ponds, particularly on the occasion of popular festivals. Sexual promiscuity and prostitution appear to have been commonplace, and in spite of Islamic prohibitions, the consumption of alcohol was common as well. Such was the case at the Nayrūz festivities in 1188. Besides the open consumption of alcohol and transgressive sexual behaviors, another popular practice during the annual Nayrūz celebration was the tradition of spraying passers-by with (sometimes dirty) water, as well as designating a common person to be the "*amīr*" of Nayrūz (al-Maqrīzī 1906: 52–53; al-Maqrīzī 1906–1908, volume 2: 32; see also Shoshan 1993: 42–44). Followed by a large crowd, the *Amīr al-Nayrūz* rode about on a horse or a donkey while collecting "debts" from people he encountered; those who refused—including the well-to-do—were splashed with water and verbally abused.

Like the suburbs, the cemeteries of Cairo were a complex social interface where binaries such as living/dead, rich/poor, and male/female were broken down. Even prior to the Fatimid era, the cemeteries exerted a strong pull on the local population, who regularly gathered there to visit tombs and shrines. The building projects implemented by the Fatimid elites, including the construction of congregational mosques such as the Jāmiʿ al-Qarāfah, as well as tombs and shrines in honor of the *ahl al-bayt*, only added to the gravitational pull, as men and woman at all levels of Egyptian society were drawn to these spaces. Taylor notes that the Jāmiʿ al-Qarāfah was one of the focal points for the celebration of the Layālī al-Wuqūd; it also drew both elites and commoners on Fridays (Taylor 1999: 24–25).

The cemeteries of Cairo and the activities that took place within them defy categories like "sacred" and "secular." Neither the practice of *ziyārah* nor the various Islamic celebrations that took place within the cemeteries were strictly religious affairs. Moreover, the construction of mosques and residences to accommodate cemetery visitation required a population dedicated to service, support, and security within those spaces. In other words, besides the regular visitors, the cemeteries were host to substantial resident populations, as well as to itinerant service providers. Taylor (1999: 60) writes: "al-Qarāfa was a place where the sacred mixed with the profane more broadly, as a host of itinerant merchants, self-appointed guides, popular entertainers, and others competed with each other to service the various needs of those living in or visiting the cemetery."

In essence, by the end of the Fatimid era, Cairo's suburbs and cemeteries had emerged not only as spaces of leisure and entertainment, but as heterotopic spaces within the landscape of the city. These distinctive spaces existed "outside of all places." Distinguished by their ambivalence and liminality, they provided space for Egyptians to challenge and subvert the normal social order. These were spaces that embodied the carnivalesque: normal social and spatial boundaries were blurred or broken as diverse social groups converged, interfaced, and engaged in behaviors and activities that defied or disrupted the social order.

Over the course of the Fatimid era, these spaces came to embody the ambivalence and ambiguity of the actions occurring within them. That is, the practice of Egyptians inscribed the liminality and ambivalence of their activities and behaviors into these physical spaces. However, these spaces, now heavy with meanings, continued to inform the habitus of Egyptians as they moved and acted within them. Thus the heterotopic nature of Cairo's suburbs and cemeteries, well-established by the time the Mamluks came to power, would persist, as generation after generation re-experienced and re-inscribed these meanings.

Importantly, professional entertainers plied their trades within these heterotopic spaces. Entertainers were themselves ambiguous and liminal personae, and their activities and behaviors situated them outside the norm—both socially and spatially. Entertainers were drawn to practice their trades in settings that made space for their unorthodox lifestyles and behaviors. Conversely, their regular presence in these spaces imparted their own marginality into the spatial reality and informed perceptions of the suburbs and the cemeteries. In this way, professional entertainers would be key to the ongoing re-inscription of heterotopic meaning into these spaces.

Mamluk Expansion

The Mamluk period witnessed substantial western and southern expansion of al-Qahirah (Figure 11). As noted earlier, the city grew westward into the new land made available by the Nile's shift in course. Much of the development of the western suburbs at this time was encouraged by the sultan al-Nāṣir Muḥammad ibn Qalāwūn, who initiated the construction of the Khalīj Nāṣirī (the Canal of Nāṣir) in 1325 (Abu-Luhgod 1971: 35–36, Behrens-Abouseif 1985: 9–15, Raymond 2000: 125–128). This canal ran on a course roughly parallel to the main Khalīj, then turned east,

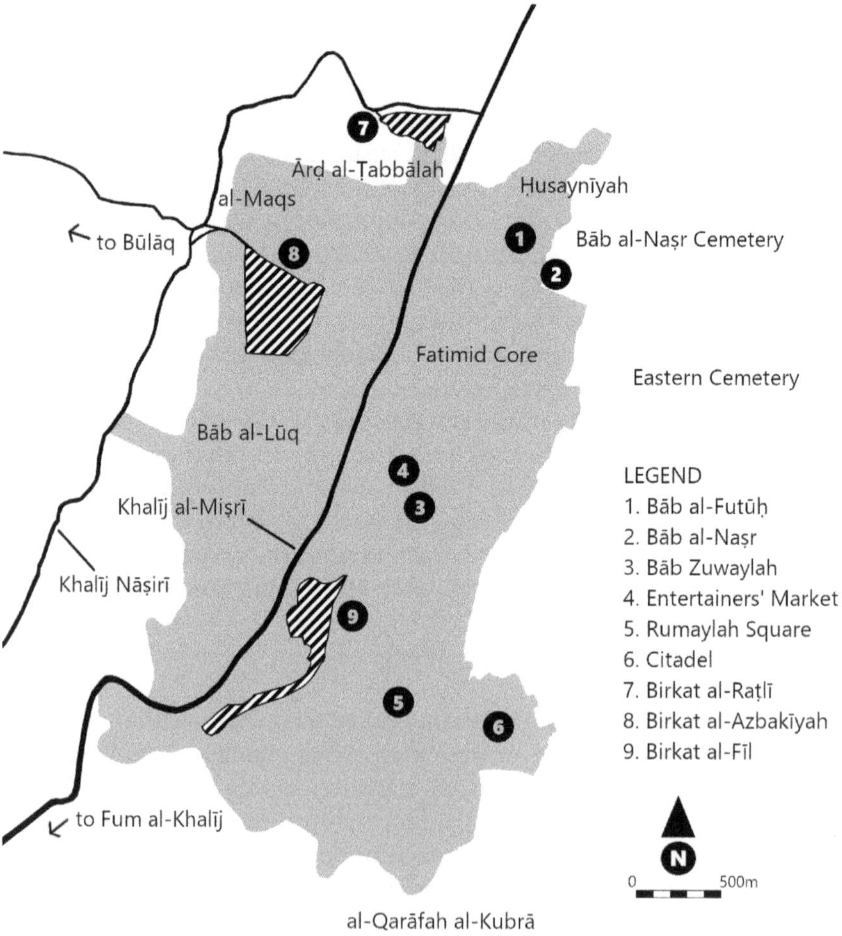

Figure 11: Mamluk Cairo (map by the author).

running north of (and helping to supply) the Birkat al-Raṭlī, then joining the primary canal at a location north of Bab al-Sha'irīyah. Sultan al-Nāṣir encouraged the urbanization of the expanse between the two canals by providing land grants to the nobility. In addition, al-Nāṣir ordered the construction of a number of additional bridges over both canals, making the area more easily accessible from the city proper. As a consequence, under al-Nāṣir, construction boomed in the area, from the vicinity of Birkat al-Raṭlī in the north to the land of al-Lūq in the south.

Sultan al-Nāṣir also encouraged settlement in the southern suburban expanse located between Bāb Zuwaylah and the Citadel (Abu-Luhgod 1971: 35, Raymond 2000: 132–135). Settlement in this area was already thriving due to the relocation of Cairo's political heart to the Citadel in the Ayyubid period. As with the western suburbs, al-Nāṣir promoted development in the area by parceling out land grants, particularly in the vicinity of the large Birkat al-Fīl, located west-northwest of the Citadel.

The construction boom of the al-Nāṣir era turned out to be somewhat short-lived, as a series of crises struck Egypt in the latter half of the fourteenth century, including multiple episodes of plague and famine, periods of misrule, and external military threats (Raymond 2000: 138–148). In general, development in the western suburbs declined, though it did not cease; perhaps the most noteworthy new construction in the western suburbs was the complex of the *amīr* Azbak (Behrens-Abouseif 1985: 19–35), which will be described below. Certain areas within the western suburbs continued to thrive, particularly along the streets leading from the northern gates of al-Qahirah to the port of Būlāq, which had supplanted al-Maqs as an important port city as the Nile receded westward.

Still, the area between the Khalīj and the Nile would retain its suburban quality for many more centuries. By contrast, the southern suburbs, as the "connective tissue" between al-Qahirah and the Citadel, continued to see growth and development. As Behrens-Abouseif points out, areas that had developed "organically and functionally" were able to weather the crises of the late fourteenth and early fifteenth centuries, while those that were intentionally promoted by al-Nāṣir tended to decline (Behrens-Abouseif 1985: 13).

One of the most substantial constructions undertaken in the western suburbs in the wake of this period of decline was the development of the complex of the *amīr* Azbak, the *atābak* (army commander-in-chief) of al-Ashraf Qāytbāy (r. 1468–1496) from 1476 to 1485. Azbak's project included excavating a large pond on the site of the pond known as Baṭn al-Baqarah, re-excavating an old canal known as Khalīj al-Dhakar to connect the new pond to the Khalīj Nāṣirī, and restoring the bridge known as Qanṭarat al-Dikkah over the Khalīj al-Dhakar. Azbak's palace was constructed on the southeastern bank of the pond. Soon, other elites were drawn to construct their own residences in this pleasant setting, and religious and commercial building soon followed suit. The area was named after its founder: Azbakīyah.

The Mamluk era was also a time of cemetery expansion. Many of the Mamluk elite preferred to be buried within the city, and they established lavish mosque-mausoleum complexes for this purpose (El Kadi and Bonnamy 2007: 33). On the other hand, beginning in the fourteenth century, many Mamluks chose burial sites in the strip of desert land located between the city's eastern wall and the Muqaṭṭam hills (El Kadi and Bonnamy 2007: 175–178). Their choice of the eastern desert, rather than al-Qarāfah al-Kubrā to the south, was likely due to a lack of space in the latter. The main overland pilgrimage route to Mecca passed through this area, with the result that a wide range of urban services already existed there. The establishment of numerous elaborate funerary complexes and their associated facilities, including lodging, religious schools, and more, ensured that, like its counterpart to the south, the eastern cemetery existed as much to service the living as to house the dead.

The Spaces of Entertainment Under the Mamluks

Within the evolving social and spatial geography of al-Qāhirah, certain public spaces continued to be firmly associated with entertainment and leisure. More importantly, these spaces carried forward the "otherness" that was established in the Fatimid and Ayyubid eras. In Fatimid times, Cairo's suburbs and cemeteries had emerged as heterotopic spaces. Socially and spatially distinct from the rest of the city, these were sites within which diverse populations converged and interfaced, and where the normal social order was challenged and occasionally upended. Throughout the Mamluk era, these spaces that constituted Cairo's landscape of entertainment continued to be set apart by their ambivalence and liminality, as professional entertainers and other marginal personae lived and worked within them.

In addition to the suburbs and cemeteries, sources from the Mamluk period reveal the emergence and integration of significant new spaces within Cairo's entertainment landscape. One of these was the Mīdān al-Rumaylah, or Rumaylah Square, located at the foot of Ṣalāḥ al-Dīn's Citadel. Over the course of the Mamluk era, this public square became increasingly important as a gathering place for Cairo's common people and as a site for both popular entertainment and state ceremonials.

Another significant entertainment-related space to emerge at this time was not a space of performance. Rather, it was a space associated with the mundane business of entertainment: the buying and selling of musical instruments. The location of this market for entertainers, near the southern gate of Bāb Zuwaylah, is significant: in the ensuing centuries, the streets and alleys to the west of Bāb Zuwaylah would continue to be strongly associated with the entertainment trades.

The Continuing Significance of the Canals and Ponds of Cairo

The canals and ponds of the city suburbs carried forward the associations with entertainment, leisure, and vice that had been established in earlier times. These sites remained important gathering places for Cairo's common people, particularly on festive occasions. Periodic attempts by the government to regulate certain popular festivals appear to have been less successful in the suburbs, an indication of just how deeply entertainment and leisure were inscribed into the suburban landscape. Various attempts to regulate or suppress the annual Nayrūz festival are recounted by al-Maqrīzī, from the Fatimid era into his own lifetime (al-Maqrīzī 1906: 48–54; 1906–1908, volume 2: 30–33). Yet, even under the heavy regulation instituted in 1378: "People abstained from these games at al-Qāhirah; however, there was some indulgence on the canals and ponds and other places of pleasure" (al-Maqrīzī 1906: 53; 1906–1908, volume 2: 32).

The Mamluk aristocracy continued to use many of the *manāẓir* that had been constructed by the Fatimid nobility. In some cases, these structures were rebuilt or remodeled. Ibn Taghrībirdī describes how al-Mu'ayyad Shaykh refurbished the Fatimid pavilion known as al-Khams Wujūh (The Five Faces), while the area around a neighboring pavilion, al-Tāj (The Crown), was repurposed for other structures:

> On the 4th the Sultan rode in a litter from the Citadel toward the Belvedere of "The Five Faces" which he had built anew near "The Crown," and which had been completed; the people call it "The Crown and the Seven Faces," but it is not that; for it has only five faces. As for "The Crown," it is in ruins, but the magnate of the Financial Government, Vizier Jamâl ad-Dîn Yûsuf, controller of the army bureau and of the privy funds, built there magnificent structures, a public fountain, a school, a garden, etc., in this our time [Popper 1957: 81].

These two pavilions were located in the vicinity of the land known as Ārḍ al-Ṭabbālah.

Ārḍ al-Ṭabbālah, and the nearby Birkat al-Raṭlī, continued to be popular sites of pleasure, recreation, and vice (Figure 12). According to al-Maqrīzī, the area experienced a temporary decline due to an outbreak of

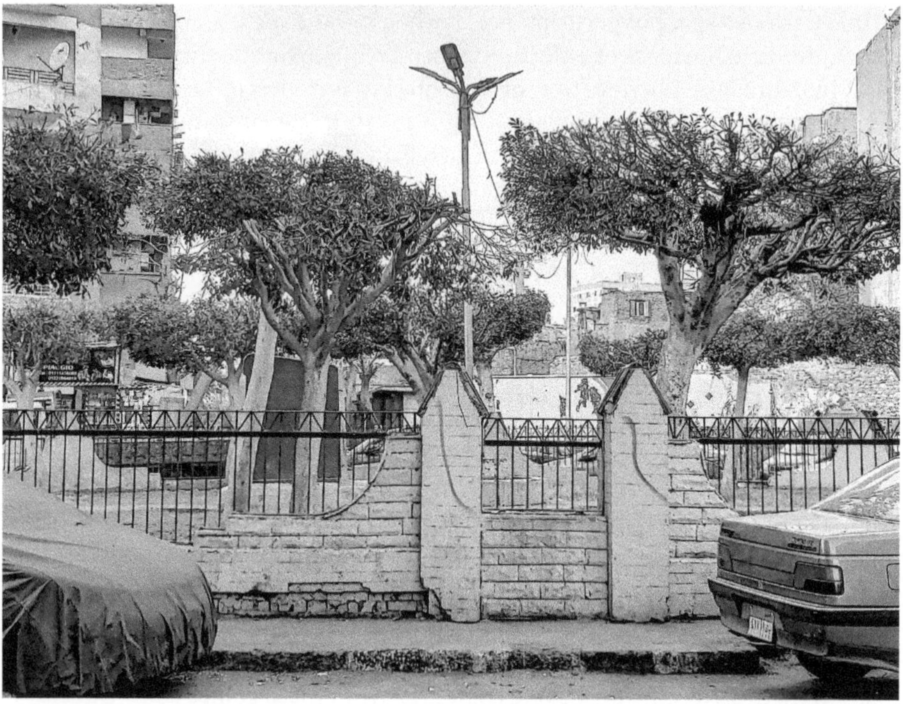

Figure 12: Former location of the Birkat al-Raṭlī (photo taken by the author in 2022).

an unidentified plague around 1296 or 1297 (al-Maqrīzī 1906–1908, volume 3: 204–205). However, the area began to thrive again following the construction of the Khalīj Nāṣirī in 1325, and it remained a popular retreat for the well-to-do until around 1375. In the ensuing decades, Ārḍ al-Ṭabbālah again experienced a decline in population and development, until most of the resident population was confined to the banks of the pond. According to al-Maqrīzī, by the mid-fifteenth century, much of the resident population consisted of "undesirables" (presumably including entertainers and prostitutes), and the place had become infamous as a site of immoral activities.

Documenting the situation at the dawn of the Ottoman conquest, Ibn Iyās indicates that some of the well-to-do maintained homes near the Birkat al-Raṭlī (Salmon 1921: 26–31). However, at the time of the Nile flood celebrations in 1516, the Dawādār (the chancellor who was managing affairs while the sultan was abroad fighting the Ottomans) restricted commerce on the lake and forbade settlements on the embankment. According to Ibn Iyās:

> Ḳāḍī Berekāt Ibn Mūsa, the Inspector of Markets, besought the Dawādār to allow the ships to enter as usual and to let the people live on the embankment; but he refused, saying that the people would corrupt the wives of the gentlemen who came with the Sulṭān for the ceremony of the opening of the Nile [Salmon 1921: 28].

As a result, the residences on the banks of the lake ended up deserted. This situation led a contemporary poet to elegize the lake and its pleasures:

> There the drunkard was in the height of enjoyment, passing round the wine-goblets on the night of the full moon.
> There were the ships, decked or open, for passengers;
> Reciters of verse came thither with players of musical instruments,
> And lutes sounding softly like the turtle dove [Salmon 1921: 30].

This situation was far from permanent, however. By the time of the French conquest, the elites had resumed building residences on the embankments, and Birkat al-Raṭlī retained its reputation as a center of pleasure and leisure (al-Jabartī 1888–1896, volume 9: 277–278; 1904, volume 4: 314–315).

The area that came to be known as Azbakīyah carried forward its earlier associations with leisure and entertainment as well. The area experienced a brief florescence in the wake of *amīr* Azbak's development. In 1485, the opening of the Khalīj was celebrated in Azbakīyah for the first time (Behrens-Abouseif 1985: 23–24). At the dawn of the Ottoman era, the common people of Cairo gathered there every Friday to enjoy popular entertainments (Africanus 1896: 874).

Nevertheless, extensive urban development, particularly by the elites, did not occur in this area until the early eighteenth century, and this lag can be attributed to the area's marginal and heterogeneous quality. The area known as Bāb al-Lūq, situated just south of the Baṭn al-Baqarah pond (what would become the Birkat al-Azbakīyah near the end of the fifteenth century), carried a reputation for marginality throughout the Mamluk era and well beyond it. During the reign of Sultan al-Ẓāhir Baybars (r. 1260–1277), this area absorbed somewhere between one and two thousand Mongol/Tatar refugees, as well as refugees from the Iraqi city of Mosul (Behrens-Abouseif 1985: 6; Richardson 2022: 35, 52–53). It is also quite clear that many of the residents of Bāb al-Lūq were people of the Banū Sāsān/Ghurabā': people who were both socially and professionally marginal (Richardson 2022: 52–55).

Richardson writes that the marginal reputation of Bāb al-Lūq developed in the wake of the influx of foreign refugees and Ghurabā' into this area (2022: 35, 53). However, I would argue that this suburban zone was positioned to receive these marginal and heterogeneous populations due to its already heterotopic nature. That is, the western suburbs of Cairo were characterized by their ambivalent and liminal qualities, as well as their association with entertainment, recreation, and vice, well before the thirteenth century. Marginal populations, such as professional entertainers, were drawn to spaces that could accommodate their outsider status. Bāb al-Lūq was such a space, and as a consequence, held a fundamental attraction toward these groups. Conversely, the influx of these populations into spaces such as Bāb al-Lūq served to re-inscribe their heterotopic qualities.

Azbakīyah would remain a marginal area until the early eighteenth century, and its social and economic heterogeneity would persist even longer. Raymond notes that the middle-class homes in the area were inhabited only during the hot season (Raymond 2000: 221), and the aristocracy preferred to build their residences elsewhere (particularly in the southern suburbs). Still, as with the Birkat al-Raṭlī, the elites continued to be drawn to the bucolic landscape of Azbakīyah and the pleasures it afforded, ensuring the continuing heterogeneity of the western suburbs.

The Expanding Role of Shrines and Cemeteries as Sites of Recreation

In the Mamluk era, the shrines and cemeteries of Cairo continued to exist as heterotopic spaces within which there was no clear boundary between the sacred and the secular. The practice of *ziyārah* continued to thrive (Lutfi 1991: 114–115). The Moroccan scholar and traveler Ibn Baṭṭūṭah, observing the practice at al-Qarāfah in the fourteenth century, writes:

> At Cairo too is the great cemetery of al-Qaráfa, which is a place of peculiar sanctity, and contains the graves of innumerable scholars and pious believers. In the Qaráfa the people build beautiful pavilions surrounded by walls, so that they look like houses. They also build chambers and hire Koran-readers, who recite night and day in agreeable voices. Some of them build religious houses and madrasas beside the mausoleums and on Thursday nights they go out to spend the night there with their children and womenfolk, and make a circuit of the famous tombs. They go out to spend the night there also on the "Night of mid-Sha'bán," and the market-people take out all kinds of eatables [Ibn Baṭṭūṭah 1953: 51].

Around the same time, the conservative Islamic scholar Ibn al-Ḥājj railed against the practice, writing:

> Observe, may God forgive us and forgive you, what the women have invented in connection with these visits. They have allocated for each shrine a specific day of the week, so that most of their weekdays are used to obtain their wicked desires.... On Mondays, they visit the shrine of al-Husain; on Tuesdays and Saturdays, they visit al-Sayyida Nafisa; Thursdays and Fridays were dedicated

> to visiting the tombs of other holy saints and the tombs of their dead [quoted in Lutfi 1991: 114].

Of tremendous significance to the religious practice of ordinary Egyptians was the rising popularity of Sufi mysticism throughout the Mamluk era (Shoshan 1993). Along with the popular adoption of Sufi thought and practice came a growing reverence for esteemed Sufi spiritual leaders. The tombs and shrines of Sufi saints were integrated into the practice of *ziyārah*, and there emerged a wide array of popular *mawālid* in their honor (Taylor 1999: 64–65).

The Mamluk era marks the rise of the popular *mawālid* as they are celebrated today (Schielke 2006: 165). As noted earlier, the Mūlid al-Nabī (the Mūlid of the Prophet), along with *mawālid* for other members of the Prophet's family, were first instituted in Egypt under the Fatimid dynasty. However, these early *mawālid* were primarily courtly affairs. In the Mamluk era, the Mūlid al-Nabī was revived and transformed into a popular festival (though with state participation). Thereafter, a number of other *mawalid* were modeled after it.

The Mamluk-era *mawālid* mingled sacred activities—recitation of the Qur'ān, *dhikr*, etc.—with a broad array of secular entertainments. The latter included music and dance, games, fortune telling, *arājūz* (puppet theater, derived from the Turkish *karagöz*), and *khayāl al-ẓill* (shadow play). These festivals drew large crowds to tombs and shrines, and many *mawālid* functioned as regional fairs where artisans and craftsmen could gather to sell their goods and services (Taylor 1999: 65). For many professional entertainers, the *mawālid* became a vital source of income.

In their secular characteristics, the *mawālid* of the Mamluk period resemble earlier popular festivals. Indeed, the rise in popularity and prevalence of the *mawālid* appears to coincide with the disappearance of certain other festivals, a point noted by Schielke (2006: 162–163). For example, the Coptic Feast of the Martyrs, discussed previously, was banned from 1355 onward (al-Maqrīzī 1895: 194–197; 1906–1908, volume 1: 110–112). Similarly, the festival of Nayrūz appears to have been permanently suppressed in Cairo in the early fifteenth century (though it persisted in the countryside for many centuries) (Shoshan 1993: 49–51).

The parallels between the *mawālid* and these earlier popular celebrations are unmistakable. Nevertheless, as Schielke (2006: 159–166) notes, it is incorrect to view the *mawālid* themselves as continuations of the earlier festivals. Rather, the *mawālid* that emerged in the Mamluk era represent the continuation of a longstanding festive tradition: "a tradition of festive culture characterised by a dramatic reversal of the everyday and/or an ambivalent combination of piety and amusements" (Schielke 2006: 161).

What is clear is that the thriving practice of *ziyārah*, together with the rise of popular *mawālid*, ensured that Cairo's shrines and cemeteries remained vital and integral to the city's landscape of entertainment.

The Growing Significance of Rumaylah Square in the Entertainment Landscape

Rumaylah Square was situated at the base of the Citadel, just northwest of the fortress (Figure 13). Shortly after the completion of the Citadel, the Ayyubid sultan al–Malik al-Kāmil (r. 1218–1238) moved a livestock market to this location. In time, the square became a bustling place of commerce (Raymond 2000: 98).

Rumaylah Square, due to its proximity to the Citadel, figured prominently in state ceremonials. Among these were the processions of the *maḥmal*, an ornate palanquin that accompanied the annual pilgrim caravan to and from Mecca (Behrens-Abouseif 1997, Shoshan 1993: 70–72). Ceremonial in nature, the *maḥmal* was typically empty; rather than carrying people or goods, it functioned as an emblem of the Mamluk sultan's power and authority, as well as his piety and devotion to the annual

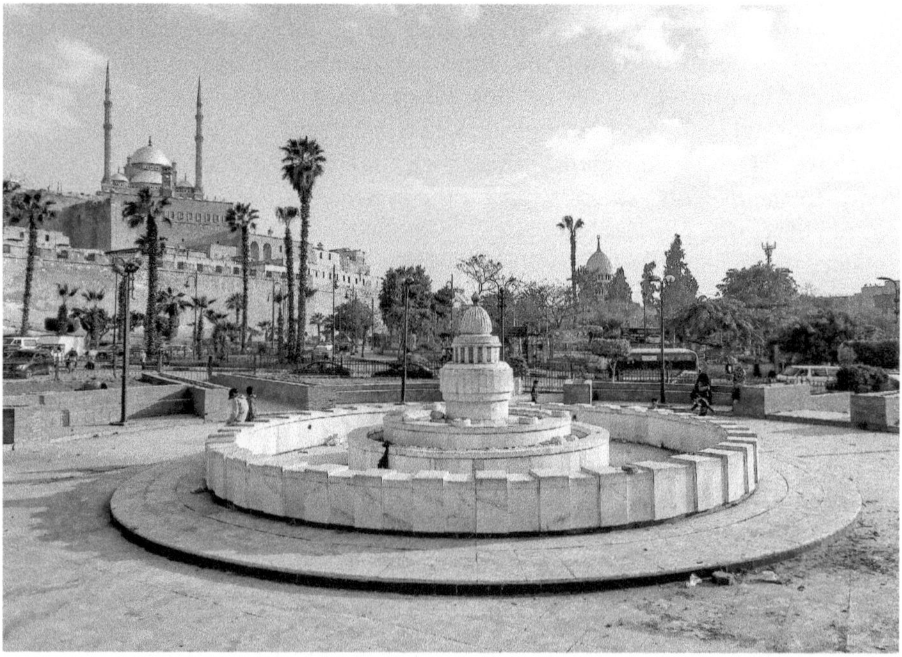

Figure 13: Mīdān al-Rumaylah (photo taken by the author in 2022).

pilgrimage. The *maḥmal* is first recorded in Egypt in association with the pilgrim caravan of 1266. The processions of the *maḥmal* commenced and concluded at Rumaylah Square, and they invariably attracted large crowds of spectators.

Ordinary Egyptians gathered at Rumaylah Square for other reasons as well. Shoshan relates the following anecdote regarding the arrest of a particularly hated *amīr*:

> When in 1338, or the following year, rumours about his arrest spread, merchants suspended business, and people, in fact whole families, gathered at the Rumaylah quarter, below the Citadel, lit candles, raised Qur'āns, waved banners, and cheered. Celebrations lasted for a whole week, music was played, performances (*khayāl*) were staged; people wrote lines of poetry (*azjāl wa-balālīq*) in which they commemorated the event [Shoshan 1993: 57].

Over time, Rumaylah became increasingly significant as a regular gathering place for Cairo's common people.

Thus, by the end of the Mamluk era, Rumaylah Square was established as a point of confluence between diverse social groups. Over the course of the Ottoman era, Rumaylah continued to be characterized by its social and economic heterogeneity, as diverse populations gathered here to engage in commerce, to participate in festivals, and to consume popular entertainment. Marginal populations, including popular entertainers, came to frequent this area, plying their trades in the square and residing in neighborhoods nearby.

Spaces of Residence and Commerce in the Entertainment Landscape

Mamluk-era sources offer some information regarding the spaces where professional entertainers lived, as well as the spaces where they engaged in the more mundane aspects of their trades, such as buying and selling musical instruments. As noted earlier, an important residential zone for professional entertainers was located in Bāb al-Lūq, in Cairo's western suburbs. Another such residential zone was the suburban neighborhood of Ḥusaynīyah, located just north of Bāb al–Futūḥ and adjacent to the Bāb al–Naṣr cemetery (Richardson 2022: 35, 52–53). Like Bāb al-Lūq, Ḥusaynīyah absorbed a number of refugees in the late thirteenth century (see Irwin 2004). Never an attractive neighborhood for urban development by Cairo's elites, the influx of these diverse populations contributed to the neighborhood's popular quality and drew socially and professionally marginal populations to the area. In the eyes of Mamluk Cairo's well-to-do, including the chroniclers who have provided the documentation of the era, both Bāb al-Lūq and Ḥusaynīyah were marginal neighborhoods.

Beyond the spaces just described, the Mamluk era witnessed the emergence and integration of a new and significant space within the entertainment landscape of Cairo: a popular market for buying and selling musical instruments. This market for entertainers was located in the vicinity of Bāb Zuwaylah. More specifically, it was accessed from an alley leading west from Jawhar's original southern gate, which was slightly to the north of the imposing stone gate later constructed under Badr al-Jamālī. The market was most likely positioned just north or just west of the mosque of al-Mu'ayyad Shaykh. A description is provided in al-Maqrīzī's history of Bāb Zuwaylah:

> This gate, when al-Qā'id Jawhar founded al-Qāhirah, consisted of two contiguous doors near the *masjid* known as Sām ibn Nūḥ [Shem, son of Noah]. It was through one of them that al-Mu'izz entered when he came to al-Qāhirah; it was the one that was contiguous to the *masjid*, of which a vault remains today, hence the name of the door of the arch which is given to it. It was popular with the public; one entered and exited by there, while the neighboring door was neglected; it was a common saying that whoever passed it never succeeded in any business.
>
> This door has disappeared today without a trace, except that it extended to the place that today is called al-Ḥajjārīn, where musical instruments like *ṭanābīr*, *'īdān*,* and the like are sold. Until today, it is said that whoever goes that way never succeeds in any business. Some say it is because one finds there the immoral instruments and the riffraff of singers. But it is not at all as they claim, because the common saying was born among the inhabitants of al-Qāhirah from the day that al-Mu'izz entered it, before there was a market of instruments and a meeting place of the debauched [al-Maqrīzī 1906–1908, volume 2: 209; 1920: 89–90].

In his day, al-Maqrīzī, indicates the Sūq al-Ḥajjārīn (Market of the Stonecutters) was also known as Sakan al-Malāhī (Place of Musical Instruments) (al-Maqrīzī 1906–1908, volume 2: 198; 1920: 73).

The information provided by al-Maqrīzī is interesting for a number of reasons. First, it offers us a concrete description of a Cairo space dedicated to the commercial aspects of the entertainment trades *other* than performance. His description, though brief, makes it clear that this market was frequented by individuals connected to these trades. Given the typical organization of neighborhoods within the city according to ethnicity or occupation, it is highly likely that besides musical instrument sellers, this market hosted workshops for the manufacture of the instruments,

---

* The musical instruments referred to here: ṭanābīr, singular *ṭunbūr*, a long-necked lute, and *'īdān*, singular *'ūd*, a short-necked lute.

the residences of the merchants and craftsmen, and perhaps even the residences of entertainers themselves, perhaps making this a third residential zone for popular entertainers in Mamluk Cairo.

Second, although al-Maqrīzī dismisses the notion that this area gained its negative reputation due to the presence of musical instruments and people connected to the entertainment trades, it is telling that his contemporaries make this connection. The popular association of the "unlucky" nature of this place with entertainment and entertainers speaks to the ambivalent attitudes of Egyptians toward the latter. It is quite clear that the presence of entertainers and the business of entertainment informed local perceptions of this space, just as perceptions of Bāb al-Lūq and Ḥusaynīyah were informed by the presence of professional entertainers and other marginal personae in those neighborhoods.

Lastly, it is critical to note that the streets and alleys near this market were firmly associated with the entertainment trades in future centuries. In fact, one of the small alleys to the southwest was one of the primary residential neighborhoods for female professional entertainers in the late nineteenth and early twentieth centuries. As with other spaces in the entertainment landscape, the ties between this space and professional entertainment that were established in these early centuries persisted in future eras.

Inscription and Re-Inscription of Meaning in Cairo's Public Entertainment Spaces

Well before the Mamluks assumed control of Egypt, Cairo's entertainment landscape had begun to take shape. Certain public spaces, most notably the suburbs and cemeteries, became firmly associated with leisure and entertainment, and defined by their heterotopic features. These were spaces where normal social and spatial boundaries were blurred, challenged, or subverted. Within them, diverse groups converged and interfaced, and Egyptians engaged in behaviors and activities that defied or disrupted the social order. Over the course of the Mamluk era, the heterotopic qualities that had come to define Cairo's suburbs and cemeteries were reified and reinforced. At the same time, new and significant spaces emerged within the entertainment landscape, and these spaces would also come to be distinguished by their heterotopic nature.

Though Cairo's southern suburbs were gradually transforming into an elite residential neighborhood, the city's western suburbs remained a marginal zone throughout the Mamluk era. By the dawn of the Ottoman period, the western suburbs were host to a range of minority populations, as well as an assortment of "undesirables," including prostitutes, entertainers, and hashish sellers. Azbakīyah was the site of regular gatherings of Cairo's common people. Yet, the canals and ponds of the suburbs continued to draw the elites during the summer season, ensuring the ongoing interfacing of these disparate populations. Thus, this area continued to exist as a zone of ambivalence and liminality, and it would retain this quality for years to come.

Cairo's shrines and cemeteries, too, remained ambiguous and liminal spaces within the city's landscape. These were sites where the sacred and the secular converged, particularly during the *mawālid*, which exploded in popularity during this period. Ibn Taghrībirdī describes the raucous mix of sacred and secular activities during the Mūlid al-Nabī celebrations at the *zāwiyah* (Sufi chapel) of Shaykh Ismā'īl al-Anbābī (d. 1388):

> I must also disapprove of the celebration that takes place still today in the chapel mentioned; and because of the immoralities practiced by the people there, its abolition would be a most meritorious act. For the celebration has become one of the people's entertainments to which they resort in droves several days before it begins; some have done so for years without even knowing where the door of the chapel itself is, for it has simply become a custom for them and those whose company they wish and others like them to go there for pleasure, without any religious purpose [Popper 1954: 58].

Like the western suburbs, Rumaylah Square emerged as a space characterized by the interfacing of disparate social groups. Its proximity the Citadel ensured its prominent role in state ceremonials, such as the processions of the *maḥmal*, which attracted both elites and commoners. However, common people came together here for other reasons as well, and over the course of the Ottoman era, this space increasingly functioned as a regular gathering place for ordinary Cairenes. At the time of Napoleon's conquest, the French described Rumaylah Square as a "perpetual fair," complete with popular entertainers (Jomard 1829: 438–440).

In these heterotopic spaces, professional entertainers found the room that they needed to live and work. These were spaces that could accommodate these marginal individuals, whose lifestyles and behaviors placed them outside the mainstream of Egyptian society. In turn, their ongoing presence in these spaces imparted their own ambivalence and liminality into the spatial reality and contributed to the heterotopic nature of Cairo's entertainment landscape.

The market for entertainers situated near Bāb Zuwaylah deserves mention here. On the one hand, this space lacked the social heterogeneity that characterized the western suburbs, the city's shrines and cemeteries, Rumaylah Square, and the socially marginal suburban neighborhoods of Bāb al-Lūq and Ḥusaynīyah. Like most typical neighborhoods within the city of Cairo, the local residents and businesses of this space appeared to have shared ties to the same trade—in this case, professional entertainment. Yet, there was a perceived "otherness" to this space. Telling is al-Maqrīzī's description, though brief. His account makes it clear that this market was frequented by individuals connected to the entertainment trades, and that popular perceptions of this space as "unlucky" were informed by the ongoing presence of entertainers and the business of entertainment. Notably, certain streets and alleys near this market continued to be associated with the entertainment trades in future centuries, and Muḥammad 'Alī Street, which was completed in the 1870s and which quickly emerged as a hub for the business of professional entertainment, intersected with these spaces.

In short, professional entertainers played a critical role in the inscription and re-inscription of heterotopic meanings into certain Cairo spaces. Entertainers, themselves ambivalent and liminal figures in Egyptian social and spatial reality, imparted these qualities into the spaces that they inhabited, both by their presence and by their practice. Contemporary documentation makes it clear that Mamluk-era popular entertainment—not only music, song, and dance, but a wide range of other amusements, including early forms of dramatic representation such as *arājūz* (puppet theater) and *khayāl al-ẓill* (shadow play) (see Badawi 1988: 10–30)—were often openly transgressive of Egyptian social norms. The practice of these popular amusements in places like Cairo's western suburbs, cemeteries, and Rumaylah Square served to reify the heterotopic nature of these spaces.

It is worth elaborating on Mamluk shadow play (*khayāl al-ẓill*) here, not only because it illustrates the transgressive nature of Egyptian popular entertainment, but because the surviving examples reveal stock characters drawn from the lowest strata of Egyptian society, including contemporary popular entertainers. Badawi (1988: 12) offers this useful description of the mechanics of the shadow play:

> In shadow plays, which were performed in the streets and market places and occasionally also at court and in private houses, the action was represented by shadows cast upon a large flat screen by flat, coloured leather puppets, held in front of a torch, while the hidden puppet master, *al-Rayyis* or *al-Miqaddim*, delivered the dialogue and songs, helped in this by associates, sometimes as many as five persons including a youth who imitated the voice of women.

Much of what is known of Mamluk-era shadow plays comes from the three surviving plays of Muḥammad Ibn Dāniyāl, an ophthalmologist from Mosul who immigrated to Cairo in the late thirteenth century (Kahle 2015). Also a renowned poet, Ibn Dāniyāl set himself apart from his contemporaries with his decision to compose a literary adaptation of what was primarily a folk genre (see Rowson 1997: 172–174).

Ibn Dāniyāl's plays are a bawdy romp through the carnivalesque. Besides being sharply satirical of contemporary Cairo society, the plays are filled with coarse language, graphic descriptions of bodily functions, and other elements of the grotesque and the obscene. Marginal characters figure prominently in the plays, and all of them include music, singing, and dancing. Notably, the second of the three plays, *'Ajīb wa-Gharīb*, features a succession of characters from the Banū Sāsān/Ghurabā': a motley array of medical practitioners, occultists, entertainers, and laborers. Even more interestingly, the language of the play is peppered with Sīn (Richardson 2022: 37–39).

Ibn Dāniyāl's familiarity with Cairo's underworld, as well as his fluency in Sīn, were not coincidental. Ibn Dāniyāl lived just inside the northern gate of Bāb al-Futūḥ (Rowson 1997: 172), and it is quite likely that most of the clients of his ophthalmologic practice were from the nearby neighborhood of Ḥusaynīyah (Richardson 2022: 36). As already noted, this was a neighborhood populated by marginal groups, including professional entertainers. Undoubtedly, Ibn Dāniyāl had interactions with a variety of marginal characters, including members of the Banū Sāsān/Ghurabā', as well as the *ḥarāfīsh* (singular *ḥarfūsh*), a collective of lower-class street toughs who also spoke Sīn (Irwin 2004: 163, Richardson 2022: 36–37). Thus Ibn Dāniyāl's work is informative not only in its content, but in what it reveals about the entertainment landscape within which Ibn Dāniyāl was creating. Ibn Dāniyāl's plays are not merely carnivalesque literature: they reflect a complex social and spatial reality within which the carnivalesque was interwoven. That is, the marginal characters and transgressive behaviors depicted in these plays were part of real life in Mamluk-era Cairo, and their ongoing presence was key to meaning-making in the medieval Cairene landscape.

Conclusion

Cairo's landscape of entertainment first began to take shape in the time of the Fatimids. In the popular imagination, certain public spaces came to be associated with entertainment and leisure: the canals and ponds of the suburbs, and the city's shrines and cemeteries. These were spaces of ambivalence and liminality, wherein the social order was defied and disrupted. Normal social and spatial boundaries were blurred or broken as diverse populations came together and engaged in transgressive behaviors and activities. In short, these were heterotopic spaces.

The heterotopic qualities of Cairo's entertainment landscape were both a product and a producer of the actions occurring within them. While these spaces informed the habitus of Egyptians as they moved and acted within them, it was the practice of Egyptians within Cairo's suburbs and cemeteries that inscribed heterotopic meanings into these spaces. Thus the heterotopic nature of Cairo's suburbs and cemeteries, well-established by the time the Mamluks came to power, was produced and reproduced, and throughout the Mamluk period, the spaces that constituted Cairo's entertainment landscape continued to be "outside of all places."

Professional entertainers were key to the inscription of heterotopic meanings into these spaces in the Cairene landscape. As ambiguous and liminal personae, their activities and behaviors situated them outside the norm, and as a consequence, they worked and resided in settings that made space for their unorthodox lifestyles and behaviors. Simultaneously, their life and work imparted their ambiguity and liminality into the spaces they inhabited, and informed public perceptions of these spaces. Perhaps the most concrete illustration of this in the Mamluk era is the entertainers' market described by al-Maqrīzī, the negative reputation of which was clearly informed by the presence of professional entertainers. In the ensuing centuries, the ties between professional entertainers—particularly male and female dancers—and these heterotopic spaces in the landscape of Cairo become increasingly explicit in contemporary sources, demonstrating that the presence of professional entertainers was fundamental to the ongoing re-inscription of heterotopic meaning in Cairo's landscape of entertainment.

This entertainment landscape persisted into the ensuing Ottoman era and beyond. Most remarkably, the meanings imparted into this landscape would endure even through the dramatic transformations of Cairo's urban geography under Muḥammad ʿAlī Bāshā and his grandson Ismāʿīl. This endurance of meaning in spite of physiognomic change makes it clear that the dialectical and mutually constituting relationship between professional entertainers and spaces of entertainment was a profoundly important force in meaning-making within the city of Cairo.

THREE

Ottoman Elaboration, Khedivial Change

On January 23, 1517, the last Mamluk sultan of Egypt was decisively defeated in a battle just north of the Cairo city gates, and Egypt passed under the rule of Ottoman Sultan Selim. At that moment, Cairo lost its status as the economic and cultural capital of an empire: the city was relegated to a provincial outpost, one among many, subservient to the Ottoman capital at Istanbul. Abu-Luhgod (1971: 50) writes:

> In such a manner did Cairo—which had ruled for almost 550 years over the prosperous and extensive Fāṭimid, Ayyūbid, and Mamluk empires, which had been an unrivaled center of world commerce, which had been the undisputed model of culture for the Islamic world, and which was still the largest city of the Middle East and Europe—pass into the hands of the Turks, to become a mere provincial capital subordinate to Constantinople.

Raymond is more measured in his assessment, noting that although administration and governance changed, there was a high degree of continuity between the Mamluk city and the Ottoman city. He writes: "Ottoman Cairo was similar to the Cairo of before 1517; the city would change much more between 1798 and the rule of Muhammad Ali" (Raymond 2000: 202).

Indeed, the French occupation from 1798 to 1801, and a few years later, the rapid ascent of Muḥammad ʿAlī Bāshā, would initiate an era of profound change in Cairo. The urban developments introduced by the French and elaborated upon by Muḥammad ʿAlī enabled the massive urban planning projects that would be undertaken by Muḥammad ʿAlī's grandson, Ismāʿīl, in the latter half of the nineteenth century. Ismāʿīl's unprecedented urban development schemes would substantially impact the geography of the city and leave their imprint on Cairo's entertainment landscape.

Nevertheless, certain spaces maintained their longstanding associations with professional entertainment, and the landscape of entertainment demonstrated remarkable continuity in the face of the many changes that were implemented during the Khedivial era. Particularly in the zone west of the Khalīj, the meanings that had been deeply inscribed since the Fatimid era persisted. Indeed, some developments in and around Azbakīyah served to reinscribe the heterotopic qualities that had long characterized this space. In particular, the rise of formalized entertainment venues in this area in the latter half of the nineteenth century reinforced its ties to professional entertainment and physically embodied the ambivalence and liminality of Cairo's western suburbs. These venues emerged as a visible and tangible manifestation of the ongoing dialectical interplay between professional entertainer and entertainment space in the Cairene landscape.

Ottoman Cairo

Although frequently characterized as a period of stagnation, the Ottoman era was in fact a time of relative stability as well as steady growth for the city of Cairo (Figure 14). However, as Behrens-Abouseif (1985: 54) notes:

> During the Ottoman period, the boundaries of Cairo did not continue to expand, as they had under the Mamluks; rather, building activity occurred within the previous boundaries. This means that the urban canvas filled in rather than stretched.

Development within the city suburbs, already underway in the Mamluk period, continued in earnest, particularly to the south of the city core. The relocation of several tanneries from south of Bāb Zuwaylah to an area near Bāb al-Lūq at the dawn of the seventeenth century opened up new areas for residential development. Cairo's wealthiest elites settled along the shores of the nearby Birkat al-Fīl, and from the mid-seventeenth through mid-eighteenth centuries, this was the primary residential district of the ruling class (Raymond 2000: 219). By contrast, urban development to the west of the city core lagged, and the area retained a suburban quality until the early eighteenth century (Raymond 2000: 221–222).

As noted in the last chapter, al-Qāhirah was initially organized on ethnic and occupational lines. Sub-group identification continued to affect the layout of the city during the Ottoman period, with city residents divided according to ethnic identity, religious affiliation, occupation, and local *ḥārāt* affiliations (Abu-Luhgod 1971: 58–62, Raymond 2000: 231–234). Abu-Luhgod notes that there was some correspondence between ethnicity and religion, and a great deal of congruence between occupation and

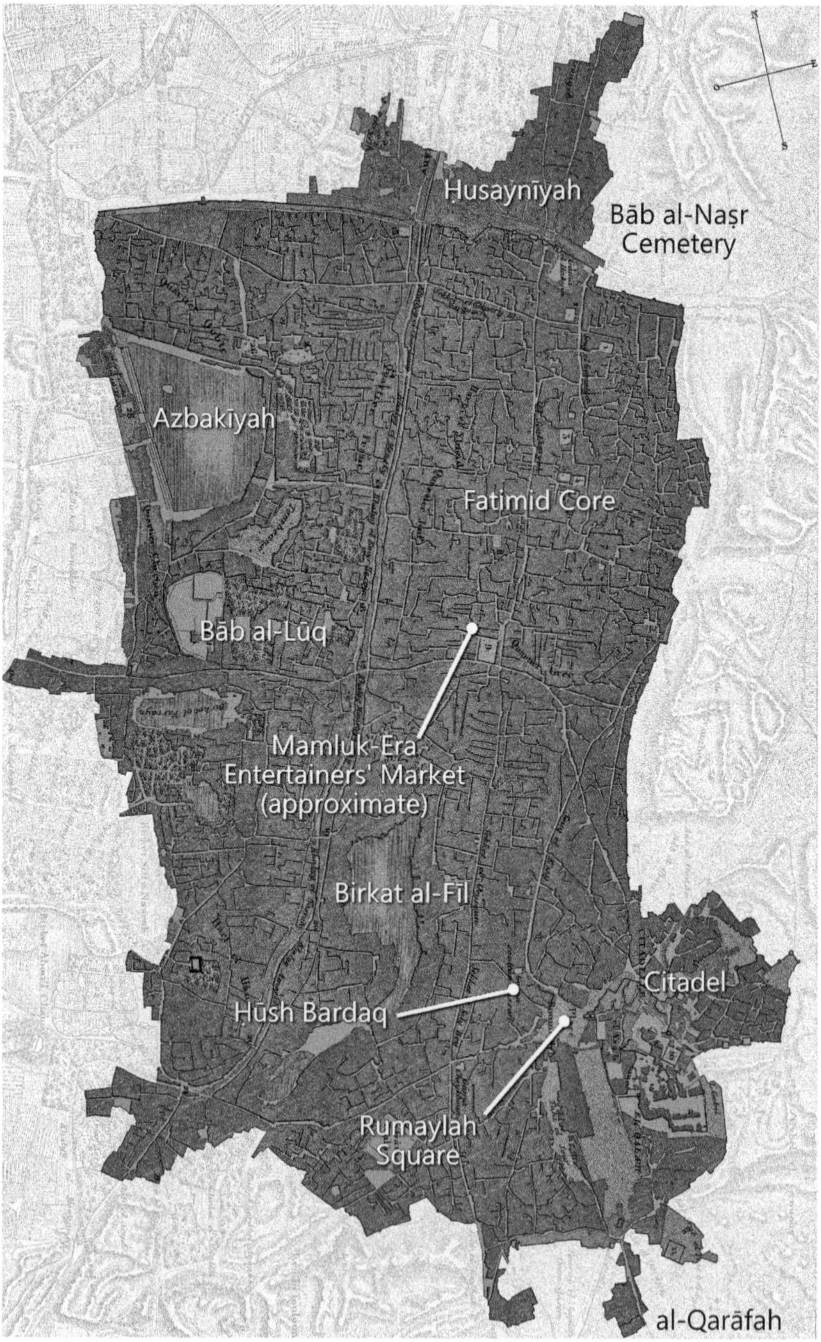

Figure 14: Map of early nineteenth century Cairo (after Dufour, 1838).

ethnic identity (1971: 59). For example, Egypt's indigenous Copts were traditionally employed in occupations tied to administration, taxation, and record-keeping: scribes, bookkeepers, customs officials and the like; consequently, the main Coptic neighborhoods of Cairo were situated near ports and administrative centers.

Wealth and class affiliation were factors in the organization of the Ottoman city as well. The grand residences of the nobility, wealthy merchants, and *'ulamā'* were generally situated in the city center and the southern suburbs. By contrast, the middle and lower classes resided in the urban *ḥārāt*, somewhat removed from the city center, or else in the suburban districts, particularly the western suburbs.

Still, many neighborhoods were characterized by some degree of socioeconomic heterogeneity. In the city center, various forms of collective residences, including the *wakālah*, the *khān*, and the *rab'*, were located along the main commercial avenues and near the markets (Raymond 1980). Their location near areas of heavy commercial activity was tied to their function: the *wakālah* and the *khān* provided temporary lodging for foreign traders, travelers, and soldiers, while the *rab'* offered affordable permanent housing to local merchants and artisans of the lower middle class. Yet, the city center also hosted costly and lavish homes of the elite, since only the wealthiest could afford to own real estate there. As a result, upper class dwellings in central Cairo were often in close proximity to these collective residences, which housed individuals and families from radically different socioeconomic backgrounds. Raymond (2000: 270) notes that the soldiers who resided in the temporary housing at the city center often engaged in illicit activities, indulging in alcohol and patronizing prostitutes, resulting in periodic crackdowns by the authorities.

Some socioeconomic heterogeneity also existed within the *ḥārāt* of Cairo (Al-Messiri Nadim 1979: 313–314, Abu-Luhgod 1971: 64). The *ḥārah* brought together the residences, manufacturing sites, and commercial locations of people tied to a particular trade, with the result that individuals of a range of means and abilities frequently lived and worked in close proximity. Nevertheless, there were "wealthy" *ḥārāt* and "poor" *ḥārāt* (see Al-Messiri Nadim 1979: 314, Raymond 2000: 271). The latter were associated with activities and occupations such as slaughtering and butchering, milling, and tanning—activities that made them undesirable to elite residents.

In the Ottoman era, perhaps the most heterogeneous area of Cairo was its western suburbs. The area was host to a wide range of ethnic, religious, and social minority groups—Copts, Levantine Christians, Europeans, and others. The western suburbs were also home to a range of activities and occupations deemed undesirable within elite neighborhoods. Nevertheless, many of Cairo's well-to-do maintained residences there; like their predecessors, they were drawn to the open landscape and cool breezes on the banks of the Birkat al-Azbakīyah.

Although Christian neighborhoods existed in both al-Qāhirah and Fusṭāṭ, Ottoman Cairo's most substantial Christian population was situated in the western suburbs, particularly north of the Birkat al-Azbakīyah in al-Maqs. For generations, the village of al-Maqs had been home to a majority Christian population. Before the westward shift of the Nile, the village was a port city. The administrative activities associated with the port, such as taxation and record keeping, guaranteed a concentration of indigenous Copts, given their specialization in these activities throughout the history of Muslim rule in Egypt (Abu-Luhgod 1971: 59, Behrens-Abouseif 1985: 4–5). The construction of Ṣalāḥ al-Dīn's wall, besides increasing security, organically tied al-Maqs to Cairo's urban center and encouraged further growth. Christian neighborhoods also existed south of the Azbakīyah pond, though they were not as extensive as the quarter of al-Maqs.

Notably, these neighborhoods were neither exclusively Christian nor exclusively Coptic. The neighborhoods north and south of the Azbakīyah pond were host to substantial Muslim and non-Coptic Christian populations as well. Moreover, there was a lack of segregation among these varied groups. Behrens-Abouseif (1985: 40) notes: "*Maḥkama* documents and Coptic *waqf* deeds of the 16th and 17th centuries indicate that Muslims dwelt near Christians without strict segregation," and some mosques were surrounded by Coptic dwellings.

The western suburbs of Ottoman Cairo were also host to a substantial European community. By the time of the French conquest, the area between al-Maqs and Qanṭarat al-Mūskī (the Mūskī Bridge) was known as the Ḥārat al-Afranj, the Frankish Quarter.* Prior to the Ottoman era, European merchants who conducted trade in Egypt were largely prohibited from settling in Cairo. This situation began to change toward the end of the Mamluk period, when al-Ashraf Qānṣūh al-Ghūrī (r. 1501–1516) established a treaty with the French that allowed them freedom of movement within Egypt (Behrens-Abouseif 1985: 41). These privileges were reaffirmed and expanded upon in agreements between the Ottoman sultan and Western powers—first the French in the 1530s, followed by several others over the course of the Ottoman Empire. These agreements, known as the Capitulations, ensured that European nationals residing and doing business in Egypt were largely outside the jurisdiction of Egyptian law

* The term *afranjī* referred to western Europeans, and would eventually come to refer to Europeans in general. By contrast, Europeans of the former Byzantine Empire, such as Greeks, were referred to as *rūmī*.

(Abu-Lughod 1971: 127). The decision to grant extraterritorial privileges to foreigners established a legal and financial imbalance between foreigners and indigenous Egyptians that would have profound implications for centuries.

There were a number of reasons why the western suburbs were attractive to Copts, Levantine Christians, Europeans, and other minority groups. On a practical level, the western suburbs had more open land available for settlement, while still retaining spatial proximity to the city center. However, population pressure was not the only factor discouraging their settlement within the urban core. Although small Christian (and Jewish) *ḥārāt* had existed within the city from the foundation of al-Qāhirah, the social climate under the Mamluks was less tolerant toward Christians. Behrens-Abouseif (1985: 38) notes:

> Both the great building activities of the Mamluks, and their generally hostile policy towards the Copts, were likely to prevent expansion of the Christian quarters within the urban core. Moreover, one may assume that after the religious riot of 721/1321 the Christian population of the capital preferred to live in the suburbs.

A range of trades that were unwelcome in elite Muslim neighborhoods thrived in the western suburbs. Since alcohol was manufactured and sold by Christians in Muslim-majority Egypt, many taverns were located in the neighborhoods west of the Khalīj (Behrens-Abouseif 1985: 40).* Prostitution was also commonplace in the area, as noted by many contemporary observers (see Africanus 1896: 874, Dankoff and Kim: 2011: 393–394). According to the Ottoman explorer Evliya Çelebi, several guilds related to the trade, including male and female prostitutes, pimps, and enforcers, were based in Bāb al-Lūq (Dankoff and Kim: 2011: 393–394). Industries that produced pollution and foul odors were also relegated to the suburbs. As the southern suburbs of Cairo became increasingly urbanized, the tanneries south of Bāb Zuwaylah were relocated westward to Bāb al-Lūq (Raymond 2000: 263).

All of these factors explain why the western suburbs were not attractive to extensive development and permanent settlement by elites—at least not initially. As noted in the last chapter, Azbak's development spurred some new construction on the southern shore of the Birkat al-Azbakīyah. Among the late Mamluk developments were a mosque and several additional structures established by the prominent jurist Shaykh ʿAbd al-Ḥaqq

---

* According to Lewicka (2005), these may not have been taverns in the European sense, where alcohol was consumed on the premises. Rather, she argues that the establishments referred to as "taverns" in medieval and early Ottoman historiography were places where alcohol was bought and sold, but not necessarily consumed.

al-Sunbāṭī on the southwestern shore of the pond (Behrens-Abouseif 1985: 40). In the sixteenth century, the wealthy and powerful Bakrī family, leaders of the Bakrīyah Sufi order, established a palatial residence nearby (Behrens-Abouseif 1985: 49–52). By the end of the seventeenth century, the influential Shaykh al-Bakrī had been placed in charge of Cairo's Mūlid al-Nabī celebrations, and the festivities were centered at the Bakrī residence in Azbakīyah.

Nevertheless, it was not until the early eighteenth century that more extensive developments were undertaken around the Birkat al-Azbakīyah. Perhaps the most significant construction of this time was the complex of the prominent *amīr* 'Uthmān Katkhudā (d. 1735). The complex included a mosque as well as a wide range of residential and commercial structures (Behrens-Abouseif 1985: 55–58). Unlike the suburban constructions of the Mamluk era, which were pioneering attempts at urbanizing a largely undeveloped area, large-scale developments like that of 'Uthmān Katkhudā occurred as a response to pre-existing economic activity and population growth. Behrens-Abouseif (1985: 58) writes:

> Unlike Azbak's quarter, 'Uṯmān's project was rather a response to increasing activity and population demands in the area west of the Ḫhalīğ. This is illustrated by the fact that on the day the mosque was inaugurated, the number of worshippers was so great that many could not be accommodated inside; they had instead to pray at the nearby Mosque of Azbak. 'Uṯmān Katḫudā's foundation is thus characteristic of its period, in which urban projects played a consolidating rather than pioneering role.

In the decades following 'Uthmān Katkhudā's project, the well-to-do were increasingly attracted to the area. Indeed, many of Cairo's elites migrated from the Birkat al-Fīl to the newly fashionable Birkat al-Azbakīyah, perhaps attracted by the open space and uncongested streets (Raymond 2000: 222–223).

These developments increased the presence of Cairo's elites in the western suburbs, but they did not erase the presence of marginal social groups there. Rather, the area remained socially and economically heterogeneous. As had been the case for centuries prior, the western suburbs of Ottoman Cairo existed as a social and spatial interface between radically diverse populations.

The Spaces of Entertainment in Ottoman Cairo

Under the Fatimids, Cairo's entertainment landscape had begun to take shape. Certain public spaces—the canals and ponds of the suburbs, as well as the city's shrines and cemeteries—became associated with entertainment and leisure in the popular imagination. These were heterotopic spaces: spaces of ambivalence and liminality, where the social order was defied and disrupted, and where the normal social and spatial boundaries of Cairo were blurred and broken. In the Mamluk era, Cairo's suburbs and cemeteries carried forward their associations with entertainment and leisure, and the heterotopic qualities that had come to define them were reified and reinforced. As new and noteworthy spaces were integrated into Cairo's landscape of professional entertainment, including the massive public square known as Mīdān al-Rumaylah, and the market for entertainers situated near Bāb Zuwaylah, these new spaces came to be characterized by their ambivalence and "otherness" as well. Ottoman-era sources demonstrate the continuity of these meanings in Cairo's entertainment landscape.

Contemporary observers of Cairo's suburban canals and ponds make it clear that under the Ottomans, these continued to be focal points for recreation, entertainment, and leisure. The most significant of these ponds was the Birkat al-Azbakīyah, which was not only an important site for popular festivals, but a regular gathering place for common people. Behrens-Abouseif (1985: 77–78) notes that by the time of the French occupation, Azbakīyah and Rumaylah were the main public squares of Cairo. The western suburbs, with Azbakīyah as their focal point, as well as Rumaylah Square, were spaces where radically disparate social groups converged, and where the "rules" of society were bent or even broken.

Cairo's shrines and cemeteries also remained integral to the entertainment landscape in the Ottoman era. The common people of the city gathered at these locations, not only on Fridays, but on the occasion of religious festivals, including the numerous *mawālid* that occurred throughout the year. Contemporary observers describe—sometimes with dismay—the raucous celebrations that took place in these spaces during the popular *mawālid*. Here, Egyptians engaged in activities and behaviors that were frowned upon in other spaces and contexts, pushing and pulling at social norms and boundaries.

In addition to Cairo's suburbs and cemeteries, Ottoman sources offer additional information regarding spaces that were tied not only to the performance of entertainment, but to other aspects of the entertainment trades, particularly spaces of residence and commerce. Like the suburbs and cemeteries, these spaces came to embody heterotopic qualities, in large measure due to their association in the public imagination with the entertainment trades and professional entertainers. Mamluk-era sources reveal that spaces of residence and commerce already existed in Bāb al-Lūq, in Ḥusaynīyah, and in an area just west of Bāb Zuwaylah. The Ottoman period yields some additional evidence regarding such spaces, including a neighborhood populated by female dancers: Ḥūsh Bardaq. Also of tremendous significance in this regard was a new type of venue for socialization and leisure: the coffee house. Coffee was introduced to Egypt in the 1530s, and soon thereafter, coffee houses became widespread throughout Cairo (Behrens-Abouseif 1985: 43–44). Over the course of the Ottoman era, these establishments became important gathering places for professional entertainers—not only for the performance of entertainment, but for the business of meeting and negotiating with customers.

Professional entertainers, including male and female dancers, were ubiquitous in all of these spaces, and throughout the Ottoman era it becomes increasingly clear that the presence of professional entertainers was fundamental to the ongoing re-inscription of heterotopic meaning into Cairo's entertainment landscape. Sources from this period abundantly demonstrate that public perceptions of these spaces were inextricably tied to their association with professional entertainers. Moreover, Ottoman-era sources are increasingly specific in their mention of singer/dancers such as *ghawāzī* and *khawalāt*. The ongoing presence of professional entertainers in these locales further etched these spaces onto the map of the city and into the minds of the local population: professional entertainers were key to the production and reproduction of Cairo's heterotopic entertainment landscape.

Azbakīyah and the Western Suburbs

Throughout the Ottoman era, the zone to the west of the Khalīj remained a largely rural area, with its landscape of gardens and ponds. The association of the suburban zone with entertainment, leisure, and vice, firmly established centuries earlier, carried forward under the Ottomans. The Andalusian diplomat and scholar Leo Africanus (1896: 884), who was present in Cairo when the Ottomans took control of the city, observes: "The cookes shops stand open very late: but the shops of other artificers shut up before ten of the clocke, who then walke abroad for their solace and recreation from one suburbe to another." Sir Henry Blount (1636: 43) describes the scene in the 1630s: "In these *Byrkhaes*, and *Calhis* [Khalīj], towards evening, are many hundreds washing themselves, in the meane while divers passe up, and down with *Pipes*, & *Roguy Fidles*, in Boats, full of *Fruits*, *Sherbets*, and good *banqueting stuffe* to sell." The bank of the Nile at Būlāq was also a popular place to gather and promenade: the Ottoman historian Muṣṭafā ʿAlī indicates that both "high and low" congregated there every Saturday (Tietze 1975: 36, 41).

The celebration of the Nile flood remained one of the most important festivals of the year, and when the dam of the Khalīj was cut, the western suburbs were alive with merriment. As in prior centuries, Cairenes gathered on the banks of the canals and ponds, and the well-to-do sailed their boats upon the floodwaters. Popular entertainers plied their trades among the populace. Both Muṣṭafā ʿAlī and Leo Africanus describe festivities lasting for seven days (Africanus 1896: 881, Tietze 1975: 36), although Evliya Çelebi suggests that the joyous atmosphere continued for three months, until the flood subsided (Prokosch 2000: 204). As in previous eras, the celebrations were raucous and transgressive: describing the flood celebration in 1799, al-Jabartī writes that local Christians, Syrians, and Greeks mocked the Muslim Mamluks by riding in pleasure boats and imitating their speech, dress, and manner of bearing arms (al-Jabartī 1888–1896, volume 6: 151–152; 1904, volume 3: 81–82).

The focal point of the western suburbs was the Birkat al-Azbakīyah (and the open plaza it created when the Nile flood receded) (Figure 15). By the dawn of the Ottoman era, Azbakīyah was well-established as a regular gathering place for Cairo's common people. A rich description is provided by Leo Africanus. According to John Pory's English translation:

> Vpon a certaine large place of this suburbe standeth a great palace and a stately college built by a certaine Mammaluck called *Iazbach*, counseller vnto

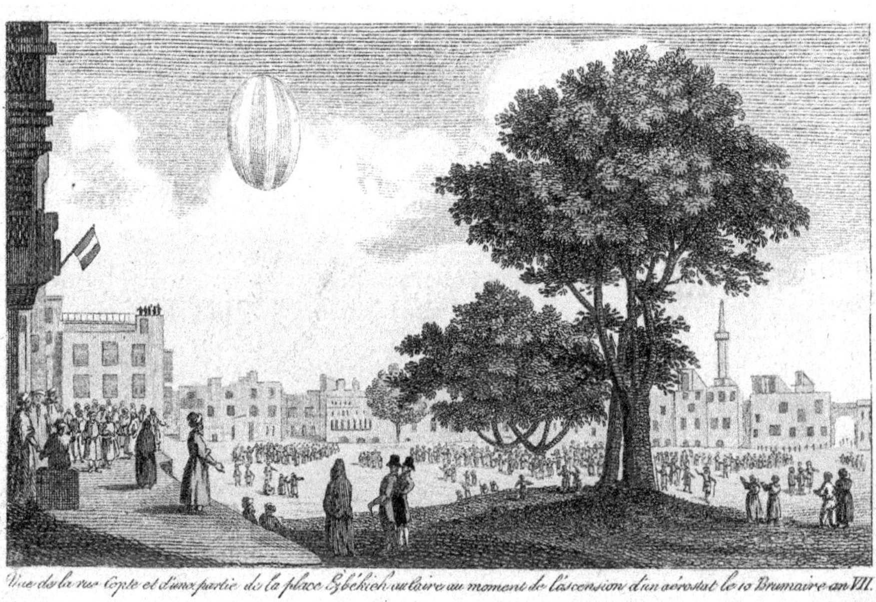

Figure 15: Azbakīyah during the French occupation (engraving of an earlier work by Luigi Mayer, from Jean-Baptiste Joseph Breton's *L'Égypte et la Syrie*, 1814).

> the Soldan of those times; and the place it selfe is called after his name Iazbachia. Hither after Mahumetan sermons and deuotions, the common people of Cairo, togither with the baudes and harlots, do vsually resort; and many stage plaiers also, and such as teach camels, asses, and dogs, to daunce [Africanus 1896: 874].

The description goes on to detail some of the entertainments that Leo Africanus personally witnessed, including dancing donkeys, fortune tellers, martial artists, and epic poets who sang of the Arab conquest of Egypt.

Pory's translation of "baudes and harlots" somewhat glosses over some details in the source text, however. In the original Italian, Leo Africanus states that people were drawn to Azbakīyah because it was the site of many "dishonest things" such as taverns and loose women (Africano 1500: 91). Similarly, Ottoman explorer Evliya Çelebi observes that Bāb al-Lūq, just south of the Birkat al-Azbakīyah, was host to many brothels, coffee houses, and *būẓah* shops (Prokosch 2000: 41). He also notes that guilds of male and female prostitutes, pimps, and enforcers were based in this area (Dankoff and Kim: 2011: 393–394). The location of these trades and their practitioners in this area should come as no surprise: recall that Bāb al-Lūq was home to socially and professionally marginal groups such as the Banū Sāsān/Ghurabā' as early as the late thirteenth century.

Among the public women who frequented the area were the female professional entertainers known as *ghawāzī*. Carsten Niebuhr, a German explorer in service of Denmark, frequently encountered the *ghawāzī* in the western suburbs, particularly in the vicinity of the Khalīj, during his visit to Egypt in the 1760s:

> At first, we never saw them but by accident, and in a public house without the city; but, towards the conclusion of our stay in Egypt, we had better opportunities of gratifying our curiosity. A great part of the houses in which the Europeans live, stand along the great canal which passes through Cairo: and those *Ghasi* accordingly derive their best profits from dancing opposite to these houses in the canal, when it is dry, before the opening of the dyke [Niebuhr 1792: 140].

Two decades earlier, Pococke (1743: 192) had observed these female entertainers in Cairo, remarking: "There are women who go barefaced about the streets, dancing, singing, and playing on some instrument."

Egypt's Ottoman-era elites continued to be drawn to the banks of Cairo's suburban ponds, and some constructed summer homes on the Birkat al-Azbakīyah. During flood season, the wealthy would sail their pleasure boats out onto the lake:

> The Lake both square and large, is but only a Lake when the River overfloweth; being joined thereunto by a Chanel; where the Moors (rowed up and down in Barges, shaded with Damasks and Stuffs of India) accustom to solace themselves in the Evening. The water fallen, yet the place rather changeth than loseth its delightfulness: affording the profit of five Harvests in a year, together with the pleasure; frequented much in the cool of the day [Sandys 1673: 94].

Yet, as previously noted, it was not until the early eighteenth century that the elites established more permanent residences in the area. Richard Pococke (1743: 30) describes the scene in the 1730s:

> Nothing can be imagined more beautiful, than to see those places fill'd with water, round which the best houses in the city are built; and when the Nile is high in the summer, it must be an entertaining prospect, to see them cover'd with the fine boats and barges of all the great people, who come out in the evening to divert themselves with their ladies: As I have been inform'd, concerts of music are never wanting, and sometimes fireworks add to the amusement; all the houses round being in a manner illuminated, and the windows full of spectators to behold this glorious sight.

Niebuhr (1792: 63) notes that "the most considerable persons in the country" preferred to live on the banks of the suburban ponds.

In the late Mamluk period, Azbakīyah was a significant site for the celebration of popular festivals. Shortly after its creation, the Azbakīyah pond became one of the primary locations for the annual celebration of the Nile flood: in 1485, the opening of the Khalīj was celebrated here for the first time (Behrens-Abouseif 1985: 23–24). When the Bakrīyah Sufi order assumed control of organizing the Mūlid al-Nabī, the festivities came to be centered at the Bakrī residence. The relocation of this important annual festival to Azbakīyah would further boost the significance of Azbakīyah as a site of entertainment. Azbakīyah remained the central site for Cairo's Mūlid al-Nabī celebrations, until Ismā'īl's developments in the area necessitated a relocation of the festivities somewhat further to the west.

The western suburbs, with Azbakīyah as the focal point, drew together individuals from vastly different sectors of Egyptian society to enjoy the pleasures it afforded. This was a zone of confluence between disparate populations: elites and commoners, Muslims and Christians, native Egyptians and foreigners, men and women—just as it had been for generations. Even as Egypt's nobility sailed their pleasure craft upon the placid waters of the Birkat al-Azbakīyah, the most marginal people in Egyptian society plied their trades on the shores. Among them were the popular entertainers, including the *ghawāzī*, who found ready audiences in the carnivalesque atmosphere of Cairo's western suburbs.

Rumaylah

In the Mamluk era, Rumaylah Square emerged as a staging point for state ceremonials such as the *maḥmal* processions and as a gathering place for Cairo's common people. By the time of Napoleon's conquest, Rumaylah had evolved into what the French described as a "perpetual fair" wherein the local population regularly engaged in both business and pleasure (Jomard 1829: 438–440). The square was frequented by merchants and shopkeepers, livestock dealers, beggars, prostitutes, popular entertainers, and even preachers and mystics (see al-Damurdāshī 1991: 115–116). There were also permanent residents who set up modest huts at the base of the Citadel.

Much like Azbakīyah, Rumaylah Square was a point of confluence among radically distinct social groups. Though situated at the doorstep of Egypt's rulers and traversed regularly by the aristocracy, Rumaylah was host to a motley assortment of individuals from the lowest echelons of Egyptian society. Evliya Çelebi lists several unusual trade guilds that were based out of Rumaylah Square, including the guild of beggars, the guild of camel meat and camel liver cooks, the guild of earth rat hunters, and the guild of henbane sherbet makers; he also notes that a guild of male prostitutes frequented the square (Dankoff and Kim: 2011: 394–395, 397–398).

Accounts from the turn of the eighteenth and nineteenth century make it clear that professional entertainers—specifically female dancers—had established residences in the vicinity of Rumaylah Square at some point during the Ottoman Era. An account is offered by al-Jabartī of a dancer "from the Rumaylah quarter" who was executed in 1799 after getting drawn into some intrigue with her lover, a Turkish servant to a French official (al-Jabartī 1888–1896, volume 6: 101–102; 1904, volume 3: 51). It is quite likely that this dancer was from a neighborhood known as Ḥūsh Bardaq, located just southwest of the mosque of Sultan Ḥassan. This neighborhood will be described in greater detail below.

In short, Rumaylah Square in the Ottoman era was a socially and economically heterogeneous space that accommodated marginal personae and marginal behaviors. Professional entertainers not only worked in this popular square, but established residences here, at the foot of the Citadel, the seat of the Egyptian government. As in the western suburbs, popular entertainers, including female dancers, found in Rumaylah a space where they belonged. In turn, the heterotopic nature of Rumaylah Square was reinforced and reified by the presence of these ambivalent and liminal populations.

Shrines and Cemeteries

Shrine and cemetery visitation remained an important part of life for the inhabitants of Ottoman Cairo. Both Leo Africanus, writing near the dawn of the sixteenth century, and Muṣṭafā ʿAlī, writing at its end, describe masses of people walking or riding to the cemeteries for *ziyārah* every Friday morning (Africanus 1896: 877, Tietze 1975: 33). Besides these weekly cemetery visits, the two primary Muslim feast days, the many *mawālid* interspersed throughout the year, and various other festivals such as ʿĀshūrāʾ provided another pretext to gather at Cairo's shrines and cemeteries. Foreign observers, Muslim and non-Muslim alike, remarked on the great frequency of festivals in Egypt. Muṣṭafā ʿAlī observes:

> They are not content with the two noble Feasts and with the splendid gatherings connected with the departure and arrival of the pilgrims. Contrary to other countries, in Cairo never a month passes without some festivity taking place, without their flocking together saying today is the day of the excursion to such and such place, or today is the day when such and such [procession] goes around [Tietze 1975: 49].

The French Orientalist Claude-Étienne Savary (1785: 285), who traveled through Egypt in the 1770s, writes:

> All these mad ceremonies that the pagan religion authorized are renewed today around the tombs of the saints, in front of the churches of the Copts, and in the fairs of which I spoke to you. The taste for pilgrimages still subsists among them. Their dances, their music are the same. Despite the shackles with which the Mohammedan religion has chained them, their nature shines through, and the inclinations of their fathers are maintained; so true it is that old habits, born of the climate, triumph at the end of all laws.

Regarding the tombs of the saints, he elaborates in a footnote: "The Mahometans go on certain days of the year to the tombs of some personages whom they regard as Saints, and celebrate their feast by indulging in joy, good cheer, and license."

A colorful account is provided by al-Jabartī of the annual *mūlid* in honor of Shaykh ʿAbd al-Wahāb, a minor Sufi saint who died in 1758 (al-Jabartī 1888–1896, volume 2: 176–179; 1904, volume 1: 224–225). A few years after the *shaykh*'s death, torrential rains in Cairo destroyed a number of tombs, including that of ʿAbd al-Wahāb. Consequently, his descendants and followers erected a newer, much grander mausoleum, as well as a kiosk and a courtyard to accommodate the horses and donkeys of visitors; the tomb and associated facilities were located in the eastern cemetery, on elevated ground not far from the complex of Qāytbāy. Upon completion of the construction, his descendants established an annual *mūlid* for the *shaykh*; al-Jabartī describes the festivities:

> Tents, kitchens, and coffee houses are set up, and the crowd congregates, made up of people of all kinds and classes. There are peasants, purveyors of amusements and games, *ghawāzī*, prostitutes, monkey trainers, and magicians.

> Fires are lit, garbage and excrement are thrown away, and natural needs are met among the trampled tombs. Day and night, they play games, they fornicate, they dance, and they beat on drums and play flutes. This continues for ten days or more. A tent is set up for the *'ulamā'* [religious scholars] and the jurists, and the emirs and the traders attend as well. No one finds fault with it, so everyone takes their share: everyone believes that these are meritorious acts and religious duties and it must be so, because otherwise the *'ulamā'* would have condemned these acts instead of taking part [al-Jabartī 1888–1896, volume 2: 178–179; 1904, volume 1: 225].

This account paints a vivid picture of a carnivalesque scene wherein social boundaries were obliterated—the living celebrated among the tombs of the dead, the secular overlapped with the sacred, and men and women mingled with impunity.

Like the Islamic scholar Ibn al-Ḥājj in the fourteenth century, many Ottoman observers were particularly troubled by popularity of *ziyārah* among Cairene women. Visitors from elsewhere in the Ottoman Empire expressed surprise that Egyptian women were free to gather at shrines and cemeteries as they pleased. Evliya Çelebi remarks that women needed no permission from their husbands, and that the latter could not question their wives about their whereabouts, as the right to visit the cemeteries was written into their marriage contracts (Dankoff and Kim: 2011: 412).

A common criticism of shrine and cemetery visits was that they provided a pretext for women to engage in rendezvous with men:

> On Fridays when people go to visit the graves of the dead that rest in Karafa and in particular the blessed sepulchres of the Imām Abu l-Laith, the Imam Shāfi'ī, and of Sitt Nafīsa, their women usually meet there with the *jundīs* [cavalrymen] that are not afraid of a bullying strong-man. Those who find no opportunity or cannot afford making the preparations for intercourse at least [use this visit] at the sacred places for making the arrangements [for a rendezvous]. Then they go to the usual places of sin and adultery [Tietze 1975: 41].

The same accusation would be made by early nineteenth-century observers as well (Michaud 1833–1835, vol. 5: 254).

What is quite clear is that Cairo's shrines and cemeteries were heterogeneous spaces that played host to socially transgressive behaviors and activities. These spaces challenged and subverted the ordinary social and spatial boundaries of Egyptian society as they drew together profoundly diverse populations. The line between sacred and secular was blurred or even broken. Within these heterotopic spaces, Cairo's professional entertainers plied their trades, and the presence of these marginal personae reinforced the ambivalence and liminality of these locales.

Spaces of Residence and Commerce in the Entertainment Landscape

In the Mamluk era, contemporary sources allude to the spaces where professional entertainers lived, as well as the spaces where they engaged in the more mundane aspects of their trades, such as buying and selling musical instruments. Many of Cairo's professional entertainers resided in Bāb al-Lūq, in the western suburbs, and Ḥusaynīyah, just north of Bāb al-Futūḥ. Another Mamluk-era residential neighborhood for entertainers may have existed in the vicinity of the musical instrument market located west of Bāb Zuwaylah.

Under the Ottomans, Bāb al-Lūq continued to be an important residential zone for professional entertainers and practitioners of other marginal trades. Similarly, Ottoman-era entertainers continued to reside in Ḥusaynīyah. Ḥusaynīyah's ongoing association with marginal people and trades, including professional entertainment, is documented by Ottoman-era chroniclers. At the dawn of the eighteenth century, the home of the *shaykhat al-maghānī*, the head of the female singers' guild in Cairo, was located in Ḥusaynīyah. Her house was targeted during 'Alī Āghā's crackdown on taverns, brothels, and other places of vice between 1703 and 1705 (al-Damurdāshī 1991: 122). During Ramadan 1814, a group of soldiers who were camped outside of Bāb al-Futūḥ first circulated through the cafés of Ḥusaynīyah, forcing the owners to open and serve them, after which they were joined at their camp by an assortment of female dancers and prostitutes (al-Jabartī 1888–1896, volume 9: 102–103; 1904, volume 4: 227–228).

Besides these spaces, another residential area for professional entertainers existed in Cairo: as noted earlier, female dancers had established a settlement near Rumaylah Square. Multiple sources describe a quarter for entertainers called Ḥūsh Bardaq, located just southwest of the Sultan Ḥassan mosque (Figure 16). The word *ḥūsh* describes a group of modest dwellings surrounding a common courtyard; Ḥūsh Bardaq began as a squatters' encampment established in the ruins of a Mamluk-era palace. John Lewis Burckhardt (1830: 148), writing of Ḥūsh Bardaq in the early nineteenth century, describes it as a settlement of *ghawāzī*: "At Cairo itself their number is but small; they live all together in a large khan, called Hosh Bardak, just below the castle." The *ḥūsh* was noted on the map of Cairo created during the French occupation (see Jomard 1829: 141).

A number of other locations recorded by the French bore names that are suggestive of associations with professional entertainers, and their location near documented entertainment and leisure spaces is telling. For example, a street called Darb Ḥūsh al-Khawal (the Lane of the *Khawal*'s

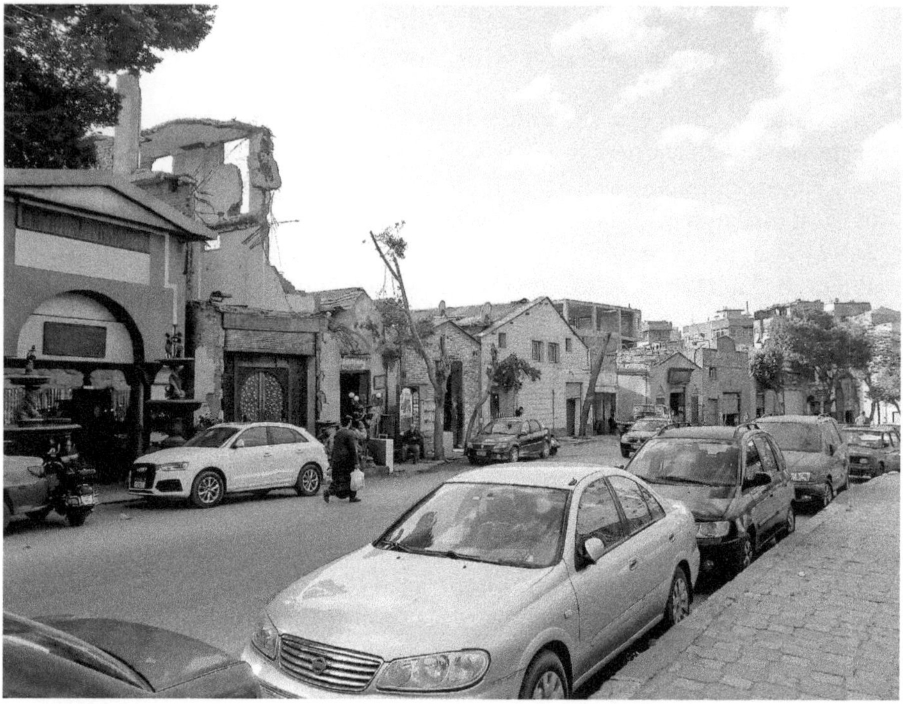

Figure 16: Former location of Ḥūsh Bardaq (photo taken by the author in 2022).

Courtyard) existed just to the south of Rumaylah Square (Jomard 1829: 154). Similarly, a street named Darb al-Bahlawān (The Acrobat's Lane) was situated to the southwest of the Birkat al-Fīl (*ibid.*, 178). Unfortunately, there is currently insufficient evidence to confirm whether these were neighborhoods of professional entertainers.

Unsurprisingly, the residential spaces described above were situated in close proximity to significant public spaces within Cairo's entertainment landscape. The neighborhood of Ḥusaynīyah was adjacent to the Bāb al-Naṣr cemetery, and a short distance from Ārḍ al-Ṭabbālah and the Birkat al-Raṭlī. The Bāb al-Lūq neighborhood, south of the Birkat al-Azbakīyah, was located at the heart of Cairo's western suburbs. From Bāb al-Lūq, it was just a short walk eastward, across the Khalīj by way of the Bāb al-Kharq bridge, to reach the musical instrument market. Ḥūsh Bardaq was adjacent to both Rumaylah Square and al-Qarāfah.

Coffee Houses

Coffee was introduced to Egypt under the Ottomans, leading to the emergence of a new type of space associated with entertainment and leisure: the coffee house (Figure 17). Coffee houses were widespread in Ottoman Cairo. By the end of the sixteenth century, there were several hundred of these establishments in Cairo; at the time of the occupation, the French documented well over one thousand (Behrens-Abouseif 1985: 44).

The coffee house was a space of gathering and socialization for local men. Muṣṭafā 'Alī indicates that "early rising worshippers and pious men" visited the coffee house early in the morning, sipping a cup of coffee in order to fortify themselves for their religious observances—a practice he found admirable (Tietze 1975: 37). On the other hand, many men lingered at coffee houses for hours, which Muṣṭafā 'Alī was quick to criticize.

Also distasteful to Muṣṭafā 'Alī was the presence of popular entertainers in Cairo's many coffee houses (Tietze 1975: 38). Indeed, it appears that it was commonplace for storytellers, singers, and musicians to gather at coffee houses to entertain the customers (Niebuhr 1792: 126). Describing three popular coffee houses at the Qanṭarat al-Mūskī, Evliya Çelebi writes:

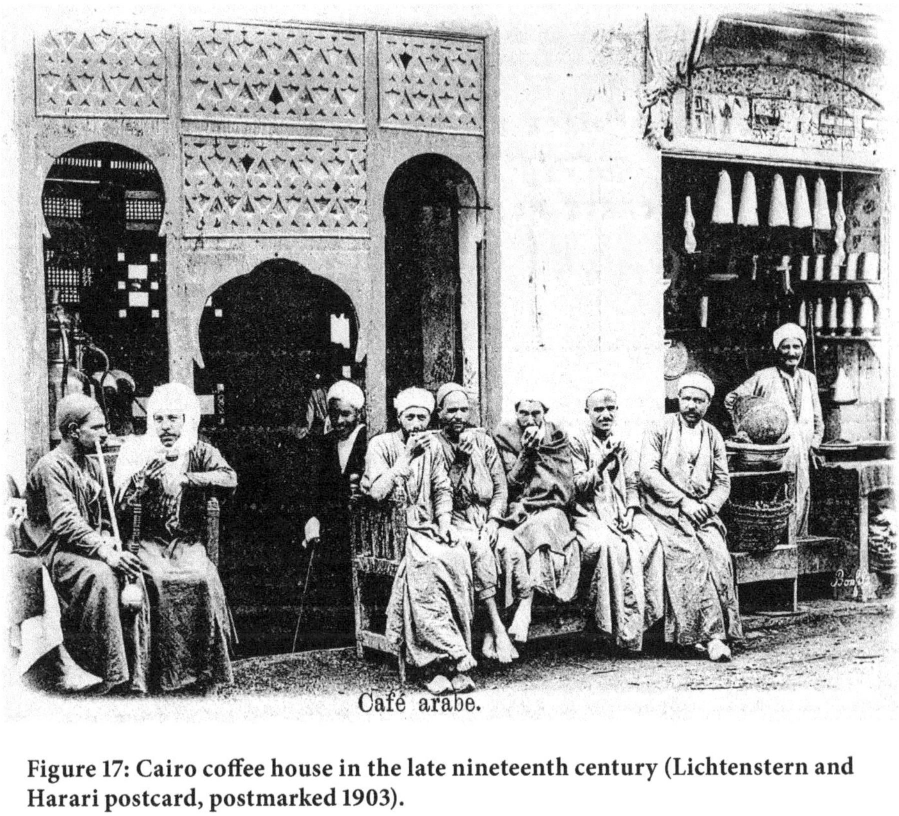

Figure 17: Cairo coffee house in the late nineteenth century (Lichtenstern and Harari postcard, postmarked 1903).

> And because this bridge is really so airy and pleasant, everything that has rank and name in musicology comes together in these coffee houses. There are merry goings-on from morning to evening, and the lively discussion never stops [Prokosch 2000: 208–209].

Coffee houses were common in the entertainment zones of Ottoman Cairo. In addition to the establishments at Qanṭarat al-Mūskī just described, Evliya Çelebi observed a number of coffee houses at and sometimes on the various bridges crossing the Khalīj (Prokosch 2000: 208–209). Coffee houses were also widespread in Bāb al-Lūq (Prokosch 2000: 41).

In his 2007 examination of Ottoman-era coffee houses in Istanbul, Cairo, and Aleppo, Alan Mikhail notes that the complexities of coffee house culture challenge traditional assumptions about urban geography in the Ottoman period. That is, coffee houses cannot be accommodated by simple binaries like public/private or male/female. Mikhail (2007: 135–136) points out that coffee houses were fluid environments with multiple overlapping functions: "Ottoman cafés were at differing moments domestic spaces, places of business and leisure, an extension of the street or market, a venue of entertainment, a space of courtship, an arena of communication, a place in which to read and a realm of distraction." Notably, he turns to Foucault's concept of heterotopia to capture the complicated reality of the coffee house:

> In [Foucault's] own words, heterotopias "have the curious property of being in relation with all the other sites, but in such a way as to suspect, neutralize, or invert the set of relations that they happen to designate, mirror, or reflect." Ottoman coffee houses did just this as spaces with connections to the neighbourhood, home and market that made them at once familiar but contemporaneously novel in the way that men could gather within them as spaces of layered functionality and a multitude of ambiences [Mikhail 2007: 137].

I would add to Mikhail's observations that the frequent presence of popular entertainers in these spaces contributed to their "otherness" and to the multiplicity of meanings and functions that they embodied. The inherent ambivalence of these spaces, together with (and related to) the ongoing presence of popular entertainment and its professional practitioners, tied coffee houses to the broader landscape of entertainment in Ottoman Cairo.

Professional Entertainers and the Continuity of Meanings in Cairo's Public Entertainment Spaces

At the outset of the Ottoman period, Cairo's suburbs and cemeteries were firmly established as heterotopic spaces within the landscape.

These were spaces characterized by their carnivalistic mésalliances: disparate groups converged and interfaced, and Egyptians engaged in behaviors and activities that defied or disrupted the social order. In these spaces "outside of all places," normal social and spatial boundaries were blurred, challenged, or subverted.

Throughout the Ottoman era, these heterotopic features of Cairo's entertainment landscape were reified and reinforced. The western suburbs, with Azbakīyah as the focal point, continued to attract individuals from vastly different sectors of Egyptian society—rich and poor, Muslim and Christian, native and foreigner, man and woman—to enjoy their pleasures. Cairo's shines and cemeteries continued to draw a diverse array of visitors into a space where the boundary between sacred and secular was blurred and broken, and where transgressive activities and behaviors were the norm. In these locales, professional entertainers, including professional dancers, found spaces that could accommodate their marginality. Their presence, in turn, reinforced and reified the heterotopic nature of the spaces where they lived and worked.

The presence of professional entertainers was key to the inscription and re-inscription of heterotopic meaning into Cairo's entertainment landscape. A good illustration of this comes, oddly enough, from al-Jabartī's obituary for the Ottoman-era *amīr* Qāsim Bik Abū Sayf, who died in 1802 (al-Jabartī 1888–1896, volume 7: 103–105; 1904, volume 3: 230–231). Qāsim Bik constructed a grand dwelling for himself in Nāṣirīyah, which took its name from a Mamluk-era pond. Nāṣirīyah was situated in the suburbs, well to the south of Bāb al-Lūq and due west of the Birkat al-Fīl. Opposite his fine mansion, Qāsim Bik established a magnificent garden. The garden was laid out in the manner of agricultural fields: these were planted with a variety of crops and irrigated by a complex system of conduits and canals. The garden could be traversed by means of a number of well-maintained paths, and trees planted along the paths and canals provided shade and added to the beauty of the setting. Qāsim Bik opened his garden to the public, and for the convenience of visitors, he provided water jugs, benches, chairs, and even latrines. Coffee houses opened within the garden as well. Qāsim Bik's garden became a popular meeting place for Egyptians from all levels of society, and soon it began to attract singers, musicians, and "loose women" (al-Jabartī uses the term *ghawānī*). Notably, according to al-Jabartī, the garden then became a place of debauchery and vice, to the point that respectable people refused to enter.

The account of al-Jabartī's is more than a little suggestive that the presence of popular entertainers contributed to the atmosphere of moral ambiguity into which the garden descended. This heterotopic space was short-lived, however: the French invaders commandeered Qāsim Bik's properties, and the Nāṣirīyah mansion and gardens became the headquarters for the Institut d'Egypte (al-Jabartī 2006: 109). Still, Qāsim Bik's garden demonstrates how a publicly-accessible leisure space was fundamentally transformed as Egyptians of various social classes converged in the same locale alongside popular entertainers. While the garden of Qāsim Bik did not remain as a public space of entertainment, other spaces—such as Azbakīyah—continued in this role, and the embeddedness of professional entertainers in those spaces enabled their heterotopic qualities to be re-inscribed over the course of many generations.

In the midst of all this continuity, some seeds for future change were sown. For centuries, the landscape to the west of Cairo's urban core had been associated in the popular imagination with entertainment, leisure and vice; from the Fatimid era onward, this area was defined by its heterotopic qualities. In the Ottoman era, this zone came to center on Azbakīyah. Already a focal point for popular gatherings, the relocation of important annual festivals such as the Mūlid al-Nabī to Azbakīyah served to increase its centrality in Cairene life. Developments in this area at the dawn of the nineteenth century further boosted Azbakīyah's importance. Over the course of the century, Azbakīyah began to eclipse other spaces in the entertainment landscape, such as Rumaylah Square, which would gradually diminish in relevance. In the mid- to late nineteenth century, the proliferation of formalized entertainment venues in and near Azbakīyah physically reinforced the association of this space with professional entertainment and destined Azbakīyah to overshadow other spaces in Cairo's entertainment landscape.

From French Conquest to Khedivial Dynasty

The invasion and ensuing occupation by Napoleon's forces at the turn of the nineteenth century dramatically affected the city of Cairo. However, as several scholars have noted, the majority of the administrative changes instituted by the French did not survive their departure in 1801 (Abu-Lughod 1971: 84–85, Raymond 2000: 291–292). In reality, the most profound impact of the occupation was that it laid the foundation for the more drastic transformations that were to take place under Muḥammad 'Alī and his descendants (Figure 18).

Napoleon established his headquarters at Azbakīyah, in the palace that the Mamluk *amīr* Alfī Bik had just completed on the western bank of the pond (Behrens-Abouseif 1985: 71, al-Jabartī 2006: 42). Behrens-Abouseif notes that this site was likely chosen for security

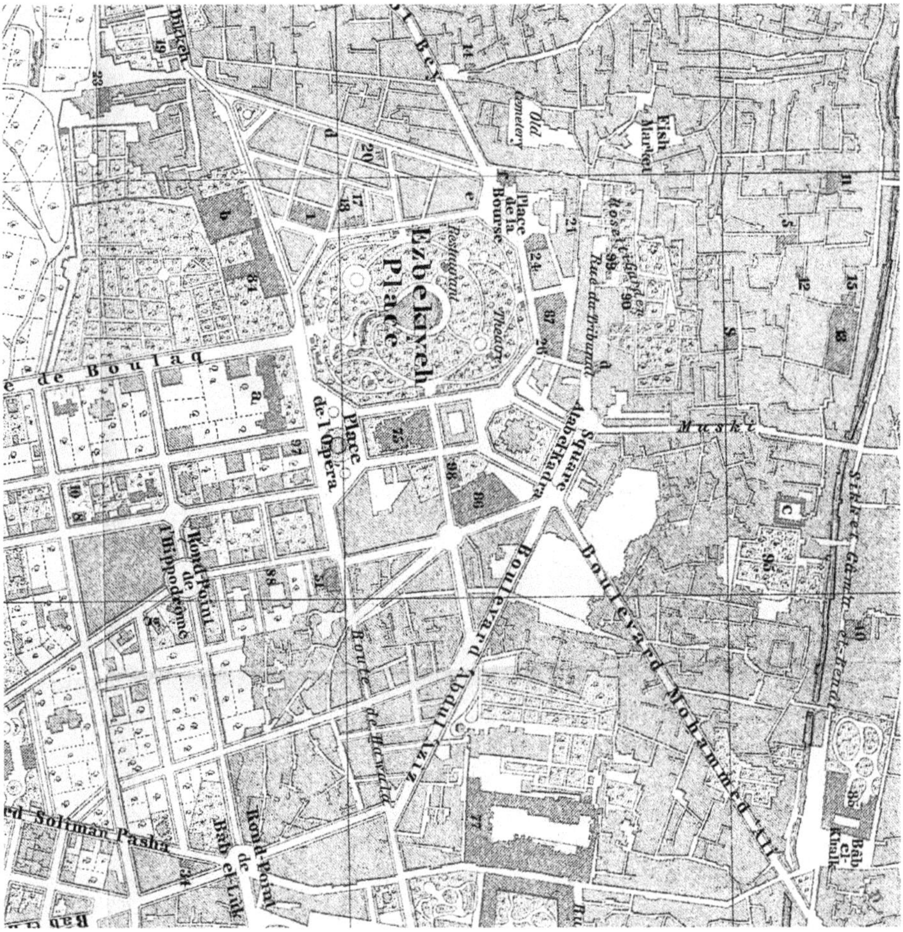

Figure 18: Detail from a map of late nineteenth century Cairo, after the construction of Muḥammad 'Alī Street, but before the completion of the northern leg of 'Imād al-Dīn Street (Wagner and Debes, 1885).

reasons: the location was remote from the urban core, yet offered easy access to the city from the north and the west, as well as to the port of Būlāq (1985: 71). Napoleon's decision to locate his command here contributed to the centrality of Azbakīyah in Cairo life.

Among the French projects that would have lasting impacts to the city of Cairo were the urban planning developments undertaken in and around the strategic headquarters at Azbakīyah. One such development was the creation of a number of large thoroughfares connecting Azbakīyah to different areas of the city (Behrens-Abouseif 1985: 74). Among these was a road connecting the area to the southeast of the Azbakīyah pond—then known as al-'Atabah al-Zarqā' (The Blue Threshold)—with the Qanṭarat al-Mūskī. This was the beginning of al-Mūskī Street.

Another noteworthy development was the establishment of European-style entertainment venues at Azbakīyah (Behrens-Abouseif 1985: 76–77, al-Jabartī 2006: 107, Sadgrove 1996: 27–31). Among these were cafés, restaurants, and taverns after the European fashion, and a Tivoli Égyptien modeled on its Parisian counterpart. At the Tivoli, situated to the east of the Azbakīyah pond and near the Ḥārat al-Afranj, the French enjoyed a wide range of amusements, including music, dancing, and games. Soon a theater was constructed, and for the first time, European-style theatrical productions were performed in Egypt. Entertainment venues of this sort would become increasingly commonplace in nineteenth-century Cairo.

Still, the overall impact of the French occupation was negligible when compared to the total transformation of Egypt that would take place under the dynasty of Muḥammad 'Alī. Muḥammad 'Alī arrived in Egypt with the Ottoman army, as the latter retook Egypt from the French. He was as a soldier of fortune, a lieutenant commander of a corps of Albanian mercenaries. The years following the expulsion of the French were tumultuous, with factions of the Ottoman army, as well as Mamluks, vying for power. Muḥammad 'Alī took advantage of the chaotic situation, maneuvering himself into a position of authority, and gaining the support of the local population, who longed for stability and security. In 1805, the Ottoman Porte, in a desire to restore order, elevated Muḥammad 'Alī to the rank of *bāshā* and appointed him *wālī* (governor) of Egypt.

Of necessity, Muḥammad 'Alī spent the first decade of his rule consolidating power (Abu-Lughod 1971: 85–87). In 1811, he organized the massacre of most of the remaining Mamluks. Only then could he turn his attention to the broader social, political, and economic reforms which would become his legacy. Among the most significant reforms undertaken by Muḥammad 'Alī were the confiscation and nationalization of agricultural lands, and the establishment of taxes on *waqf* deeds. These actions essentially gave the Egyptian government a monopoly on cultivable land and broke the power of the local elites. To maximize agricultural production, Muḥammad 'Alī ordered the reconstruction of Egypt's irrigation system of canals, and Egypt's rural peasantry was conscripted to complete this work.

Among the other substantial reforms were the establishment and training of a European-style bureaucracy and military. He sought out European expertise, both by importing European specialists in various fields and by sending Egyptians abroad to study. He also established European-modeled schools and factories, and imported European industrial technologies.

In the initial years of his reign, Cairo was not substantially impacted by Muḥammad ʿAlī's reform projects, with the exception of a reorganization of government administration and a restructuring of police and military forces in the city (Abu-Lughod 1971: 87). However, in the latter two decades of his rule, Muḥammad ʿAlī turned his attention to Cairo, and the result would be many significant morphological changes to the city. Many of the developments undertaken by Muḥammad ʿAlī in Cairo were rooted in hygienic and aesthetic concerns (Behrens-Abouseif 1985: 83–84). For example, large rubbish mounds that existed both within and without the city were leveled. The majority of Cairo's ponds were then filled in using the materials excavated from the rubbish heaps; they were believed to be a source of pestilence, particularly when the water levels fell. Among the ponds that disappeared was the great Birkat al-Azbakīyah. Wilkinson (1847: 115), describing Azbakīyah in the 1840s, writes:

> The entrance to Cairo from Booláḵ is by the gate of the Uzbeḵéëh, an extensive square, containing about 450,000 square feet; nearly the whole of which used to be, during the inundation, one large sheet of water. In the following spring it became a cornfield, with the exception of that part appropriated to a military esplanade. Within the last few years a canal has been cut round it, in order to keep the water from the centre, though from the lowness of its level much still oozes through to its surface, during the high Nile; and it has been laid out partly as a garden, and partly as fields, with trees planted on the banks of the canal that surrounds it. A broad road leads through the centre, from the entrance to the opposite side, passing over a bridge at either end; and it is in contemplation to establish a Turkish café on one side, and a European one on the other, for the convenience of the natives and the Franks.

Besides leveling the rubbish heaps and filling the ponds, cemeteries located within the city were razed, including a sizable cemetery located at the southeast corner of the Birkat al-Azbakīyah (El Kadi and Bonnamy 2007: 35).

Muḥammad ʿAlī was also concerned with improving circulation within the city. In 1845, a city plan (*tanẓīm*) was drafted: within the *tanẓīm*, two new thoroughfares were proposed (Abu-Lughod 1971: 95–97, Raymond 2000: 302–303). The first would extend al-Mūskī Street eastward to al-Azhar. The second would cut a path from Azbakīyah southeastward to the Citadel. The process of acquiring properties and demolishing buildings for these massive undertakings began in 1845, but these projects would only be fully realized under Muḥammad ʿAlī's grandson, Ismāʿīl.

The urban development projects of Ismāʿīl exceeded Muḥammad ʿAlī's vision and were to have a much more profound impact on the geography of the city. Ismāʿīl had ambitions for the transformation of Cairo even before his fateful visit to the Paris Exposition Universelle in 1867 (Abu-Lughod 1971: 103–104, Raymond 2000: 311–312). He organized a Ministry of Public Works to coordinate his urban planning efforts, and he made the first attempts toward the establishment of water and gas utilities in Cairo in 1865. Outside the city center, he completed the construction of the Ismā'īlīyah Canal, while simultaneously filling some of the smaller remaining canals. These canal projects were particularly significant, because they opened up the land that would be crucial to Ismā'īl's massive developments in the western suburbs.

In Paris, Ismā'īl was introduced to the contemporary urban planning projects of the Baron Haussmann. Indeed, Ismā'īl was received personally by Haussmann and was given extensive tours of the newly "Haussmannized" city. Abu-Lughod (1971: 105) notes:

> This was, of course, not his first visit to the French capital. As a young man he had attended the military academy of Saint Cyr and in 1854 had returned to that city on a mission for Sa'īd Pasha. These trips, however, predated the revolutionary changes introduced by Haussmann. That Ismā'īl was deeply impressed by the city's reconstruction is attested by reports in contemporary French journals. Thus, while his trip of 1867 cannot be credited with being Ismā'īl's first introduction to a European capital nor even with creating his interest in city development—which predated his trip—the visit did give Ismā'īl renewed inspiration and motivation, a fact that can be surmised from the events which directly followed it.

With the opening of the Suez Canal planned for November 1869, Cairo was set to play host to dignitaries from throughout the Western world. Ismā'īl resolved that they would be greeted by a city to rival any European capital; he returned from Paris determined to remake Cairo in the Haussmannian mode.

The period from 1867 to 1869 was a time of frenetic development. Realizing that neither the time nor the resources were available to transform the Fatimid city, Ismā'īl turned his attention to the western suburbs. A new city plan was developed based on the Haussmannian model: it consisted of a network of broad boulevards intersecting at a series of public squares. The new street system barely encroached upon the medieval city, with two notable exceptions. The eastward extension of al-Mūskī Street was finally completed; known as Sikkat al-Jadīdah (New Street), it cut a path from Azbakīyah to al-Azhar. The second, first envisioned by Muḥammad 'Alī, would become his namesake: Muḥammad 'Alī Street, finally completed in the early 1870s, sliced its way southeast from Azbakīyah to the Citadel.

Ismā'īl's engagement and eventual entanglement with Western powers ensured a steady influx of foreigners into Cairo. Though the western suburbs had already been host to some foreign residents (primarily Greeks, Italians, and French), from Ismāʿīl's reign onward, the population of foreigners in the zone west of the Khalīj increased steadily. Europeans were drawn to settle in this area because of the presence of an established European population, the availability of real estate, and the presence of familiar amenities and infrastructure. The French and the British became an increasingly wealthy and influential presence, particularly in the administrative and financial sectors. Besides the resident foreign population, the rise of mass tourism in the late nineteenth century brought a flood of visitors to the city. The increasing number of foreigners in the zone west of the Khalīj led to the creation of a range of foreign institutions in the area, including consulates, schools, hotels, and restaurants (Behrens-Abouseif 1985: 86). The famous Shepheard Hotel was established on the site of the Alfī Bik palace (Napoleon's former headquarters) in 1849 (Behrens-Abouseif 1985: 87).

Foreigners—particularly Europeans—who visited Cairo in the wake of Ismāʿīl's urban planning projects tended to describe Cairo as a "dual city" (see Ahmed 2005). The areas on either side of the Khalīj were contrasted according to neat binaries such as European/Oriental, Western/Eastern, and modern/traditional. The "old" city east of the Khalīj was portrayed as a timeless and pristine relic of a more primitive era, in direct contrast with the progressive and forward-looking "new" city. Travel guide books encouraged visitors to hasten through the new "European" city in order to experience the true "Oriental" city: "It need hardly be added that the traveller in search of Oriental scenes will not care to devote much time to this modern and almost entirely European quarter, but will hasten to make acquaintance with the Arabian parts of the city" (Baedeker 1878: 257).

Those same guide books were quick to outline the range of European-style amenities available in the "European" quarter. The "new" city provided a convenient and comfortable staging point for excursions into the "old" city, allowing foreign visitors to Cairo to experience the latter in much the same manner as visiting a museum in London or Paris. After a visit to the "museum," visitors found reprieve in the familiar comforts provided by the European-style hotels, restaurants, and entertainment venues located to the west of the canal.

The narrative of the "dual city" has persisted into the modern era: both Raymond (2000) and Abu-Lughod (1971) describe the city post–Ismāʿīl as two Cairos—one ancient and traditional, one progressive and modern—existing side by side. Behrens-Abouseif (1985: 99) writes: "A new city was growing parallel to historic Cairo, and the Mūskī bridge was only a thin connection between the two worlds." There were certainly important distinctions between the areas to the east and the west of the Khalīj. Following Ismā'īl's developments, the western zone became host to a foreign presence that was much more substantial and increasingly more influential than in previous eras. The population of foreigners as well as indigenous elites in this zone made it the epicenter of power, wealth, and business activity in Cairo: the undisputed downtown of the turn-of-the-century city. The Egyptian government, from Ismā'īl onward, poured resources into the "new" city and increasingly neglected the "old." Raymond (2000: 334) writes that "its streets were neglected, cleaning was haphazard, water supply was only partial, and the sewers were poor or insufficient."

However, recent scholarship has challenged the discourse of the "dual city" (see Alsayyad et al. 2005, Hanna 2002). As Heba Farouk Ahmed writes (2005: 167): "Giving the city a facelift and developing new quarters to reflect a new age did not mean giving it a new identity." Though real differences existed between the two areas, defining Ismā'īl's "modern" development strictly in opposition to the city's "medieval" core ignores the pre-existing relationship between these two areas of the city, a relationship that had developed over the course of centuries. In short, the "dual city" discourse ignores the continuity of meanings in Cairo's "new" downtown. Ismā'īl's downtown was constructed in what had been the city's western suburbs, a zone that had long been characterized by its social and economic heterogeneity. As amply demonstrated in the last chapter, the area to the west of the Khalīj was a space of confluence between radically diverse populations. In spite of the seeming "Europeanness" of this area in the late nineteenth century, it continued to be a zone of heterogeneity: the dominance of Europeans in the area—both in terms of population and in terms of wealth—should not obscure the ongoing presence of Egyptians of all social classes in this zone (see Hanna 2002). Moreover, the long historical association of this area with entertainment, leisure, and vice continued, as will be discussed below. The urban development projects of Ismā'īl did not erase the meanings that had been deeply inscribed into certain Cairene spaces.

The Spaces of Entertainment in the Khedivial City

Without question, the developments undertaken by Muḥammad 'Alī and Ismā'īl profoundly impacted Cairo's entertainment landscape. Perhaps the most dramatic transformation was the disappearance of most of the city's canals and ponds in the 1830s. These features had been integral to the social and spatial reality of Cairo's inhabitants for centuries, and suddenly they were no more. Though the celebration of the Nile flood continued to be observed (Didier 1860: 238), the disappearance of the ponds that had once figured so prominently in the festivities—most notably, the Birkat al-Azbakīyah—meant that the celebrations came to be largely confined to the banks of the Nile and the Khalīj.

Yet, what is perhaps more remarkable than the disappearance of these geographic features is that the spaces they occupied in the Cairo landscape continued to be firmly associated with recreation and entertainment. More importantly, these spaces remained "outside of all places" in the Cairo landscape: their heterotopic qualities persisted, in spite of all the change. These meanings had been so deeply inscribed into these locales that even the physical modification of the landscape could not erase them. Indeed, these meanings would endure even after Ismā'īl's Haussmannization of the western suburbs, and by the beginning of the British occupation, Azbakīyah was their hub.

Cairo's main cemeteries—al-Qarāfah al-Kubrā, Bāb al-Naṣr, and the eastern Mamluk cemetery—were, at least in morphological terms, initially unaffected by the urban transformations instituted by Muḥammad 'Alī and Ismā'īl. Shrine and cemetery visitation continued throughout the nineteenth century as it had for centuries prior. Notably, the construction of Ismā'īl's boulevards led to the destruction of numerous structures within the city core, and some of the displaced residents settled in the cemeteries.

Indeed, the broad boulevards known as Sikkat al-Jadīdah and Muḥammad 'Alī Street created knife-like incisions into the fabric of the Fatimid city. Yet, even in these transformed spaces there was a persistence of meaning. The construction of Muḥammad 'Alī Street was completed in the early 1870s, and this broad boulevard quickly became the focal point of the business of professional entertainment in Cairo. By the dawn of the twentieth century, this street was home both to professional entertainers as well as to businesses associated with entertainment, such as musical instrument manufacturers and sellers. Yet, as discussed in the last chapter, a market for musical instruments existed in this part of the city long before the construction of this street. It is likely that the pre-existing associations of nearby neighborhoods with entertainment, combined with the street's easy proximity Azbakīyah, provided a strong draw for people in the entertainment trades.

Within the entertainment zones of nineteenth-century Cairo, certain venues associated with entertainment and leisure abounded. Coffee houses, introduced in the Ottoman era, were commonplace. As noted earlier, these establishments were important spaces for socialization and leisure for local men. In addition, these were spaces where professional entertainers gathered and interacted with their clientele. Besides coffee houses, however, the nineteenth century witnessed the emergence of a variety of new venues specifically dedicated to entertainment and leisure: theaters, music halls, and *cafés chantants*. For convenience, I will periodically refer to these venues collectively as entertainment halls. Importantly, most of Cairo's entertainment halls were located in the zone west of the Khalīj: specifically, in Azbakīyah and vicinity. These venues would be the scene for profound changes in Egyptian traditional entertainment—including belly dance—at the turn of the nineteenth and twentieth centuries.

The Ascendance of Azbakīyah

The centrality of Azbakīyah in Cairo life was well established by the time that Muḥammad 'Alī decided to drain the pond and commission a park on the site. At the outset of the Ottoman era, Azbakīyah was a regular gathering place for Cairo's common people, as well as a central location for the celebration of popular festivals. Even after the transformation of the space, Azbakīyah continued in this role (Wilkinson 1847: 116). With the continued growth of Būlāq and Shubrā, it also functioned as an important thoroughfare between the urban core and the developing suburbs. Additionally, the Cairo terminus of the Cairo-Alexandria railway, constructed in the early 1850s, was located just to the northwest at Bāb al-Ḥadīd. In short, Azbakīyah was a focal point of life in Cairo in the early-to-mid nineteenth century.

Charles Didier (1860: 9–10) describes the scene in the early 1850s, prior to the completion of the railway:

> The Esbékieh is a continual passage of donkeys, camels, pedestrians and horsemen, without counting the carriages; because it is by there that one goes on one side to Boulak by the gate of Elfi, on the other to Choubrah by the new Bab-el-Hadid gate. The Esbékieh is, moreover, haunted by buffoons and entertainers who amuse the people with their tricks and their jokes.... Furthermore, there are quite a large number of cafés established in the shade of the sycamore trees, and where the Arabs come to drink their favorite beverage, smoke and play dominoes, a European innovation which was then all the rage in Cairo. One of these cafés, more fashionable than the others, was frequented in the evening by one of those storytellers of whom I shall speak later and who always gathered around him a large audience.

Until Ismā'īl's developments in the latter half of the nineteenth century, Azbakīyah continued to be the central site for Cairo's annual Mūlid al–Nabī celebrations, and the jarring intersection of sacred and secular activities during this event caused Didier (1860: 353) to remark:

> The profane and the sacred were mixed together in such a straightforward way that it ceased to be shocking. Here stood a vast blue tent where litanies were sung and prayers chanted, and beside it the magic lantern, Kara-Gueuz, delighted the crowd with fabulous obscenities; there howling dervishes uttered their holy barks in unison, and quite near the Arab Polichinelle spouted his bawdy *lazzi* to onlookers, for the theater of Guignol is not the exclusive privilege of the Champs-Élysées. The Orientals, whom one imagines in Europe to be so serious, so grave, have pushed back the limits of indecency.

As Didier's accounts illustrate, popular entertainers were a common sight in Azbakīyah. However, beginning with Muḥammad 'Alī's proscription in the 1830s, "public women"—female professional dancers and female prostitutes—largely disappeared from public view. Contemporary observers note the conspicuous absence of the *ghawāzī* at festivals such as the Mūlid al-Nabī, where the female dancers had previously been one of the most popular attractions: "The Ghawázee have lately been compelled to vow repentance, and to relinquish their profession of dancing, etc.; consequently there are now none of them at the festival [Mūlid al-Nabī of 1834]. These girls used to be among the most attractive of all the performers" (Lane [2005 (1836): 437]).

In spite of government restrictions, it is quite clear that both female dancers and prostitutes continued to ply their trades in secret, and it appears that many lived and worked in the vicinity of Azbakīyah. Didier indicates that clandestine brothels existed at mid-century in the Coptic quarter (north of Azbakīyah) and the Frankish quarter (east of Azbakīyah); his account implies that Bāb al-Lūq was no longer a center for prostitutes (Didier 1860: 330). Similarly, Didier's lengthy account of an encounter with a dancer named Ghazāl makes it clear that female professional dancers continued to operate in the area in secret (Didier 1860: 331–341). After their initial meeting on the road to Qaṣr al-'Aynī, Didier followed Ghazāl to a house in the Coptic quarter north of Azbakīyah, where they arranged a performance that, due to her fear of the authorities, was to take place at night on a boat on the Nile. Sadly for Ghazāl, she was arrested before the performance could take place, flogged, and deported to Upper Egypt.

Male dancers were unaffected by Muḥammad 'Alī's action against female dancers and prostitutes, and numerous foreigners remarked upon their popularity (Clot-Bey 1840: 94–95; Lane 1860: 381–382; Lane 2005 [1836]: 376–377; Lane-Poole 1846: 65–66, 71–72). Indeed, Clot-Bey suggests that the popularity of the *khawalāt* and the *jink* increased in the wake of the ban on public performances by female dancers. These dancing men were ubiquitous at popular festivals, and they appear to have been commonplace in the coffee houses of Azbakīyah (Kennard 1855: 125, Nerval 1884: 87–89).

Azbakīyah was further transformed under Ismāʿīl, but its centrality in Cairene life and its long association with entertainment, recreation, and vice would persist. Azbakīyah became the hub of Ismāʿīl's grand urban development projects, with several of his new broad boulevards radiating from the Azbakīyah Gardens. The Gardens themselves were redesigned between 1868 and 1872: Ismāʿīl employed the French landscape architect Jean-Pierre Barillet-Deschamps to design a lush setting styled after the public parks and pleasure gardens of Britain and France. The new gardens were much smaller than their predecessor—Ismāʿīl sold a substantial portion of the old park in order to capitalize on European demand for real estate in the area (Behrens-Abouseif 1985: 92)—and were encircled by a gate.

Simultaneously, Ismāʿīl established a variety of government-controlled entertainment venues near the Gardens (Mestyan 2017: 99, Sadgrove 1996: 45–66). A French-style variety theater (Théâtre de la Comédie), a grand Italian-style opera house (Théâtre Khédivial de l'Opéra), and a circus (the Cirque Rancy) were all inaugurated in 1869. A hippodrome and the Azbakīyah Garden Theater opened the following year. The circus, the hippodrome, and the French theater were short lived (demolished in 1872, 1881, and 1887, respectively); the opera house and the Azbakīyah Garden Theater would remain part of the Azbakīyah landscape for many decades to come. Toward the end of the century, a number of privately-own entertainment halls began to emerge in the vicinity of the Gardens as well.

All of these developments continued to position Azbakīyah centrally in the lived experience of Cairenes and to reaffirm the area's association with professional entertainment. Popular entertainers continued to ply their trades in the area, though governmental restrictions on female dancers and prostitutes persisted. Foreign visitors in the 1860s and 1870s remarked on the ongoing regulation of "public women" (see, for example, Blanc 1876: 137, Knox 1879: 509, Leland 1873: 130–131). Leland, who visited Cairo in the early 1870s, observes:

> The dancing-girls are obliged by law to remain at one or two places on the Nile. Formerly they strayed through the streets of Cairo and other towns, and a resident assured me that he had seen them perform on the verandah before Shepheard's Hotel. The result of the moral restriction has been to confine familiarity with their feats to the wealthy, since it is still the fashion for the well-to-do, when they give "fantasias" in their houses, to send for Ghawâzi, who are invariably procured from somewhere [Leland 1873: 130–131].

At the same time, Leland notes that female singers performed at a *café chantant* within the Azbakīyah Gardens:

> I had not been many nights in Cairo before I went with a friend to the Arab *café chantant*, in the Esbekiah Gardens, where, as I was told, good singing could be heard. There was a kiosk or round place for musicians, such as is usual in Europe, but it was jealously shut in with thin curtains, behind which the 'Awalim were singing [Leland 1873: 128].

This same venue was documented by Charles Dudley Warner, also in the 1870s:

> There is a *café chantant* on one side of the open, tree-grown court of a native hotel, in the Ezbekeeh where one may hear a mongrel music, that is not inexpressive of both the morals and the mixed condition of Cairo to-day. The instruments of the band are European; the tunes played are Egyptian. When the first strain is heard we say that it is strangely wild, a weird and plaintive minor; but that is the whole of it. The strain is repeated over and over again for a half hour, as if it were ground out of a coffee-mill, in an iteration sufficient to drive the listener insane, the dissolute scraping and thumping and barbarous dissonance never changing nor ending.
>
> From time to time this is varied with singing, of the nasal, fine-tooth-comb order, with the most extraordinary attempts at shakes and trills, and with all the agony of a moonlit cat on a house-top. All this the grave Arabs and young Egyptian rakes, who sit smoking, accept with entire satisfaction. Later in the evening dancing begins and goes on with the strumming, monotonous music till at least the call for morning prayer [Warner 1900: 101–102].

Warner's account suggests that dancers performed in this café as well, and additional accounts from the period confirm this. For example, the observations of Belgian botanist Gustave Delchevalerie regarding the various activities and amenities at the Azbakīyah Gardens were recorded in contemporary horticultural periodicals:

> A European restaurant is open there in a chalet surrounded by halls of greenery, as well as a European café chantant where small troupes of French or Italian operettas are heard in the summer in the evening, while the Tam-Tam and the Almées resound and dance in the Arabic café chantant [Linden 1884: 52, see also Morren 1881: 365].

The appearance of female professional entertainers in a venue like this as early as the 1870s is significant. As will be discussed below, the proliferation of *cafés chantants*, theaters, and music halls in Azbakīyah and vicinity in the late nineteenth century signaled the start of an era of profound change in Egyptian traditional entertainment. These entertainment halls represented a new way for Egyptians to experience familiar entertainments like music, song, and dance: not in the traditional social contexts of weddings, festivals, and the like, but in structures that existed solely for the display of professional entertainment. These venues enabled female dancers to continue to ply their trades in spite of heavy regulation, and maintained the presence of these marginal figures in the Azbakīyah landscape.

Indeed, the creation of these structures lent a new physicality to the meanings that had long pervaded this landscape. It was as if an inscription that was previously drawn in ink was now engraved in stone. In the second half of the nineteenth century, the rise of these formalized entertainment venues in and around Azbakīyah tangibly reified and reinforced the association of this space with professional entertainment. Over time, the proliferation of entertainment halls in this zone ensured that Azbakīyah and vicinity would eventually eclipse other spaces in Cairo's entertainment landscape.

Rumaylah

In the early nineteenth century, Rumaylah Square continued to function as a staging point for state ceremonials, such as the *maḥmal* processions, which are described in detail by Edward Lane (2005 [1836]: 432–436, 478–481). Notably, in his description of the *maḥmal* procession accompanying the departure of the pilgrims' caravan to Mecca, he writes: "As this procession is conducted with less pomp in almost every successive year, I shall describe it as I first witnessed it, during my former visit to Egypt [in the 1820s]" (Edward Lane [2005 (1836): 478]). Lane's statement here suggests the *maḥmal* processions were already in decline prior to mid-century. With the opening of the Suez Canal in 1869, pilgrims were able to travel to Mecca by steamship; consequently, the annual overland pilgrim caravan and the associated parading of the *maḥmal* further declined. However, as Egypt continued to supply the Kiswah, the ceremonial cover for the Ka'bah in Mecca, *maḥmal* processions continued into the first half of the twentieth century, though the processions were no longer associated with Rumaylah Square (see McPherson 1941: 264, 323–324).

Rumaylah Square remained an important gathering place for Cairo's common people throughout much of the nineteenth century. The fair-like atmosphere described by the French during Napoleon's occupation persisted into mid-century. Michaud (1833–1835, vol. 5: 249) writes: "On the square of Roumeyleh, located at the base of the citadel and near the mosque of Hassan, a fair is held every day to which jugglers and entertainers of all kinds come; they have monkeys, bears, and other animals trained in tricks." Several decades after Michaud, a settlement of professional entertainers still existed at Ḥūsh Bardaq (Newbold 1856: 292, Von Kremer 1864: 264).

Still, by the close of the century, mentions of Rumaylah Square and its "perpetual fair" become less frequent in contemporary sources, suggesting the declining relevance of the square, at least within the landscape of entertainment. Undoubtedly, the completion of the grand new ʿĀbdīn Palace in 1874 (Abu-Lughod 1971: 113, Raymond 2000: 316), and the subsequent relocation of the administrative center there, contributed to Rumaylah's decline as one of Cairo's main public squares. The waning popularity of the *maḥmal* processions was likely a factor as well. Perhaps most important of all, however, was the massive gravitational pull of Azbakīyah, which by the end of the nineteenth century was at the core of Cairo's entertainment landscape.

Shrines and Cemeteries

The practice of shrine and cemetery visitation was abundantly documented by foreign visitors throughout the nineteenth century (Figure 19). As in prior centuries, weekly *ziyārah* was popular, particularly among Cairene women. In addition, Cairo's shrines and cemeteries were alive with activity during festivals.

The two primary Muslim feast days, Īd al-'Aḍḥā and Īd al-Fiṭr, were occasions for massive public gatherings at the cemeteries. As they had in past generations, these celebrations provided the usual mix of sacred and secular activities. Multiple observers describe the scene at the Bāb al-Naṣr cemetery. Edward Lane (2005 [1836]: 475) writes:

> The great cemetery of Báb en-Nasr, in the desert tract immediately on the north of the metropolis, presents a remarkable scene on the two 'eeds. In a part next the city gate from which the burial-ground takes its name many swings and whirligigs are erected, and several large tents, in some of which dancers, reciters of Aboo-Zeyd, and other performers, amuse a dense crowd of spectators; and throughout the burial-ground are seen numerous tents for the reception of the visitors of the tombs.

Joseph François Michaud observed the celebration of ʿĪd al-Fiṭr in 1831. Desiring to witness the popular celebrations, he made his way through the crowded streets, and after passing through the Bāb al-Futūḥ:

> ... we found outside the walls a great multitude of people which were devoted to all kinds of amusements; almées danced under tents filled with spectators; the ring game, the swing amused the crowd; at each step one met a paladin surrounded by an attentive troop; curious people, mounted on camels, circulated peacefully in the midst of all these spectacles, and seemed to be in the front row to see everything [Michaud 1833–1835, vol. 5: 253].

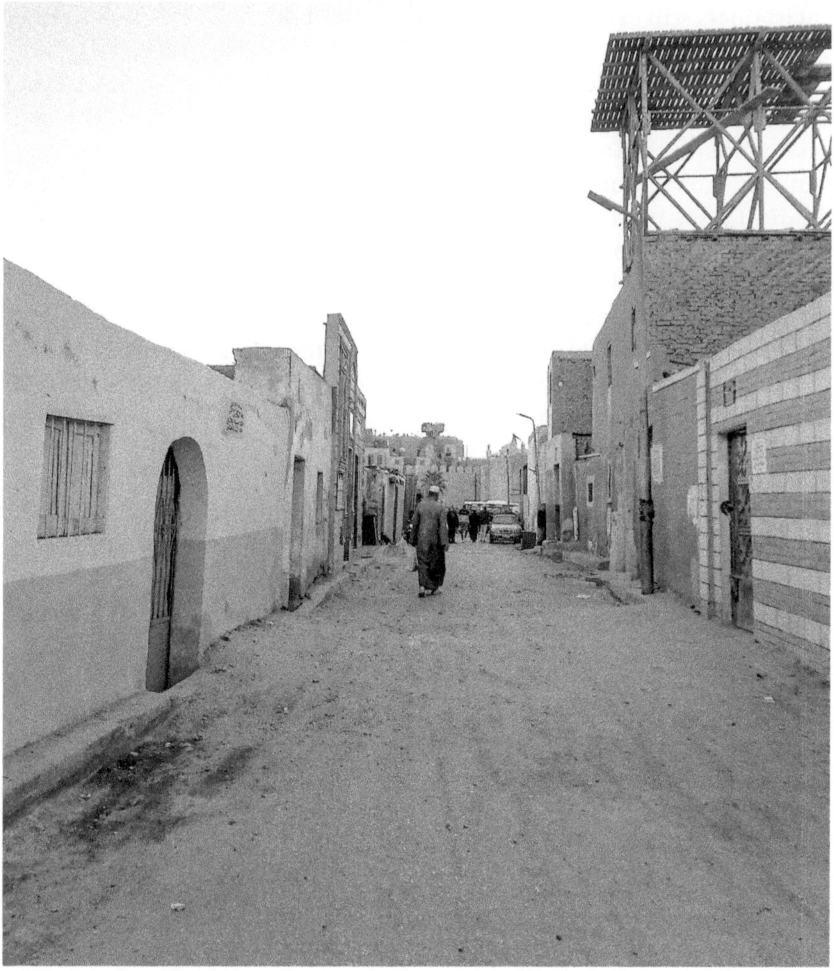

Figure 19: Cemetery of Bāb al-Naṣr (photo taken by the author in 2022).

Eventually, while caught up in the crowd, Michaud encountered groups of women and children picnicking: he failed to realize that he had wandered into the cemetery:

> The women who had gathered in this way were celebrating the festival of Beyram; there was as much joy among the tombs as in the liveliest quarters of the city, for all these women were convinced that the dead rejoiced with them, and that they took part in all the pleasures of the feast [Michaud 1833–1835, vol. 5: 253–254].

Echoing earlier accounts, Michaud goes on to suggest that the cemetery was a site for rendezvous:

> Before leaving this field of the dead, we saw magnificent tents erected among the tombs; many women spend the three days of the Beyram under these tents; amorous rendezvous take place there, and places consecrated to the mourning of death sometimes become a veritable place of prostitution. I dare not repeat to you all that the scandalous chronicle says on this subject, and what the two angels of the sepulcher, Nadir and Moukir, saw [Michaud 1833–1835, vol. 5: 253–254].

Beyond the two Īd celebrations, a variety of other festivals drew crowds to the shrines and cemeteries. The *mūlid* of Sayyidah Zaynab attracted revelers to her shrine, where they could participate in both sacred and secular aspects of the festival. Lane, describing the *mūlid* in the 1820s, writes: "In a street near the mosque I saw several reciters of the Aboo-Zeyd, Háwees, Kureydátees, and Dancers, and a few swings and whirligigs" (Lane 2005 [1836]: 461). Similarly, the festival of 'Āshūrā' on the tenth day of Muḥarram, due to its association with the martyrdom of Ḥusayn, drew crowds to the area around Ḥusayn's shrine. Lane describes gatherings of *ghawāzī* near the mosque during 'Āshūrā' in the late 1820s:

> The avenue to this mosque [Ḥusayn], near the Kádee's court, were thronged with passengers, and in them I saw several groups of dancing-girls (Gházeeyehs), some dancing and others sitting in a ring in the public thoroughfare, eating their dinner, and (with the exclamation of "Bi-smi-llah!") inviting each well-dressed man who passed by to eat with them ... so it is that on the occasion of all the great religious festivals in Cairo, and at many other towns in Egypt, these female warriors against modesty (not always seductive, I must confess) are sure to be seen [Lane 2005 (1836): 423–424].

After public performances by female professional entertainers were banned, male entertainers could still be seen at the festivals. Lane describes male dancers at the *mūlid* of Ḥusayn in 1834:

> The nearer I approached the building, the more crowded did I find the streets. In one place were musicians; before a large coffee-shop were two Greek dancing-boys, or "gink," elegant but effeminate in appearance, with flowing hair, performing to the accompaniment of mandolins played by two of their countrymen, and a crowd of admiring Turks, with a few Egyptians, surrounding them. They performed there also the evening before, and, I was told, became so impudent from the patronage they received as to make an open seizure of a basket of grapes in the street [Lane 2005 (1836): 453].

Throughout the nineteenth century, Cairo's shrines and cemeteries remained integral to Cairo's landscape of entertainment. Diverse populations converged in these heterotopic spaces, where they engaged in transgressive activities and behaviors. Yet, beginning in the late nineteenth century, certain factors signaled imminent changes to the function and the significance of these spaces. First, the Comité de Conservation des

Monuments de l'Art Arabe, a governmental body established in 1881 for the purpose of safeguarding Islamic and Coptic monuments in Cairo, was increasingly intolerant of cultic activities such as shrine visitation within the cemeteries (al-Ibrashy 2005). The Comité's activities were focused on architectural preservation based strictly on historic and artistic merit, the latter defined according to the interests of the Western tourist consumer. Accordingly, the Comité was frequently at odds with the local inhabitants, visitors, and supporters of the shrines.

Second, although the cemeteries had always been host to a modest residential population (most notably, the caretakers and guardians of tombs and shrines), the twentieth century would bring a massive influx of new residents into the cemeteries (El Kadi and Bonnamy 2007: 257). Along with this new population came infrastructural changes, such as the extension of Cairo's public transportation system (at least partially) into the cemeteries. As a result, the cemeteries took on an increasingly residential character. Though weekly *ziyārah* and popular festivals continued to take place at Cairo's shrines and cemeteries, the significance of these spaces in the landscape of entertainment was destined to be eclipsed by Azbakīyah, where formalized venues dedicated to professional entertainment proliferated by the dawn of the twentieth century.

Spaces of Residence and Commerce in the Entertainment Landscape

Primary sources from as early as the Mamluk era have provided glimpses into the spaces where Cairo's professional entertainers lived and where they conducted the more mundane aspects of their trades—buying and selling musical instruments, negotiating with customers, and so on. In the nineteenth century, there is evidence of the ongoing association of certain Cairo spaces with these aspects of the entertainment trades. Entertainers continued to reside in neighborhoods such as Ḥūsh Bardaq, for example. Von Kremer (1864: 264) affirms the existence of this settlement in the mid-nineteenth century. Newbold (1856: 292) refers to it as Ḥūsh al-Ghajar.

On the other hand, Bāb al-Lūq may have declined as a residential neighborhood for entertainers. Didier's observations at mid-century suggest that "public women" such as female entertainers and prostitutes were based in neighborhoods just north and east of Azbakīyah, rather than in Bāb al-Lūq (Didier 1860: 330). Notably, at the dawn of the twentieth century, the main brothel districts of Cairo were located just north and northeast of the Azbakīyah Gardens (Moseley 1917: 206, Sladen 1911: 61).

After its completion in the 1870s, Muḥammad ʿAlī Street was destined to become central to the background business of professional entertainment (Figure 20). The street linked Azbakīyah and Rumaylah, Cairo's main public squares and important hubs for professional entertainment. In fact, the southeast terminus of the street was just a few hundred feet from Ḥūsh Bardaq. In addition, Muḥammad ʿAlī Street bordered on a neighborhood with long historical associations with the entertainment trades. Recall that a market for musical instruments existed in the vicinity of Bāb Zuwaylah as early as the Mamluk era. The center of the newly-completed boulevard passed just to the southwest of this neighborhood.

Muḥammad ʿAlī Street's easy proximity to both Azbakīyah and Rumaylah Square, together with the existing associations of nearby spaces with professional entertainment, ensured that professional entertainers and businesses connected to the entertainment trades would gravitate to the newly established boulevard. In the early decades of the twentieth century, this street was a hub for entertainers and central to the business of professional entertainment. The golden age of this famous street will be detailed in the next chapter.

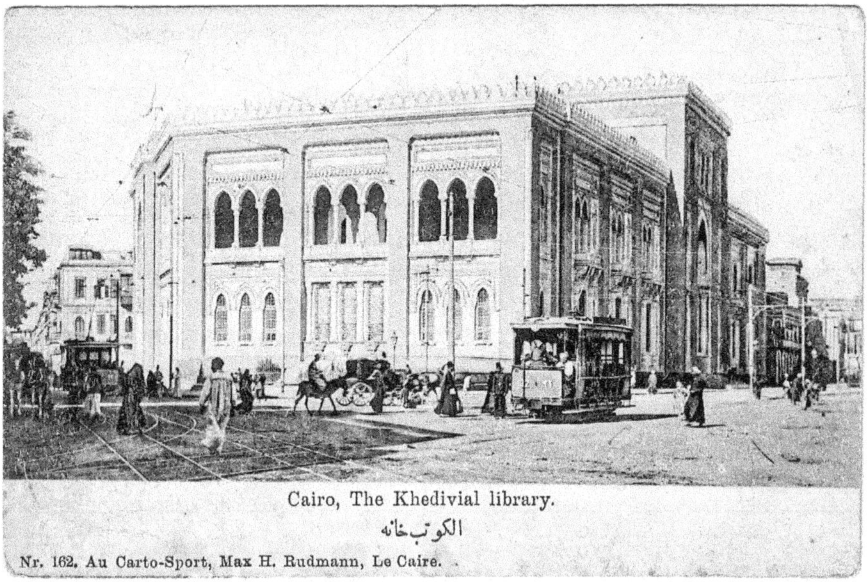

Figure 20: Intersection of Muḥammad ʿAlī Street and Būr Saʿīd Street at the turn of the nineteenth and twentieth centuries (Max H. Rudmann postcard, *circa* 1900).

Coffee Houses and Entertainment Halls

Coffee houses remained an important part of Cairene social life, particularly for Egyptian men. For foreigners, these venues, and the professional entertainers who frequently congregated within them, inspired both revulsion and fascination. Michaud visited Egypt in 1830 and 1831, before Muḥammad ʿAlī instituted restrictions on female entertainers and prostitutes, and he sought out one coffee house in particular because female entertainers typically gathered there (1833–1835, vol. 5: 251):

> There is a cafe where the jugglers and the almées usually meet; I wanted to see it; two stone benches are at the door; within the enclosure rises a large platform, and at the back is a sort of courtyard with three masonry obelisks. We chose our time badly; Ramadan had just ended, and the main cafes were deserted; two or three almées of very mediocre beauty, a few storytellers neglected by the public, that's all we could see.

Unfortunately his account offers no details regarding the coffee house's exact location.

Gérard de Nerval, on the other hand, visited Egypt in the 1840s, when female dancers and prostitutes were prohibited from public exercise of their trades. Upon visiting a coffee house on al-Mūskī Street, he was shocked by a performance by *khawalāt* (1884: 87–89). The British author Adam Steinmetz Kennard, who toured Egypt in the early 1850s, indicates that dancing boys frequented the coffee houses of Azbakīyah (Kennard 1855: 125).

In addition to coffee houses, a variety of entertainment halls—theaters, music halls, and *cafés chantants*—emerged in Cairo. Importantly, most of the city's entertainment halls were located in the zone west of the Khalīj: specifically, in and around Azbakīyah. Though the first such venue in Cairo was established under the French occupation, and a scattering of European theaters existed in Egypt in the early decades of the nineteenth century (e.g., Sadgrove 1996: 37–39), it was not until the second half of the century that entertainment halls began to thrive in Cairo.

Initially, these establishments were created to satisfy the demands of both the resident foreign population as well as European and American tourists for European-style entertainment. Even the government-sponsored venues established by Ismāʿīl near the Azbakīyah Gardens, most notably the opera house, catered to the tastes of foreigners and of the Egyptian elite. However, by the end of the century, Cairo was host to a variety of entertainment halls catering specifically to indigenous Egyptians, including Egyptians of the lower and middle classes, and many of these venues would come to incorporate belly dancers into their programming.

The emergence and eventual proliferation of entertainment halls set the stage, so to speak, for profound changes in Egyptian traditional entertainment (see Ward 2018). Prior to the introduction of these specialized venues, professional entertainment was embedded in social occasions: most ordinary Egyptians experienced professional entertainment only at weddings, during popular festivals, and informally in markets, squares, and coffee houses. By contrast, venues like theaters and music halls existed specifically for the display of professional entertainment, including song, dance, and theater.

Professional entertainment was thus cut loose from the social occasions that previously justified its performance, and for the price of admission, entertainment could be sought out and enjoyed for its own sake. Detached from ordinary social settings, the entertainment halls of Cairo emerged as a kind of liminal space, where the indigenous met the foreign, and tradition interfaced with modernity. Entertainment halls enabled Egyptians to experience professional entertainment in a new way, and in these settings, Egyptian traditional entertainment was destined to be transformed.

At a time when public performance by female professional dancers continued to be heavily regulated, it is clear that the entertainment halls of Cairo provided a space where these women could continue to ply their trades. Already noted above are the accounts confirming that female dancers were performing within at least one Azbakīyah *café chantant* as early as the 1870s. By the end of the century, belly dancers had become a common sight in the entertainment halls of Azbakīyah.

Significantly, the meanings that had long pervaded the Cairene landscape west of the Khalīj came to be physically embodied in these structures. That is, these venues lent a new physicality to this zone's heterotopic qualities. In the second half of the nineteenth century, the rise of these formalized entertainment venues in and around Azbakīyah tangibly reified and reinforced the association of this space with professional entertainment. Moreover, the ubiquity of belly dancers within these venues ensured their ongoing presence in and connection to the Azbakīyah landscape.

Continuity and Change in Cairo's Public Entertainment Spaces

Well before Ismā'īl's developments in the late nineteenth century, the stage had been set for shifts in Cairo's landscape of entertainment. By the end of the Ottoman era, Azbakīyah was already the focal point of the western suburbs. In the early nineteenth century, developments by the French and then by Muḥammad 'Alī in this area only served to increase its centrality to Cairene life. While it is undeniable that Ismā'īl's projects profoundly altered the physiognomy of Cairo, the meanings that had been inscribed into the western suburbs were not erased. At the beginning of the twentieth century, the western suburbs, with Azbakīyah as their hub, carried forward not only their associations with entertainment and leisure, but their deeply embedded ambiguity and liminality. Simultaneously, other spaces in the entertainment landscape began to wane in significance. Towards the end of the century, Rumaylah Square steadily declined in relevance as a popular gathering place. The city's cemeteries took on an increasingly residential character, and the role of shrines and cemeteries in the entertainment landscape became increasingly ephemeral.

Within the western suburbs, venues associated with entertainment and leisure abounded. These included coffee houses, which had been introduced earlier in the Ottoman era, as well as new venues specifically dedicated to the performance of professional entertainment. These new establishments—theaters, music halls, and *cafés chantants*—became the scene for profound changes in Egyptian traditional entertainment at the turn of the nineteenth and twentieth centuries. The creation of formalized entertainment venues in the zone west of the Khalīj imparted a new physicality to the meanings that had long characterized this space. Importantly, these venues allowed female dancers to continue practicing their trades in spite of ongoing regulation, and maintained their presence in the Azbakīyah landscape.

Alongside these developments, the completion of Muḥammad 'Alī Street had important implications for Cairo's landscape of entertainment. This broad boulevard quickly became central to the business of professional entertainment in Cairo. At the beginning of the twentieth century, it was home to professional entertainers as well as to an array of businesses associated with the entertainment trades. Yet, like other locations within the entertainment landscape, this space carried forward meanings that had been established in prior eras. A market for musical instruments had existed in this part of Cairo long before the construction of Muḥammad 'Alī Street. In the Mamluk era, the presence of entertainers here contributed to popular perceptions of this area as "unlucky." It is likely that professional entertainers at the turn of the twentieth century were drawn to Muḥammad 'Alī Street by the pre-existing association of nearby neighborhoods with entertainment, as well as the street's easy proximity Azbakīyah.

Conclusion

Throughout the Ottoman period, Cairo's suburbs and cemeteries carried forward the meanings that had been inscribed within them over the course of many centuries. These spaces remained firmly associated with entertainment and leisure in the popular imagination. Within them, diverse populations converged, and normal social and spatial boundaries were blurred, challenged, or even subverted. These were heterotopic spaces, and their liminal and ambivalent qualities were reinforced in practice by the Egyptians who lived and worked within them.

In these locales, professional entertainers, including professional dancers, found spaces that could accommodate their marginality. Their presence, in turn, served to re-inscribe the heterotopic nature of these spaces. Indeed, it becomes increasingly clear throughout the Ottoman era that the presence of professional entertainers was key to the ongoing re-inscription of heterotopic meaning into the entertainment landscape. Ottoman-era sources provide frequent and specific mentions of singer/dancers, and they demonstrate that public perceptions of these spaces were tied to their association with professional entertainers.

While the nineteenth century brought profound changes to Cairo's landscape of entertainment, the meanings that had been deeply inscribed in earlier centuries were not erased. Rather, many of the developments, particularly in the zone west of the Khalīj, actually served to reinforce the heterotopic qualities of certain spaces, as well as their association with professional entertainment. By the end of the century, developments in and around Azbakīyah, already the focal point of the Western suburbs, ensured its centrality in Cairo's landscape of entertainment. The proliferation of formalized entertainment venues in the area reinforced its ties to professional entertainment; these venues embodied the heterotopic qualities long associated with this part of Cairo. The widespread presence of belly dancers in these spaces ensured their continued connection to the landscape west of the Khalīj. At the outset of the twentieth century, Azbakīyah and vicinity, together with neighboring Muḥammad 'Alī Street, formed the heart of Cairo's landscape of entertainment.

FOUR

Entertainment Halls and Occupation

In his efforts to rival European powers, Ismāʿīl inadvertently ensured the gradual subordination of Egypt to the West (Abu-Lughod 1971: 113 Raymond 2000: 316–317). His grand urban planning projects were costly, and over the course of the 1860s, Ismāʿīl contracted a series of debts to European creditors—debts which the Egyptian government found itself unable to pay. In 1875, a fateful moment in Egyptian history, Ismāʿīl sold Egypt's shares in the Suez Canal to the British government, giving the British a direct interest in the financial affairs of Egypt. The following year, Egypt's debts were consolidated and placed under the oversight of a commission of financial control. Shortly thereafter, this commission was replaced by the system of Dual Control, with the British overseeing revenues and the French auditing expenses. In 1878, the British and the French assumed positions within the Egyptian cabinet: a Briton was appointed minister of finances, and a Frenchman minister of public works. Ismāʿīl attempted resistance, dismissing his cabinet in April 1879; just a few months later, the Europeans pressured the Ottoman Sultan to depose him in favor of his son Tawfīq.

The events of the latter decades of the nineteenth century mark the beginnings of an Egyptian nationalist movement, although there is some disagreement about the precise timing and the specific triggers. Mestyan (2017) has argued that prior to the 1890s, nationalism in the sense of "an ideology of solidarity, organized around the idea of 'the nation' (based on birth, *natio*) in a sovereign political unit," did not exist in Egypt (Mestyan 2017: 2). Muḥammad ʿAlī Bāshā and his descendants had tread a careful line, demonstrating their allegiance to the Ottoman Porte while simultaneously asserting Egypt's autonomy. The dynasty propagated an ideology of patriotism—solidarity and connection to a homeland, but without the demand for a sovereign polity—an ideology that could coexist with

Egypt's unique position as a semi-autonomous Ottoman province. Egyptian intellectuals like Rifāʿah Rāfiʿ al-Ṭahṭāwī embraced and promoted this patriotic ideology.

However, to focus only on the perspectives of the ruling class and the elite intelligentsia is to disregard the nationalistic spirit that was blossoming among the lower and middle classes even before the commencement of the British occupation. As Fahmy (2011: 51–55) observes, foreign interference in the Egyptian government, together with fiscal mismanagement and high taxation, led to widespread popular discontent under both Ismāʿīl and Tawfīq—discontent that found its expression in the colloquial press. These factors, together with state centralization, the development of the Egyptian railroad and postal systems (what Fahmy terms "centralization technologies"), and the development of print media, enabled the emergence of a modern territorial nationalist movement. Nevertheless, as Jankowski (1991: 244) notes, due to the European imperial menace, both territorial nationalism and loyalty to the Ottoman Empire were able coexist in Egypt for some time: "A continuing connection with the still independent Ottoman state came to be perceived as a useful instrument for resisting European imperialism as the latter first menaced and eventually engulfed Egypt."

The nationalist tendencies that were brewing over the course of the 1870s came to a dramatic climax with the ʿUrābī revolt. Aḥmad ʿUrābī was a junior officer in the Egyptian army who, along with other native Egyptians, had come to resent the structural inequalities that existed within the army. The higher ranks of the Egyptian military were reserved for members of the Turco-Circassian elite. In the 1870s, native Egyptians could rise only to the rank of colonel (a small improvement from earlier in the century, when they could only ascend to the rank of captain) (Toledano 1990: 178). In 1881, this inequity, coupled with cuts to the military budget, led ʿUrābī and several other junior officers to petition the leadership for change, who responded by stripping the officers of their ranks and arresting them (Fahmy 2011: 55–59). ʿUrābī and the others were confined in Qaṣr al–Nīl.

In response, members of the Khedivial Guard marched to Qaṣr al–Nīl and freed the officers, who, accompanied by a mass of soldiers and civilians, marched to ʿĀbdīn Palace. There, ʿUrābī thanked the soldiers for freeing him and made a series of demands, including his reinstatement. Tawfīq acceded to all of ʿUrābī's demands, and soon thereafter, military salaries and benefits were increased. These events galvanized military support for ʿUrābī, and soon, bolstered by the Egyptian press, he gained the support of the Egyptian masses. In early 1882, a shake-up in the Egyptian government led to the formation of a new, pro-ʿUrābī cabinet, and ʿUrābī was promoted to major general and appointed minister of war.

Both the local Turco-Circassian elite and the European powers were uncomfortable with the nativist direction of the new cabinet. The British and French deployed warships off the coast of Alexandria and demanded the cabinet's dissolution. Tawfīq complied, setting off anti-foreigner riots in Alexandria. The violence and instability provided the pretext for the British army to invade, and in the summer of 1882, the British occupation of Egypt began.

Under the occupation, the nationalist movement grew in earnest. At the turn of the century, it found its voice in figures like Muṣṭafā Kāmil, the young lawyer and journalist and founder of al-Ḥizb al-Waṭanī (the National Party), who leveraged print media to mobilize support for the cause. Activists like Kāmil were able to rally significant popular support in the wake of the Dinshawāy Incident of 1906, an event which came to emblemize the atrocities, injustices, and humiliations of the occupation (Fahmy 2011: 92–95).

In the rural village of Dinshawāy, British military officers outraged the village residents by hunting their domestic pigeons, an important local food source. In the altercation that followed, a British officer fled the scene and died, most likely due to heat stroke. Even though the villagers were probably not responsible for the officer's death, the British, fearing insurrection, used the death as a pretense to make examples of the Dinshawāy villagers. After a cursory trial, several villagers were given punishments ranging from death by hanging to flogging and imprisonment. The Dinshawāy Incident was widely publicized in political newspapers such as Kāmil's, and Egyptians took to a variety of other popular media, including literature, music, and theater, to vent their outrage.

At the outset of World War I, a series of factors further galvanized the nationalist movement, transforming it into an independence movement. On November 2, 1914, the British placed Egypt under martial law. Three days later, the British declared war on the Ottoman Empire, and the Protectorate of Egypt was announced. Shortly thereafter, the anti-British Khedive ʿAbbās Ḥilmī was deposed in favor of his more pliable uncle, Ḥusayn Kāmil, who was declared Sultan of Egypt. Simultaneously, the British actively suppressed the al-Waṭanī Party and other nationalist sympathizers, and press freedoms were harshly curtailed. Compounding these factors, wartime shortages, unemployment, and inflation led to widespread popular discontent.

All of these factors came to a head in 1919, with the arrest and exile of the Egyptian politician Saʿd Zaghlūl (Fahmy 2011: 138–139). At the end of World War I, Zaghlūl and two of his colleagues formed a delegation (*wafd*) that met with British high commissioner Sir Reginald Wingate; in this meeting, the delegation demanded an end to the Protectorate and its replacement by a treaty of alliance. This marked the formation of the pro-independence Ḥizb al-Wafd, or Wafd Party. Zaghlūl and the Wafd enjoyed widespread popular support, and the British decision to exile Zaghlūl and several members of the Wafd to Malta was the spark that lit the fuse of revolution. In the spring of 1919, demonstrations and riots broke out all over Egypt.

The Revolution of 1919 was an all-encompassing popular movement, involving Egyptians of all social classes, genders, and religious confessions. When the British, in an attempt to quell the discontent, freed Zaghlūl on April 7, spontaneous celebrations erupted in Cairo. Contemporary observers described elite women parading in cars while waving flags, their lower-class counterparts singing and dancing in donkey-drawn carts, and Muslim, Christian, and Jewish religious officials asserting their solidarity as Egyptians (Fahmy 2011: 140–141).

By 1920, Zaghlūl was the *de facto* leader of the independence movement, and he was heavily involved in negotiating terms with the British. As demonstrations and disorder continued in Egypt, the British once again deported Zaghlūl; simultaneously, the British unilaterally declared the end of the Protectorate. Zaghlūl was released and returned to Egypt in triumph. In Egypt's first election under the new constitution, Zaghlūl became prime minister.

While Egypt nominally achieved independence in 1922, the British continued to exert control in administrative, fiscal, and political matters for several more decades. Further, under the new constitution, the Egyptian monarchy retained the right to dissolve Parliament, ensuring the ongoing power of the royal family. These unresolved issues would continue to bubble under the surface of Egyptian social and cultural life, eventually bursting forth again at mid-century.

Cairo Under Occupation

The British occupation was a time of massive growth for the city of Cairo—both in terms of urban development and in terms of population. Yet, the structural foundation for a great deal of the growth that was to take place under the occupation was laid by Ismā'īl. Ismā'īl's developments in the western suburbs—the leveling of rubbish heaps, the filling of ponds and canals, the establishment of basic utilities and a street system—ensured that the city's initial expansion was westward.

Ismā'īl's developments were elaborated upon under occupation (Figure 21). The remaining ponds and canals were filled, including, most dramatically, the filling of the Khalīj in 1898 (Abu-Lughod 1971: 125). The bed of the

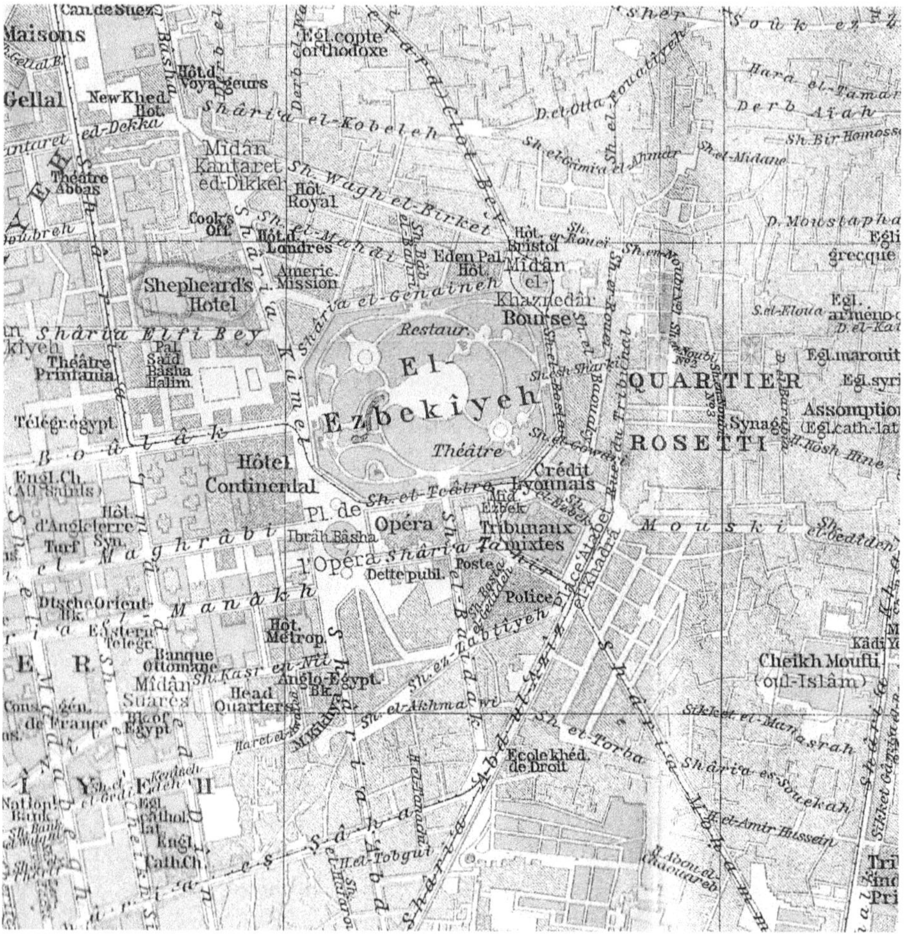

Figure 21: Detail from a map of early twentieth century Cairo (Wagner and Debes, 1911).

Khalīj was converted into a street, Khalīj Street, today's Būr Saʿīd Street (Figure 22). Municipal utilities, including gas and water, were expanded, and the beginnings of a sewer system were completed in 1915 (Raymond 2000: 326–327). Between 1894 and 1917, a tram system was constructed (Raymond 2000: 324), the first mass-transit system in Cairo, with the initial hub at al-ʿAtabah al-Khaḍrā' at the southeast corner of the Azbakīyah Gardens. The arrival of automobiles in 1903 also enhanced transportation in the city, though initially automobiles were largely confined to the broad boulevards of the western suburbs (*ibid.*). The completion of the first Aswan dam in 1902 stabilized the Nile shoreline in Cairo and enabled further developments, most notably a number of bridges (Raymond 2000: 324–326).

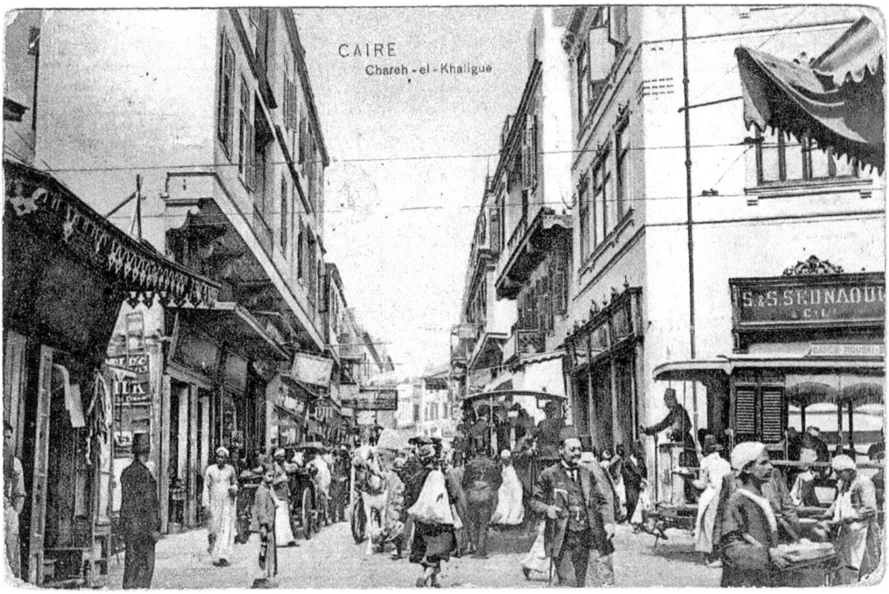

Figure 22: Khalīj Street, today's Būr Sa'īd Street, in the early twentieth century (postcard, *circa* 1910).

In the early decades of the twentieth century, the population of Cairo began to grow exponentially. A variety of factors contributed to this increase, including an influx of foreigners, as well as rural-to-urban migration. However, as Abu-Lughod notes, one of the most significant factors leading to Cairo's dramatic population growth was the declining death rate due to improved sanitation and public health measures (1971: 119). In the fifty-year period from 1897 to 1947, the population of Cairo tripled, whereas the overall population of the country only doubled. Much of the demographic growth was absorbed in the areas west, south, and north of the Azbakīyah Gardens. Growth also occurred in the city cemeteries, which increasingly functioned as affordable housing for rural-to-urban migrants and the urban poor (El Kadi and Bonnamy 2007: 257–260).

In the midst of all this growth and change, the legacy of prior eras persisted—most notably, in Azbakīyah and vicinity, the area that now constituted Cairo's downtown (*wusṭ al-balad*). Abu-Lughod's (1971: 114) characterization of Cairo west of Khalīj Street as "a self-contained colonial city" disregards the longstanding relationship between the zones on either side of the old Khalīj. Well before Ismā'īl's developments, the occupation, and the influx of foreigners into the city, the area to the west of the Khalīj had existed "outside" the Fatimid city: not just in terms of geography, but in its very nature. Over the course of centuries, this part of the city had been established as a heterotopic space, a space "outside of all places." This was a zone of ambivalence and liminality, where the normal social and spatial boundaries of Egyptian society were blurred, challenged, or even upended as people from radically different social contexts converged, engaging in behaviors and activities that defied or disrupted the social order. This space had come to embody the carnivalesque interactions and behaviors that were performed here for generations, and these inscribed meanings continued to inform Cairene's experience of this place.

Cairo's turn-of-the-century downtown, encompassing the neighborhoods of Azbakīyah, Tawfīqīyah, and Ismā'īlīyah, was an area that had long been characterized by the confluence of diverse populations—elites, commoners, Muslims, Christians, native Egyptians, foreigners, men, women—all drawn together in a space firmly associated with entertainment, leisure, and vice. In the time of the Fatimids, the ruling class relaxed in their luxurious *manāẓir*, while the common people of Cairo gathered nearby on the banks of the ponds and canals, as both enjoyed the music and song provided by popular entertainers. Hundreds of years later, the Egyptian aristocracy rubbed shoulders with European diplomats and businessmen in the grand opera house, while just across the Azbakīyah Gardens, Egyptians of the lower classes were visiting modest music halls and theaters like the Dār al-Tamthīl al-'Arabī (Arabic Playhouse), where they enjoyed indigenous music, song, and dance and theatrical presentations in colloquial Egyptian Arabic.

Focusing on the "Europeanness" of this area obscures the ongoing social and economic heterogeneity of this space and the persistence of meanings from earlier eras. This myopic approach is illustrated in the following passage, written by the Egyptian scholar Aḥmad Amīn in his 1953 *Dictionary of Egyptian Customs, Traditions, and Expressions*:

> During the occupation by the English, our people got accustomed to "freedom." As this word "freedom" became a slogan on everyone's lips, the garden of Azbakiyya became the symbol of this freedom, understood by the people to mean prostitution, liquor, hashish, and gambling.... The Azbakiyya garden became the meeting place of debauchees and was crowded with taverns and dance cabarets with male and female singers, hashish houses, and gambling dens. People of every vice flocked to it until the word Azbakiyya became synonymous with licentiousness and debauchery of every kind.
>
> At 4 o'clock in the afternoon, men and women, old and young, pressed at the gates to get their share of luck and pleasure. Prostitutes wandered its paths; at sunset the Greeks opened their taverns, and the musicians arrived.

> After dark, the lanterns and lamps were lit; each band of musicians took its place and the seats were arranged. At some places, the prostitutes sat, each at a separate table, clad in frivolous and transparent dresses and using licentious language. They walked in all parts of the garden, swaying their hips to provoke desire.... Each band of musicians was composed of the players of the instruments, and in their middle a woman, called an "*ālima*," played all the tricks of coquettery and provocation on the rich heirs who came every night. She would throw glances at them, so that everybody thought himself the chosen one [quoted in Behrens-Abouseif 1985: 99–100].

The idea that Azbakīyah suddenly became a den of vice during the British occupation is belied by centuries of history of Cairo's western suburbs. From the Fatimid period onward, generation after generation associated the western suburbs of Cairo—and, eventually, Azbakīyah—with leisure and vice. Recall the moralistic laments of Ibn Sa'īd al-Maghribī in the late Ayyubid/early Mamluk era, who described the Khalīj zone as follows: "It is constricted on both sides by numerous pavilions greatly populated by people given over to merriment, to banter, and to bawdiness, so that people of respectable morals and the great do not allow themselves to cross it in a boat" (quoted in al-Maqrīzī 1920: 58–59).

Remember that prostitution thrived in this area for centuries: both Leo Africanus and Evliya Çelebi abundantly documented the practice in Azbakīyah and nearby Bāb al-Lūq in the Ottoman area, and Didier describes the clandestine brothels just north and east Azbakīyah in the 1850s (Africano 1500: 91, Africanus 1896: 874, Dankoff and Kim: 2011: 393–394, Didier 1860: 330, Prokosch 2000: 41). The presence of popular entertainment and prostitution in Azbakīyah during the British occupation was the continuation of centuries-long practice in this area.

Over the course of the occupation, venues dedicated to professional entertainment multiplied in this area of the city (see, for example, Cormack 2021). Initially, these establishments were clustered in and around Azbakīyah. However, beginning in the 1910s, theaters and music halls multiplied along 'Imād al-Dīn Street just to the west, and soon the latter rivaled Azbakīyah proper as the most sought-after destination for entertainment. The earliest of Cairo's entertainment halls were created to satisfy the demands of Western residents and tourists, and throughout the era of the occupation, venues oriented toward European and American consumers continued to exist. However, from the late nineteenth century onward, Cairo was also host to an array of entertainment halls catering to the tastes and interests of indigenous Egyptians, including those of the lower and middle classes, and the nationalistic sentiment of the time frequently found expression on their stages (Fahmy 2011, Gitre 2019).

As noted in the previous chapter, the entertainment halls that proliferated in Azbakīyah and vicinity enabled profound changes in Egyptian traditional entertainment. Theaters, music halls, and the like represented a new way for Egyptians to experience familiar entertainments like music, song, and dance: not in traditional social contexts, but in structures that existed solely for the display of professional entertainment. The entertainment halls of Cairo existed as a liminal space, where the indigenous intersected with the foreign, and where tradition met with modernity. Within their walls, Egyptian artists and entertainers drew upon and experimented with foreign ideas and technologies, while simultaneously asserting their connection to traditional Egyptian aesthetics, interests, and values in the face of the ongoing British occupation. Indeed, Cairo's theaters and music halls were spaces where the current social order was interrogated and challenged, and where existing structures of class, gender, and power were defied, sometimes openly (see Fahmy 2011, Gitre 2019). Considering all this, it should come as no surprise that these venues—ambivalent and liminal sites that enabled experimentation and innovation in traditional Egyptian entertainment—were primarily sited in the heterotopic zone west of Khalīj Street.

Importantly, in spite of ongoing regulation of female professional dancers, by the 1890s, belly dancers were commonplace in the entertainment halls of Azbakīyah. The venues of ʻImād al-Dīn Street followed suit, as the stage version of the local belly dance became increasingly popular on Cairene stages. Belly dancers thrived in these new settings, and soon *raqṣ sharqī* and its professional practitioners were inextricably bound—both in reality and in popular perception—to the entertainment halls of Cairo. By the end of the 1930s, many dancers had achieved celebrity status. Many female professional belly dancers owned and managed their own venues, ensuring that these women played a key role in shaping the early-to-mid twentieth century Cairo entertainment landscape.

The creation of structures dedicated to professional entertainment lent a new physicality to the meanings that had been inscribed within the Cairene landscape west of the Khalīj. The proliferation of these formalized entertainment venues in Azbakīyah and vicinity tangibly reified the association of this space with professional entertainment and reinforced the centrality of this space within Cairo's landscape of entertainment. These venues embodied the ambivalence and liminality that had long characterized this part of Cairo; they were physical manifestations of this area's heterotopic qualities. The ubiquity of belly dancers within these venues ensured their ongoing connection to the landscape west of the Khalīj, and the presence of these marginal figures served to re-inscribe the heterotopic nature of the spaces where they lived and worked.

Azbakīyah and the zone west of Khalīj Street, populated by these physical manifestations of meanings that had defined the region for centuries, came to overshadow other spaces that had previously figured significantly in Cairo's entertainment landscape, such as Rumaylah Square and the city's massive cemeteries. By the end of the nineteenth century, Rumaylah had steadily declined in relevance. The relocation of Egypt's administrative center away from the Citadel, the waning popularity of the *maḥmal* processions, and the rise of Azbakīyah, all contributed to the square's decline as a popular gathering place. Simultaneously, Cairo's cemeteries took on an increasingly residential character. Though weekly *ziyārah* and popular festivals continued to take place in these spaces, their entertainment function was ephemeral. That is, Cairo's shrines and cemeteries served as temporary festive spaces, in contrast to the zone west of the old Khalīj, where entertainment was always available in the innumerable venues that existed solely for its enjoyment. From the turn of the century until the 1960s, Azbakīyah and vicinity, together with neighboring Muḥammad 'Alī Street, formed the beating heart of Cairo's landscape of entertainment.

From Azbakīyah to 'Imād al-Dīn Street

At the dawn of the twentieth century, Azbakīyah was firmly associated in the popular imagination with entertainment, leisure, and vice, just as it had been for centuries prior (Figure 23). Until the 1910s, most of Cairo's entertainment halls were situated in and around Azbakīyah. In addition, Azbakīyah was the site of Cairo's two main brothel districts. As it had been in centuries past, Azbakīyah was a site of carnivalistic mésalliances, where socially heterogeneous groups interfaced, and where Cairenes engaged in transgressive and counter-normative behaviors and activities. Men, women, Egyptians, foreigners, wealthy, poor, Muslim, Christian, all converged within this vibrant and complex zone.

The Azbakīyah Gardens were a popular place for promenading. A fee was required for entry, and police officers patrolled to maintain order (Behrens-Abouseif 1985: 92, Mestyan 2017: 87). Within the Gardens were both European and Arabic *cafés chantants*, a European restaurant, and a variety of concession stands offering snacks, tobacco, photographs, and games (Behrens-Abouseif 1985: 93). In al-Muwayliḥī's *Ḥadīth 'Īsā Ibn Hishām*, the central characters of the *'umdah*, the playboy, and the merchant first appear in the Azbakīyah Gardens (al-Muwayliḥī 2015: 13–17). The playboy brings his companions to the Gardens in search of female companionship, only to discover that the government has cracked down on such rendezvous. Consequently, the trio wander off to seek amusements (and female companionship) elsewhere in Azbakīyah.

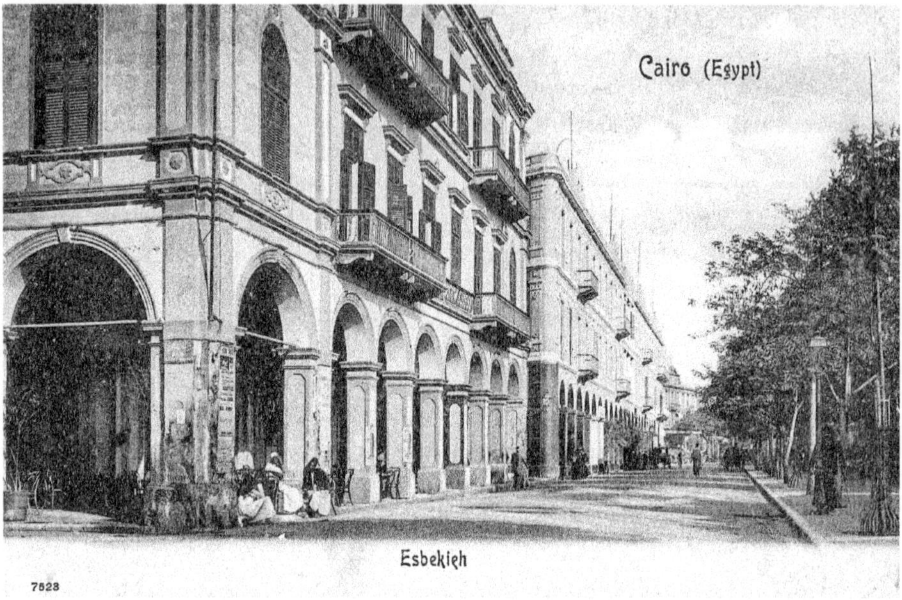

Figure 23: Turn-of-the-century Azbakīyah, looking east along the street today known as 'Alī al- Kassār Street (postcard, *circa* 1900).

Those amusements were to be found in the streets and alleys bordering the Azbakīyah Gardens. While the areas to the south and to the west of the Gardens were largely dominated by the opera house, government buildings, and the Continental and Shepheard's Hotels, the streets to the north and to the east were populated by a dizzying array of popular entertainment venues, including cafés, bars, music halls, theaters, and brothels. Much of the activity was centered on Wajh al-Birkah Street, which extended from Mīdān al-Khazindār to Mīdān Qanṭarat al-Dikkah. The new El Dorado entertainment hall was located on this street (see below). Another important venue, Salāmah Ḥijāzī's Dār al-Tamthīl al-'Arabī, was located nearby on Bāb al-Baḥrī Street, a small north-south cross street of Wajh al-Birkah. Douglas Sladen (1911: 109) paints a vivid picture:

> In the Sharia Bab-el-Bahri are the principal Arab theatre, and other places of amusement, and there are always piano-organs or bands playing the latest music-hall or comic-opera airs. The whole street is a blaze of electric light. Its ends are taken up with cafés, and its pavements are crowded with vendors of tartlets, sweetmeats, meat on skewers, and sago in teacups; while the cigarette-sellers have stalls that are works of art.

To the east of the Azbakīyah Gardens, the Thousand and One Nights Theater was tucked away on the Ḥārat al-'Usaylī. To the southeast, the al-Miṣrī Theater (Egyptian Theater) was located on 'Abd al-'Azīz Street, just off al-'Atabah Square.

Prostitution had been commonplace in the zone west of the Khalīj for centuries; by the mid-nineteenth century, it was concentrated just north and east of Azbakīyah, and at the turn of the nineteenth and twentieth centuries, prostitution continued to be centered in these areas. During the occupation, Wajh al-Birkah Street was the primary location of Cairo's unregulated foreign brothels.

> The Sharia Wagh-el-Birket is a more dissipated street, though it is not so noisy or glary. For the whole of one side of it is taken up with the apartments of the wealthier courtesans, each with its balcony, over which its denizens hang in negligés of virgin white. In the half-light the tall, Eastern-looking houses, with their tiers of balconies with houris hanging over them in all sorts of fantastic garments and postures, loom up weird and romantic. Here you may see an occasional "scene" or fracas, but it is the exception. The opposite side of the street is arcaded—and under its arcades are a succession of cafés, most of them filled with Arabs consuming strong liquors indirectly forbidden by their religion [Sladen 1911: 110].

The heavily regulated native brothels were located to the northeast of the Azbakīyah Gardens, in an area known variously as the Wāsa'a ("wide area") or the Fishmarket, so named because of the area's earlier function (Dunn 2011).

> Not far from the Clot Bey end of the Sharia Wagh-el-Birket lies the Fishmarket, the worst of the purlieus of the Esbekiya, the gay quarter of Cairo.... I have never seen such a repulsive place; the houses are squalid; the women are most of them appalling; they positively flame with crimson paint and brass jewellery and have eyes flashing with every kind of mineral decoration and stimulant, and far too much flesh. If you walk through the Fishmarket when they are prowling for victims, your clothes are nearly torn off in the agonised attempts to secure your attention. There are the usual accompaniments of drink and mechanical music, and police [Sladen 1911: 61].

The ubiquity of brothels in these areas may explain the gradual migration of theaters and music halls elsewhere. With the onset of World War I and the stationing of British troops in Cairo, the brothel districts drew large numbers of soldiers to Azbakīyah, and their rowdy behavior created an environment that was increasingly unstable. Journalist Sydney Moseley expressed his concern regarding the unrestrained behavior that he observed in what he described as the "plague spots" of Cairo:

> They would go to music-halls, sit in any seats they preferred, despite the remonstrances of the nervous attendant, interrupt the performance, throwing sallies of considerably heavy brilliance at the performers, and enter into indignant altercations with foreign members of the audience who resented

> this behaviour. Sometimes, I am afraid, our military men were the culprits, and one saw the spectacle of Tommy up in the "gods" looking down below where his trainers and commanders were making public nuisances of themselves [Moseley 2017: 204].

Occasionally, what began as rowdy behavior escalated into violence and bloodshed. Such was the case during the infamous "Battle of the Wozzer" on April 2, 2015. On this day, a conflict that began at a brothel on the tiny Darb al-Muballāt off Wajh al-Birkah Street soon escalated into a riot involving as many as 2,000 ANZAC (the Australia and New Zealand Army Corps) soldiers (Dunn 2011). The riot was put down by British and Australian troops, though not before multiple local businesses were burned to the ground. A similar, though smaller-scale, riot occurred a few months later. These issues help to explain why entertainment venues began to migrate westward.

As early as the 1890s, another center for popular entertainment existed at Rūḍ al-Faraj, located to the northwest, along the east bank of the Nile. Sources indicate that entertainment venues were commonplace in this area by the end of the nineteenth century, and thriving throughout the 1910s. In 1891, *al-Ahrām* newspaper published a complaint from residents of the Muḥarram Bik neighborhood of Rūḍ al-Faraj, who were concerned with "disreputable" dancers gathering and performing at cafés in their neighborhood (*al-Ahrām* 10 April 1891: 3). Yet, the *cafés chantants* of Rūḍ al-Faraj, as well as its single open-air theater, appear to have held a particular attraction for Cairene women in the 1910s. Hector Dinning (1920: 240) writes:

> Here women do congregate. You will see them in no *café-chantant* in Cairo. But the thing you are to remember about Rod-el-Faraq is that it is pure Arab untrammelled by European. We were the only people not Arab who used to visit it. So the Egyptians allow their women to come here. As you approach the cafés from the tram-terminus you will see the queue of gharries that have brought Egyptian women from Cairo to sit here and sip coffee and listen to the music.

Some qualifications of Dinning's observations are in order: Rūḍ al-Faraj may not have been as "pure Arab" as Dinning suggests, for Douglas Sladen (1911: 114–115) observes: "Rod-el-Farag, the lower port of Cairo, has a row of cafés on the banks of the Nile where dancing goes on, but here the performers are European, though the danse à ventre is generally part of their programme." Also, while it is true that, with the exception of the performers, women were an uncommon sight in Cairo music halls in the 1910s, some Egyptian women did attend Cairene theaters, and women certainly visited music halls as early as the 1920s (see, for example, *al-Ahrām* 28 November 1924: 7).

After this brief florescence, however, Rūḍ al-Faraj was destined to fade in significance, as the broad north-south boulevard known as 'Imād al-Dīn Street became a central destination for popular entertainment in Cairo (Figure 24). 'Imād al-Dīn Street was established towards the end of the nineteenth century, beginning with the portion extending south from Būlāq Street (today's 26 July Street), later including the segment running from Būlāq Street northward to Ramses Square.* By the end of the 1910s, a variety of entertainment venues had been established on 'Imād al-Dīn Street, as well as on its cross streets, such as Alfī Bik, in the newly developed neighborhood of Tawfīqīyah. Among the earliest venues were the 'Abbās Theater and the Casino de Paris, located across the street from one another on 'Imād al-Dīn Street proper, the Egypsiana Theater, just north of the Casino de Paris, and the Abbaye des Roses and the original Printania Theater, neighboring one another on Alfī Bik Street. By the end of the 1920s, 'Imād al-Dīn Street was lined with theaters, music halls, cinemas, bars, and cafés. Popular venues included Yūsif Wahbī's Ramses Theater, the Majestic Theater, the new Printania

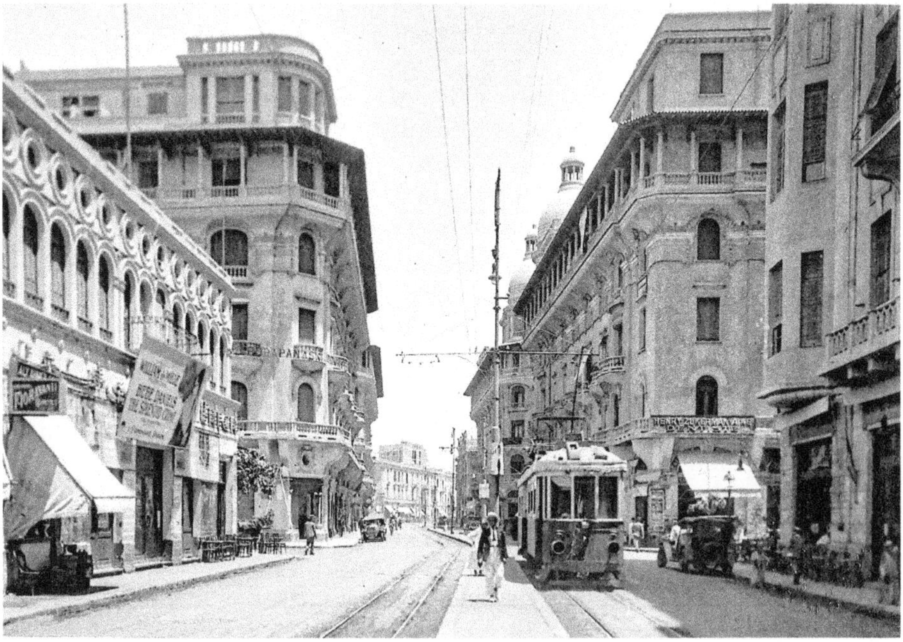

Figure 24: 'Imād al-Dīn Street in the early twentieth century (photo, *circa* 1920s, copyright Dr. Edouard Lambelet, Lehnert & Landrock—Egypt).

* The length of 'Imād al-Dīn Street south of Būlāq Street was later renamed Muḥammad Farīd Street, in honor of the nationalist politician of the early twentieth century.

Theater, and Ṣālat Badī'ah Maṣābnī, the first of Badī'ah's many entertainment establishments.

Although the theaters and music halls of 'Imād al-Dīn Street were somewhat spatially removed from Azbakīyah, they remained enmeshed in the moral ambiguity that characterized the latter. Like Azbakīyah, 'Imād al-Dīn Street was a heterogeneous space, frequented by disparate social groups. The mixing of genders, classes, religious confessions, and nationalities in the street's popular entertainment venues created an environment that challenged the social order. Moreover, these diverse populations were gathering together to enjoy performances that were frequently transgressive of social norms. Cormack (2021: 111) notes: "In the press, critics sarcastically renamed the street, calling it Fasad al-Din ('corruption of religion') rather than Emad al-Din ('pillar of religion,' the name of the Sufi sheikh buried at one end of it)."

Also like Azbakīyah, this street had its underworld. Prostitution thrived here as well, though not as overtly as in the brothel districts of Azbakīyah. Alcohol and hashish were readily available, as were hard drugs like heroin and cocaine. Protection rackets were widespread, and many business owners and professional entertainers found themselves plagued by local street gangs demanding protection money (Cormack 2021: 105–109). The costs of running afoul of the gangs could be severe: the dancer Imtithāl Fawzī was stabbed to death for refusing to comply with the demands of one such gang (Cormack 2021: 284–287).

In short, the area west of Khalīj Street continued to embody the meanings that had been inscribed within it in prior centuries. Cairo's twentieth century downtown carried forward the association with entertainment, leisure, and vice that had long characterized this part of the city. Further, downtown Cairo, encompassing the vibrant pleasure centers of Azbakīyah and 'Imād al-Dīn Street, continued to exist as a zone of ambivalence and liminality. Here, the normative social and spatial boundaries of Egyptian society continued to be blurred and bent as people from radically disparate social contexts converged. Here, Egyptians continued to engage in behaviors and activities that defied or disrupted the social order. Throughout the era of the occupation, downtown Cairo remained a space "outside of all places," a heterotopic space, and the gravitational center of the city's landscape of entertainment.

It is unsurprising that the majority of Cairo's entertainment halls were situated in this heterotopic zone west of Khalīj Street. These venues were ambivalent and liminal sites that enabled experimentation and innovation in traditional Egyptian entertainment. As such, they embodied the heterotopic qualities of Azbakīyah and vicinity. The proliferation of these structures provided a physical manifestation of the meanings that had been inscribed into the Cairene landscape west of the Khalīj. Within these venues, Cairo's female professional belly dancers were able to thrive, ensuring their continued presence and influence in Cairo's landscape of entertainment.

Anatomy of a Turn-of-the-Century Entertainment Hall

For convenience, I use the term "entertainment hall" to capture the broad array of formalized entertainment venues—theaters, music halls, and *cafés chantants*—that sprang up in Cairo in the late nineteenth and early twentieth centuries. The earliest such venues were created with Western consumers in mind (recall that the first theater in Cairo was built by the French to entertain the troops during Napoleon's occupation), and venues oriented toward a European and American clientele continued to flourish in Cairo. However, by the end of the nineteenth century, entertainment halls catering to indigenous Egyptian audiences abounded, and most such venues were located in the zone west of the Khalīj. These Egyptian-oriented venues are the focus of the current discussion.

Cairo's formalized entertainment venues included theaters in the contemporary European sense—these establishments were often referred to by designations such as *masraḥ* (theater) or *tiyātrū* (theater, from the Italian *teatro*). As with their Western counterparts, seating was arranged in boxes and stalls. The grand Azbakīyah Garden Theater boasted orchestra stalls, two tiers of box seating, and a third-floor gallery. The Egypsiana Theater was humbler, but offered stalls, a row of boxes on either side, and a high rear gallery (Dinning 1920: 273).

Some theaters, including the Egypsiana, were roofless, a point occasionally remarked on by foreign visitors (Dinning 1920: 273, Worrell 1920: 136). Some of these open-air theaters were seasonal and only opened during the summer months (Sladen 1911: 119). At others, a temporary roof of Egyptian tent fabric was installed in the winter; this was the case with the Egypsiana (Dinning 1920: 273). Tickets for theaters were generally sold via a box office window, and advance purchase was encouraged (e.g., *al-Ahrām* 1 September 1926: 7, *al-Ahrām* 15 May 1927: 6).

Other Cairo entertainment halls were more akin to European music halls or American vaudeville halls—these venues were referred to by a wide range of designations, including *ṣālah* (hall, from the French *salle*), *maḥall* (shop), and *kāzīnū* (casino, from Italian). A popular such venue at the turn of the century was El Dorado, which is described in numerous contemporary accounts (Figure 25) (see, for example, Loewenbach 1908:

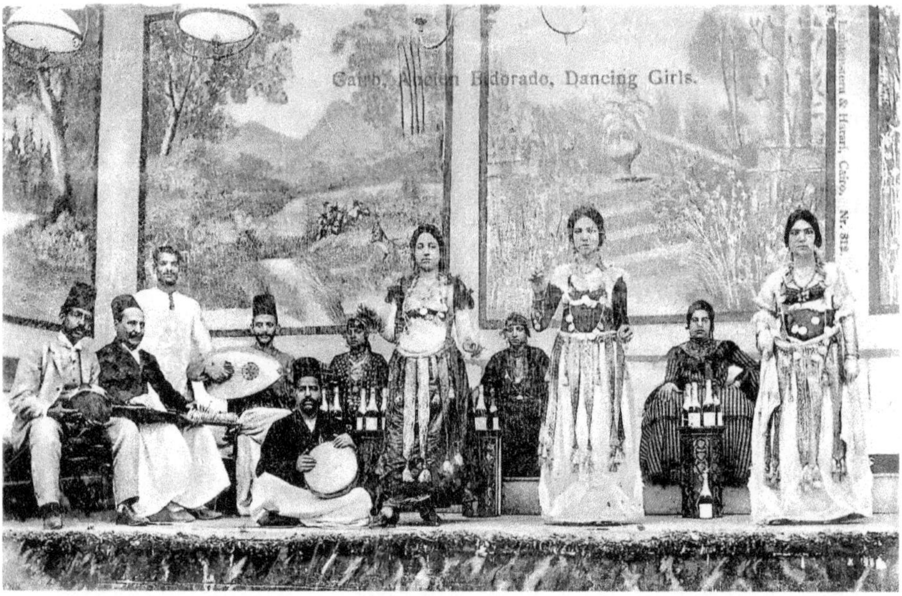

Figure 25: Dancers onstage at Cairo's El Dorado entertainment hall (Lichtenstern and Harari postcard, postmarked 1905).

218–220). Typically, these establishments consisted of a large hall with a raised stage at one end; on the stage, divans or chairs were arranged for the comfort of musicians, singers, and dancers. Audiences sat around tables, and beverages—sometimes alcoholic—were served. The humbler of these halls were barely more than coffee houses (and went by the same name—*qahwah*, i.e., café), though most differed from the latter by scheduling professional entertainment and charging admission (see, for example, *al-Zuhūr* November 1913: 359–362). In general, these venues charged admission at the door. Some establishments allowed free entry, and recovered their costs through drink purchases. By the end of the 1930s, Cairo's music halls had evolved into what would now be recognized as nightclubs and cabarets.

It is tempting to view these two general categories of entertainment halls as not only structurally but also functionally distinct from one another. Certainly, the programming at the theater-style venues tended to center on theatrical productions, and that of the music halls generally focused on music, song, and dance performances. Yet, the reality of these establishments was much more ambiguous. Even the humblest of music halls sometimes presented plays and comic skits, and at theaters, music, song, dance, and other variety entertainment was frequently offered both before and after plays, during intermissions, and sometimes during the plays themselves (Gitre 2019: 46, 81; Cormack 2021: 30–31). In general, Cairo's entertainment halls were united by their embrace of a variety show format in the style of European *cafés chantants* and music halls and American vaudeville theaters, but targeted toward an Egyptian clientele.

It is also tempting to distinguish these venues according to class. Indeed, some venues, such as the Azbakīyah Garden Theater, were targeted toward a more elite clientele. However, audiences at many venues were often quite heterogeneous, with a mix of social classes, genders, ethnicities, and religious confessions. Douglas Sladen, describing the audience at a popular Cairo theater—most likely Salāmah Ḥijāzī's Dār al-Tamthīl al-ʿArabī—notes that men were seated according to social class, and women were present, but hidden away in the boxes: "Half the boxes here had harem-grills like Sicilian nuns' churches. There were hardly any women visible; only tarbûshes in front and turbans behind" (Sladen 1911: 115). Roughly a decade later, Hector Dinning describes an even more diverse scene at Najīb al-Rīḥānī's Egypsiana Theater:

> There is a simple division of the house: a row of boxes on the ground each side of the stalls; benches for the bourgeois behind the stalls; large and high rear gallery for the herd.... The herd is there, setting the pace in the clamour—with a large proportion of Bints. This is the only Egyptian theatre in which I have seen the yashmak [face veil] in force. The whole front row of the gallery is peopled by yashmaks and gleaming eyes. The fine, white, transparent yashmak of the aristocrat is scattered up and down the boxes; it is mostly the unveiled Syrians and Italians and French that sit with their men in the stalls—with their men and their families [Dinning 1920: 273–274].

Dinning's account indicates that the gallery was populated by Egyptian men and women of the lower and middle classes, while a scattering of upper class Egyptians were seated in the boxes, and Syrians and resident Europeans sat in the stalls. He also makes it clear that whole families were in attendance: he describes (with disdain) parents and children snacking on cakes and toffees during the show (Dinning 1920: 274).

The heterogeneity of the audiences in many of Cairo's entertainment halls was enabled by a number of factors. First, entry fees were generally low enough to make both theaters and music halls affordable to a broad cross-section of the Egyptian public. Fahmy observes that the price of admission for most plays in the 1910s was 5 piasters, though some venues charged higher fees for first-class and second-class seating (Fahmy 2011: 122). Citing Najīb al-Rīḥānī's diary, he indicates that al-Rīḥānī's theater in 1917 (probably the Egypsiana) had a 10-piaster second-class section and a 15-piaster first-class section. Interestingly, admission prices remained remarkably stable for many decades. Around 1890, first-class admission to an entertainment hall called The Louvre was 10 *ṣāgh* (another term for the *qirsh*/piaster coin), while second class cost just 5 *ṣāgh* (*al-Zuhūr* November 1913: 359–360). Thirty-plus years later, the entry fee for the November 28, 1924, show at the Kāzīnū al-Būsfūr was just 5 *ṣāgh* (*al-Ahrām* 28 November 1924: 7). Similarly, the admission fee for the November 24, 1931, show at Ṣālah Su'ād Maḥāssan was 5 *ṣāgh* (*al-Ahrām* 24 November 1931: 9). In May 1929, the door charge for the Sunday matinee at the Kit Kat Cabaret was 5 piasters, though admission for the dinner/show at the Kit Kat's restaurant was pricier, at 25 piasters (*al-Ahrām* 1 May 1929: 6).

Second, spatial and temporal strategies—such as the establishment of dedicated seating areas for women and families, and the scheduling of ladies-only and families-only shows—to adjust the entertainment hall setting to Egyptian social norms meant that Egyptian women and children could enjoy Cairo's music halls and theaters as well. Many entertainment halls specifically marketed themselves as woman-friendly and/or family-friendly settings. The Kāzīnū al-Būsfūr had special seating areas reserved for families (*al-Ahrām* 28 November 1924: 7). Many venues advertised ladies-only or families-only shows (e.g., *al-Ahrām* 16 September 1919: 3, *al-Ahrām* 1 October 1930: 6; see also Fahmy 2011: 122, 207 n. 116). Dinning describes whole families attending and enjoying the show at the Egypsiana Theater (Dinning 1920: 273–274).

The mixing of classes and genders that took place in Cairo's entertainment halls was a source of concern for some. Muḥammad al-Muwayliḥī, in *Ḥadīth 'Īsā Ibn Hishām*, uses a fictional account to debate the merits of turn-of-the-century Cairo theater (al-Muwayliḥī 2015, volume 2: 163–181). Three of the main characters, 'Īsā Ibn Hishām, the resurrected Bāshā (whom 'Īsā is trying to educate about present-day Egypt), and their unnamed Friend, attend a performance at a popular Cairo theater. Immediately, the narration highlights the flirtation between the women in the boxes and the men in the stalls, as well as the rowdy behavior of the mixed "horde" in the gallery (*ibid.*, 163–165). 'Īsā tries to argue for the positive, educational aspects of the theater:

> This is a theater, something that Western peoples acknowledge as having educational and corrective qualities. It encourages virtues, exposes evil traits, and portrays the deeds of former generations so that people can be educated and learn lessons from them [*ibid.*, 167].

The Bāshā retorts:

> What I've seen here is just a repeat of what I've observed in the dance hall—drinking wine, flirting with women, portraying amorous situations in a highly suggestive manner, one that's designed solely to arouse people's passions, make things more accessible and easy, and stir up lustful emotions [*ibid.*, 169].

The Friend, at the end of the long discussion, provides the last word:

> Passions cannot be cooled by enflaming them in the first place; moderation does not emerge from recklessness. We have a minor illustration right in front of us. If the woman who draws back the curtains in her box to flirt with men actually learned about chaste behavior from the play, she would be using her hand to pull the curtains closed again. But how can we claim she has learned something when the gaps in the curtains grow ever wider? [*ibid.*, 177]

These concerns are also captured in the novelist Najīb Maḥfūẓ's *Cairo Trilogy* (Mahfouz 2001). The *Trilogy* traces the life history of one Egyptian family, using it as a microcosm for the changes undergone by the Egyptian nation from the 1919 revolution to the 1952 revolution. The family's patriarch, al-Sayyid Aḥmad ʿAbd al-Jawwād, enacts harsh and strict discipline within his household, while he regularly engages in forbidden pleasures like music, dance, and sexual liaisons with popular *ʿawālim*. A particularly conservative man, even more so than other middle and upper class men of his day, al-Sayyid Aḥmad expects the women of his family to live a cloistered life. When his eldest son, Yāsīn, takes his young wife out one evening to visit the theater of Najīb al-Rīḥānī, al-Sayyid Aḥmad is outraged:

> He said, "Don't you know that I forbid my wife to leave the house even if only to visit al-Husayn? How could you have given in to the temptation to take your wife to a bawdy show and stayed there with her until after midnight? You fool, you're propelling yourself and your wife into the abyss. What demon has hold of you?" [Mahfouz 2001: 336–337]

Notably, Yāsīn's wife, Zaynab, is dumbfounded by his reaction, since her own father had taken her to the cinema more than once (*ibid.*, 335–336).

The mixing of Muslims, Christians, and Jews in popular entertainment venues was also a cause for concern. The Interior Ministry spy Muḥammad Saʿīd Shīmī Bik, in his notes to Khedive ʿAbbās Ḥilmī, decried the friendly multi-confessional atmosphere that he observed in Cairo's bars and music halls. "You see a Muslim drink a glass to the health of some Christian as if the Noble Quran had allowed him to drink wine just like the Christian religion does" (quoted in Cormack 2021: 42, see also HIL/15/81 in *Abbas Hilmi II Papers*).

As already noted, Cairo's entertainment halls enabled profound changes in Egyptian traditional entertainment. In these venues, Egyptians were able to experience familiar popular entertainments like music, song, and dance in a new way: not in the traditional social contexts of weddings, *mawālid*, and the like, but in structures that existed solely for the display of professional entertainment. Cairo's theaters and music halls were liminal spaces, where the indigenous interfaced with the foreign, and where tradition intersected with modernity. These venues were spaces within which Egyptians were able to experiment and innovate even as they asserted their ties to tradition.

Indeed, Egyptian artists and entertainers freely adopted and adapted foreign ideas and technologies toward Egyptian aesthetics and agendas, creating hybrid forms that found broad appeal with the Egyptian public. Over the course of the British occupation, Egyptians created hybrid cultural expressions in music, song, dance, and theater (Abou Saif 1973, Danielson 1997, Fahmy 2011, Gitre 2019, Ward 2018). Yet, even the most innovative of these hybrid creations bore a strong connection to traditional entertainment and reflected the desire of Egyptian audiences for performances with ties to indigenous aesthetics and concerns. Egyptian artists and entertainers of the late nineteenth and early twentieth centuries operated at the nexus of tradition and modernity, demonstrating their ties to the former even as they embraced the latter (see Armbrust 2001).

For example, the Egyptian actor and playwright Najīb al-Rīḥānī built his career on the hybridization of indigenous and foreign comic traditions. In crafting his earliest comedies, al-Rīḥānī merged the organizational, structural, and musical elements of French farce with the existing Egyptian comedic tradition of *faṣl muḍḥik*, creating a new style christened "Franco-Arab" (Abou Saif 1973). Yet, most of his stock characters were Egyptian and reflected contemporary Egyptian values and sensibilities, and his most famous creation, the character Kishkish Bik, was beloved by Egyptians of all ages and social classes (Abou Saif 1973, Fahmy 2011: 124).

Similarly, on the stages of Cairo's occupation-era entertainment halls, Egyptian belly dancers created a new, theatrical form of Egyptian belly dance, *raqṣ sharqī*, through the hybridization of the indigenous belly dance with elements derived from foreign dances (Ward 2018). Over time, the new dance came to incorporate a variety of technical elements from European and American music and dance, as well as from other Middle Eastern and North African dance traditions. By the mid-1930s, *raqṣ sharqī* had integrated the Western features of choreographed group dance and chorus lines, and dancers were increasingly accompanied by large musical ensembles that included a mix of indigenous and Western instrumentation.

Aspects of Western dance posture and alignment were absorbed into the dance by the 1930s; other non-native elements that eventually became part of *raqṣ sharqī* include elaborate traveling steps and complex arm movements generally considered to be derived from ballet and ballroom dance technique. Nevertheless, *raqṣ sharqī* continued to share core aesthetic and technical elements with the traditional belly dance of the *'awālim* and the *ghawāzī*. Most notably, these styles of dance were united by their fundamental movement vocabulary, the importance accorded to effective improvisation by a solo performer (even after the introduction of choreography into the dance), and the value placed on effective and emotive interpretation of Egyptian musical accompaniment.

Ties to earlier modes of traditional entertainment persisted in other ways. Though entertainment halls established a structural and social division between performers and their audiences, the easy and informal interaction between entertainers and spectators that had long characterized poplar entertainment in traditional settings could not be entirely eliminated. Entertainers frequently broke the "fourth wall" during performances, pausing to interact directly with audience members or with one another (Dinning 1920: 274–276). Audiences, for their part, expressed themselves by applauding, exclaiming, or throwing small coins or bouquets of flowers at the performers (Dinning 1920: 274–276, Giffin 1911: 39).

In some venues, a *muṭayyib*—an individual whose role was to loudly and repeatedly proclaim the excellence of the performance—was sometimes present (*Hopkinsville Kentuckian* 30 May 1899: 7). The profession of *muṭayyib* was rooted in traditional entertainment; Lagrange notes that during the latter half of the nineteenth century, the *muṭayyib* played an important role at private musical performances, where he acted as an intermediary between the audience and the performers (Lagrange 1994). In spite of efforts by theater managers and even the government to guide audiences toward Western-style theatergoing behaviors—sitting quietly, applauding at appropriate times, etc. (see Gitre 2019: 57–59), such interaction continued, particularly among lower-class audiences, who maintained much closer ties to traditional entertainment culture.

Offstage interactions occurred in the entertainment halls as well, particularly between female entertainers and male audience members in music halls, and these interactions were similarly rooted in traditional modes of entertainment. First, there is evidence of female dancers occasionally moving through their audience to collect tips. This practice is documented at El Dorado (Loewenbach 1908: 220, *Star* 20 September 1902: 2), and it likely took place at other venues as well (see *al-Zuhūr* November 1913: 359). Second, many female entertainers engaged in a practice known as *fatḥ* (literally, "opening," referring to opening bottles of alcohol), in which they sat with customers, drinking and socializing, in order to encourage spending. Van Nieuwkerk details the ubiquity of this practice in the entertainment halls of the 1920s and 1930s (1995: 43–45). However, it is clear that *fatḥ* was a well-established practice by the end of the nineteenth century (*al-Zuhūr* November 1913: 361). In fact, *fatḥ* was so common at the turn of the century that it was referenced in popular music (e.g., *Raqṣ Shafīqah* 1908).

The entertainment hall practices of tipping and *fatḥ* were formalized, structured evolutions of earlier traditional practices. Lane describes how early nineteenth-century *ghawāzī* were plied with brandy and tipped with gold coins:

> In some parties where little decorum is observed, the guests dally and sport with these dancing-girls in a very licentious manner. I have before mentioned (in a former chapter) that on these occasions they are usually indulged with brandy or some other intoxicating liquor, which most of them drink to excess. It is a common custom for a man to wet with his tongue small gold coins and stick them upon the forehead, cheeks, chin, and lips of a Gházeeyeh [Lane 2005 (1836): 494–495].

With *fatḥ*, the old custom of providing beer, brandy, or other spirits to female entertainers was turned to the financial advantage of the entertainment hall owner, as well as of the entertainers themselves, who received a portion of the profits from this activity.

At the intersection of foreign, indigenous, traditional, and modern, Cairo's entertainment halls were not merely spaces for experimentation and innovation in arts and entertainment. They were spaces within which Egyptians interrogated and challenged the social order, and even the notion of "Egyptianness," by means of music, song, dance, comedy, and drama. The acts presented on Cairo stages embodied contemporary social concerns, as well as the nationalistic sentiment that was growing among the Egyptian public. Overt expressions of Egyptian nationalism and resentment of the British occupation became common on entertainment hall stages in the years leading to the 1919 revolution. Fahmy notes that Najīb al-Rīḥānī's comedies frequently included explicitly nationalistic messages directed at the audience. For example, one of the songs featured in his play *Ish* (*Wow*) included a direct appeal for Egyptian national unity (Fahmy 2011: 127). Similarly, *Qūlūluh* (*Tell Him*) dealt specifically with the events of the 1919 revolution and included nationalistic songs composed by Sayyid Darwīsh (Fahmy 2011: 161).

The significance of these performances was not lost on contemporary foreign observers:

> With the lifting of the curtain on Egypt in 1919 we discover in Cairo a rude sort of musical comedy or operetta—though there is, in fact, no plot—in pure vernacular, sung throughout, with orchestral accompaniment, satirizing Cairo life. Although offered by the nationalist paper *Wadī-an-Nīl* and *al-Afkār* it has a nationalistic significance more profound than the demonstrations of agitators or the fulminations of Syrian editors. It is Egyptian in subject, language, presentation, and reception, without mentioning the flag-waving Fātima at the close [Worrell 1920: 135].

The relevance—and risk—of these performances was also recognized by the Egyptian government. The British authorities, with the support of members of the Egyptian elite, relied on censorship of the press and of the entertainment industry to stifle these expressions of Egyptian nationalism. A press censorship law, previously enacted in 1881, was revived in 1909 (Fahmy 2011: 103–105). Additional repressive measures were added during World War I, including restrictions on public gatherings (Fahmy 2011: 117–119). Until 1919, the censorship of the entertainment industry was more limited than that imposed on the Egyptian press. Nevertheless, entertainers risked censorship or suppression if they performed acts viewed as seditious. Sladen notes the existence of nationalistic theatrical performances that would cease if a European entered the room (Sladen 1911: 116–117). Nuzhat al-Nufūs, the coffee house where the famous singer Munīrah al-Mahdīyah performed in the 1910s, was frequently closed by the British due to the nationalistic character of the performances (Danielson 1997: 46–47, al-Ḥifnī 2001: 87). This sort of repression intensified during the revolution; theatrical activities were suspended for roughly one month in spring 1919 (Fahmy 2011: 160). During this time, many entertainers participated in demonstrations.

Besides giving voice to nationalistic sentiment, the acts presented in Cairo's entertainment halls also challenged the contemporary social order through subversive language and counter-hegemonic role reversals. Fahmy observes how comic sketches at the turn of the century satirized and mocked both the Egyptian aristocracy and the religious elite, portraying both groups as out of touch with the realities of ordinary Egyptian life (Fahmy 2011: 71). Lagrange details how the *taqtūqah* (plural *taqātīq*), a type of light song that was massively popular in the 1910s and 1920s, debated issues of gender and family structure in Egyptian society:

> *Taqātīq*, ostensibly "light" entertainment, in fact addressed such serious themes as the reconstitution of family around the nuclear model, the dangers of polygamy, the right to get acquainted to the bride or the groom before marriage, the dangers of girls' autonomy for a family's wealth, the minimum age of marriage, the way spouses should deal with their husbands' misconduct, working women and women in the police and the army [Lagrange 2009b: 229].

Rather than merely providing light entertainment, the acts presented on turn-of-the-century Cairo stages were important mechanisms through which Egyptians navigated and negotiated the realities of contemporary Egyptian society. Much like the shadow plays of Ibn Dāniyāl centuries before, turn-of-the-century Egyptian popular entertainment employed transgressive and counter-normative discourse variously to satire, spoof, critique, and interrogate Egyptian life.

Belly Dance and Its Professional Practitioners in Cairo's Entertainment Halls

By the end of the nineteenth century, belly dancers were a common sight in the entertainment halls of Azbakīyah. These venues enabled Cairo's female belly dancers to continue working, in spite of the ongoing and increasingly obtrusive government regulation of their trade. There is anecdotal evidence that male belly dancers sometimes performed in these spaces as well (see Chapter One). In this new performance setting, *raqṣ sharqī*, the new theatrical incarnation of the indigenous belly dance, gradually evolved—though the term *raqṣ sharqī* was not firmly associated with the new dance until the late 1920s or early 1930s (see Ward 2018: 63–65). At some turn-of-the-century cafés and music halls, *raqṣ sharqī* appears to have been the main attraction. According to a 1913 article in the Arabic-language magazine *al-Zuhūr*, there were nineteen venues dedicated to Egyptian dance in Cairo (*al-Zuhūr* November 1913: 359–360). Interestingly, the article asserts that the female dancers performing in these establishments were not only Egyptians, but Syrians, Persians, Moroccans, and Tunisians; however, all were performing Egyptian belly dance—the author uses the terms *raqṣ miṣrī* (Egyptian dance) and *raqṣ baladī* (indigenous dance) (*ibid.*).

One such venue was El Dorado, an establishment with an interesting and somewhat complicated history. El Dorado first appears in the historical record around 1870 (see Académie Royale des Sciences, des Lettres et des Beaux-Arts de Belgique 1870: 51). Sources at the time describe it as a *café chantant* situated on the tiny Ḥārat al- Ruway'ī, just off Mīdān al-Khazindār and to the northeast of the Azbakīyah Gardens (Hugonnet 1883: 290–291). In its early years of operation, El Dorado presented European-style variety entertainment targeted at a Western clientele. Various sources mention music (performed by an orchestra of European women), dance, theatrical performances (especially operettas), acrobats, and gambling. As early as 1878, there were plans to relocate the venue (Baedeker 1878: 229); by 1885, this relocation had taken place (Baedeker 1885: 231). The new El Dorado music hall was located just to the west of its predecessor, on the east end of Wajh al-Birkah Street (today known as Najīb al-Riḥānī Street), in one of the colonnaded buildings on the south side.

Immediately after the relocation, the venue continued to offer European-style variety shows (see *The Queenslander* 27 February 1886: 336), but this situation was soon to change. Multiple sources indicate that Egyptian singers and dancers were performing at El Dorado as early as the

1890s, and by the end of the century, Egyptian music, song, and dance were the venue's primary entertainment (although sources also indicate that the venue had a cinematograph for showing motion pictures) (Baedeker 1898: 24, Delmas 1896: 55–56, Loewenbach 1908: 218–220, Reynolds-Ball 1898b: 12). Interestingly, at some point around 1905 or 1906, the old El Dorado was resurrected; it operated as Ancien El Dorado, and the two El Dorados coexisted for some time. It appears that both venues presented similar entertainment, making it somewhat unclear which El Dorado is being described in sources from the 1900s and 1910s.

Both the old and the new El Dorado were owned by Greeks. The proprietor of the new El Dorado was Antoine Christou, while Ancien El Dorado was owned by Nikita Nikitaidis (the Egyptian Directory and Advertising Company, Limited 1907: 1062; Poffandi 1896: 77, 1901: 83, 1904: 92; Société Anonyme Égyptienne de Publicité 1912: 1267). As noted in Chapter One, many (if not most) of the entertainment halls that presented Egyptian dance in the 1890s and 1900s were owned and/or managed by foreigners—particularly Greeks and Italians.

These foreign-owned venues held a particular attraction for Egyptian dancers because of the protections afforded to them under the Capitulations. For additional legal and financial security, some female entertainers married these foreign proprietors. It appears that this was the strategy pursued by Tawḥīdah, the star of the Thousand and One Nights Theater (Mille et Une Nuits), a music hall located on Ḥārat al-'Usaylī, just east of the Azbakīyah Gardens. Tawḥīdah married the owner, a Greek named Manoli Ioannidis, and took over the establishment after his death (Cormack 2021: 267–268; Danielson 1991: 295; The Egyptian Directory and Advertising Company, Limited 1907: 1062; Poffandi 1901: 83, 1904: 92; Société Anonyme Égyptienne de Publicité 1912: 1267).

Music halls like El Dorado, and the women who plied their trades within them, were frequently portrayed in an unfavorable light, both by Egyptians and by foreign observers; al-Muwayliḥī compares the music hall to a battlefield, where "swaying buttocks and waists were like attack and retreat" (al-Muwayliḥī 2015, volume 2: 69):

> You observe every bare-breasted girl as she shouts, "Who's going to join us and compete?" Then she makes the rounds, prancing and strutting. Every man who desires to be in her company throws darting glances at her. She steers them all toward the wine casks, which proceed to gush forth with blood-red wine; she then splits open people's pockets which pour forth the blood of golden coins.... In the midst of this battlefield you could see a lewd tart in her dancing finery slithering around like a snake in its skin. She would toss her victims into an abyss, and you could watch people flattened like the stumps of desolate palm trees [*ibid.*, 71].

For al-Muwayliḥī, an educated journalist with ties to Egypt's aristocracy, the female singers and dancers of the music hall were temptresses who led respectable men to part with their money and with their morality. Nearly five decades later, Aḥmad Amīn echoed al-Muwayliḥī's representation of Azbakīyah's female entertainers (see above).

In general, foreign observers characterized Cairo's "native" music halls as seedy establishments, and just as in prior decades, foreigners were both repelled and captivated by the female professional entertainers who performed on their stages. While accounts generally depict the "dancing girls" as vulgar and unattractive—even grotesque—it is quite clear that they held an enduring fascination for foreigners, and the latter actively sought them out in the city's entertainment halls:

> Cairo abounds in Egyptian cafés, where dances by the *soidisant* members of the Ghawazee tribe are the sole attractions. They are, however, altogether lacking in local colour, and are, in fact, run by enterprising Greeks and Levantines for European visitors, and the performance is as banal and vulgar as at any *café chantant* in Antwerp or Amsterdam. The whole show consists of a few wailing musicians sitting on a raised platform at one end of the café, accompanying the endless gyrations of a stout young woman of unprepossessing features, who postures in particularly ungraceful and unedifying attitudes. Then her place is taken by another, equally ill-favoured and obese, who goes through the same interminable gyrations, to be relieved in her turn; and this goes on hour after hour. This strange "unvariety show" is, nevertheless, one of the established sights of Cairo, and is frequented in great numbers by tourists [Reynolds-Ball 1898a: 191–192].

As already noted, many of Cairo's entertainment halls were indeed owned by "Greeks and Levantines." However, Reynolds-Ball's assertion that these cafés were targeted at European visitors is belied by the numerous accounts of those European (and American) visitors, who generally observed that the audiences were dominated by native men (see, for example, Delmas 1896: 55–56, Loewenbach 1908: 218–220).

There are accounts which paint an entirely different picture than those just described. A particularly interesting anecdote was recorded by a woman named Etta Josselyn Giffin, an American librarian and pioneering advocate for the blind. Giffin visited Egypt in the course of her work for the American Association of Workers for the Blind, and she observed the following at a Cairo music hall:

> Several of us visited a native music hall where Egyptian girls danced and sang to the accompaniment of native musicians. The audience of native men smoked cigarettes, seldom speaking, except when specially pleased, when they would raise both hands toward the stage and call "Allah!" "Allah!" sometimes tossing coins to the singer who was a beautiful girl—who smiled and sang

> again and again. There were no words—only ah, or oh—or oo—but the tunes were full of suggestions and memories that charmed the initiated. To me they were sweetly clear, high notes with a peculiarly haunting, plaintive melody. There was no drinking and no boisterous behavior [Giffin 1911: 39].

Giffin, unlike the journalist al-Muwayliḥi, had no vested interest in Egypt's internal social and political conflicts. Moreover, her role as an advocate for a marginalized population seems to have prepared her to be a bit more tempered in her reactions to the people and activities that she encountered in the music hall than the average foreign tourist. Giffin's anecdote reminds us that many Egyptians—as well as some foreigners—did not share the moral qualms of individuals like al-Muwayliḥi regarding these venues and their performers.

Belly dancers were not limited to cafés and music halls. As noted previously, even in theaters, music, song, dance, and other variety acts were commonly included in the program. Dance performances (sometimes *raqṣ sharqī*, sometimes other styles) were often presented before or after the main act, during intermissions, or sometimes embedded within a play. This style of programming had become commonplace by the 1920s. A 1927 observer of Egyptian plays remarked: "In Egypt muscle dances and native songs are presented between the acts" (*The Brooklyn Daily Eagle* 23 April 1927: 3). Dinning describes a child performer who sang and danced during the intermissions at the Egypsiana:

> There is a little girl of eight amongst them—the pet of the company. She takes her part in dancing and in solo work during a succession of solos. She is petted in the most obvious way at the height of the performance in an informal manner that is inconceivable on the English stage. She likes it, and responds to it with childlike abandon. Between the acts she is often sent before the curtain to sing. This she does with a mature rhythmical body-motion that brings down the house. Then the house pets her; and she responds to that [Dinning 1920: 276].

Dinning's description of the child's "mature" movements suggest that she may have been performing *raqṣ sharqī*. During the same production, men comically imitated women's dancing:

> When the men's ballet that impersonates Bints comes on, the real Bints on the stage can never resist it. And certainly there is something irresistibly comic in the spectacle of men, with men's gestures and guttural voices, wearing yashmaks and attempting a falsetto voice to accompany their belly-dance, which none but a Bint can do [Dinning 1920: 275–276].

In advertisements for venues where dance was presented during intermissions or before/after the main act, the dancers are frequently identified by name, suggesting a higher level of fame or prestige for these performers.

Some of the dancers mentioned by name in advertisements from the 1920s include Līnā, Blanche Hānim, Afrānza Hānim, and Fatḥīyah al-Maghribīyah (*al-Ahrām* 19 December 1924: 7, 6 June 1925: 6, 3 April 1927: 5, 15 May 1927: 6, 1 June 1927: 6).

Without question, by the end of the 1930s, many female belly dancers had achieved celebrity status, and these women were a powerful force in shaping the Cairo entertainment landscape. They were not only multi-talented artists who sang, danced, and acted; they were entrepreneurs who owned and/or managed their own entertainment venues. Female artists like Badīʿah Maṣābnī, Bibā ʿIzz al-Dīn, Mārī Manṣūr, Imtithāl Fawzī, and the sisters Ratībah and Inṣāf Rushdī owned and managed popular venues on or near ʿImād al-Dīn Street (Van Nieuwkerk 1995: 46). These establishments were a step beyond the humble music halls of the 1900s and 1910s. Badīʿah Maṣābnī's Casino Opera, her last entertainment venture before leaving Egypt for Lebanon in 1950, boasted a theater, an "American" style bar, a rooftop terrace, and a restaurant (Figure 26). This grand multi-storied venue was situated just to the southwest of the opera house on Ibrāhīm Bāshā Square. Under new management (first Bibā ʿIzz al-Dīn, later Ṣafīyah Ḥilmī), this venue continued to thrive for many more decades, even after the temporary setback of the Cairo fire of 1952 (see next chapter).

Egypt's celebrity belly dancers, and the venues where they performed,

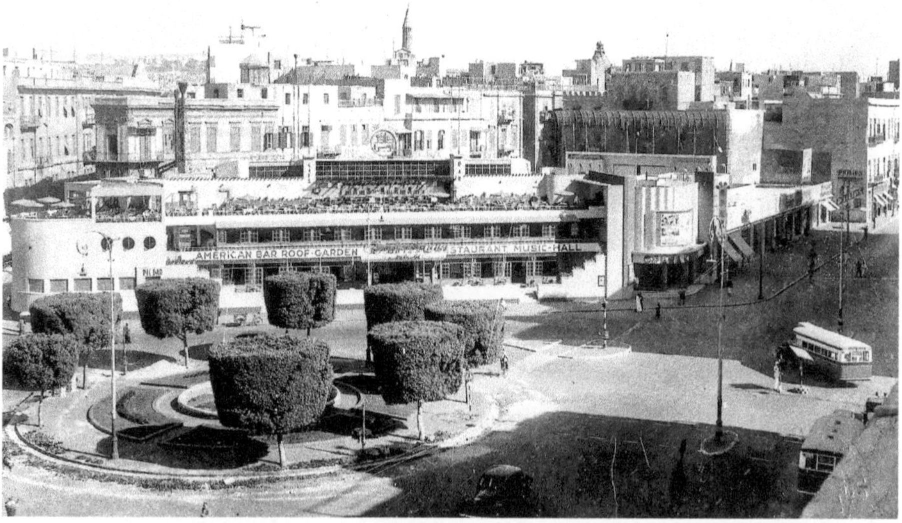

Figure 26: The Casino Opera (photo, *circa* 1940, copyright Dr. Edouard Lambelet, Lehnert & Landrock—Egypt).

came to figure centrally in the new medium of cinema. Egyptian films from the 1930s through the 1960s frequently included scenes that offered pretexts for dance performances, and many of these scenes were set in Cairo's popular nightclubs. Some of the biggest female stars to emerge in the early decades of Egyptian cinema were belly dancers who began their careers in the entertainment halls of urban Cairo: examples include Taḥīyah Carioca, Sāmiyah Jamāl, among many others. Egyptian films, as well as the many popular entertainment magazines that emerged in the 1920s and 1930s, shone a continual spotlight on famous belly dancers and the venues where they performed. Through films and magazines, many Egyptians who would never set foot inside a Cairo nightclub were able to imagine the experience, as well as to form opinions about these venues and the dancers who performed within them.

Muḥammad ʿAlī Street: A Rose Not Yet Fully Blown

In the early-to-mid twentieth century, the background business of Cairo's dancers, musicians, singers centered on Muḥammad ʿAlī Street. Finally completed in the 1870s, this broad boulevard's proximity to the entertainment zones of Azbakīyah, ʿImād al-Dīn, and vicinity, as well as the existing associations of nearby spaces with professional entertainment, attracted both professional entertainers and businesses with ties to the entertainment trades. Sayyid Ḥankish alludes to this reality in his recollections of his father, who started working as a musician in the 1940s: "My father first started working with the *ʿawalim*. They were living here in [Muḥammad ʿAlī Street] because it is near Azbakiya Gardens, Clot Bey Street, and the Downtown nightclubs" (Van Nieuwkerk 2019: 51). By mid-century, the street was lined with businesses connected to the entertainment trades: costumers, musical instrument manufacturers and sellers, record producers, and more. Professional entertainers resided on or near the street, and coffee houses provided gathering places for people of the trades. The majority of the entertainment-related businesses and residences of the twentieth century were located on the northern half of the street, extending from ʿAtabah Square southeast to the intersection with Būr Saʿīd Street (Khalīj Street).

The coffee houses of Muḥammad ʿAlī Street were crucial to the business of professional entertainers (Puig 2001, 2006). In these spaces, musicians and singers—and sometimes *ʿawālim* (Van Nieuwkerk 1995: 50)—gathered to wait for work as well as to negotiate with customers. These were also spaces where professional entertainers networked with one another and established their reputations. As Puig (2006: 518) writes,

"Musicians' cafés were initially the urban crossroads from which the musical and professional norms of the time were disseminated." Musicians who were launching their careers had to frequent the coffee houses in order to establish themselves among their peers. It was necessary to become a *ṣāḥib kursī*, literally, "owner of a chair," by regularly occupying a space in one of the local cafés (Puig 2006: 518–520).

Musicians gathered in coffee houses according to their music style and the type of instruments that they played (Puig 2001, 2006: 518). In general, there were two categories of cafés. The first were patronized by musicians from small brass ensembles known as Ḥasab Allāh bands (after the founder of the first such group). In the first half of the twentieth century, these bands were commonly hired to lead wedding processions. The second were frequented by musicians specializing in traditional Arabic instruments such as the *'ūd*, the *qānūn*, and the *ṭablah*. Initially, musicians specializing in Western instruments, such as the violin, had their own coffee houses in Tawfīqīyah (Puig 2001)—that is, in the vicinity of 'Imād al-Dīn Street.

The residences of Cairo's early twentieth-century *'awālim*, the popular female singer/dancers who entertained the urban lower and middle classes, were located along Muḥammad 'Alī Street and its neighboring streets and alleys (Figure 27). The majority of the *'awālim* resided in the alley that became their namesake: the Ḥārat al-'Awālim. Today known as Darb al-Madbaḥ, this tiny street starts at the busy intersection of Muḥammad 'Alī Street and Būr Sa'īd Street and runs southeast for a short way from there. This street existed *before* the establishment of Muḥammad 'Alī Street. In the late Ottoman period, it was known as 'Aṭfat al-Shaykh Baṭīkhah

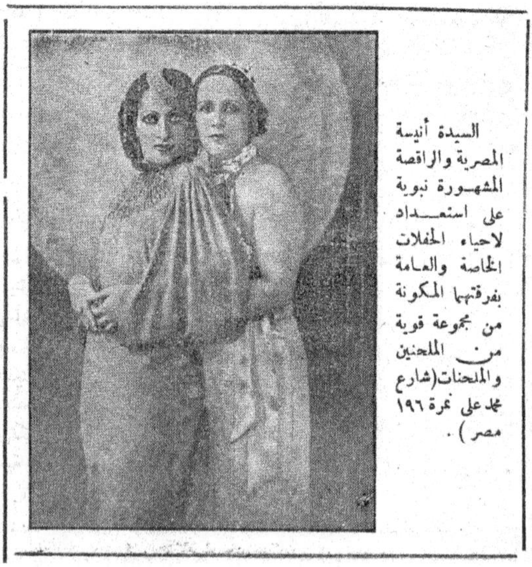

Figure 27: An advertisement for the *'awālim* Anīsah al-Miṣrīyah and Nabawīyah (Nabawīyah Muṣṭafa, who eventually transitioned to dancing in films), indicating their business address on Muḥammad 'Alī Street

(Jomard 1829: 151). Notably, it is situated just south of the site of the market for entertainers that was documented in the Mamluk era.

The *'awālim*, or else their male assistants, met with customers in an office or reception room (*salāmlik*) on the lower floor of their residence, or else in a local coffee house. Some famous *'awālim* owned substantial buildings in the area. After achieving success in the trade, the *'ālmah* Zūbah al-Klūbātīyah purchased a multi-story apartment building on Muḥammad 'Alī Street, just south of the Ḥārat al-'Awālim; the building came to be known as Ḥūsh Zūbah (Zūbah's Courtyard) (Riḍā Ḥankish, personal communication, February 1, 2022). This building still exists; it is partially owned by the Ḥankish family. The *'awālim* of Muḥammad 'Alī Street announced their services in signs hung outside their residences, as well as in advertisements posted in newspapers and magazines.

Many of the most famous *raqṣ sharqī* performers of the early-to-mid twentieth century hailed from Muḥammad 'Alī Street. Some of these dancers were *'awālim* who transitioned into the new performance circuit of entertainment halls and cinema. Such was the case with Nabawīyah Muṣṭafa, daughter of a popular *'ālmah* from Muḥammad 'Alī Street (*al-Muṣawwar* 1958). Others who may have had connections to the *'awālim* disavowed any association with these lower-class entertainers once they achieved celebrity. Na'amat Mukhtār, who grew up on Muḥammad 'Alī Street in a flat rented from the *'ālmah* Zūbah al-Klūbātīyah, denied any relationship to the *'awālim* (*About Naemet Mokhtar* n.d.).

Muḥammad 'Alī Street would remain at the heart of the business of professional entertainment in Cairo throughout the mid-twentieth century. At that time, the seeds of the street's decline were sown. From the 1960s onward, a perfect storm of social, political, and economic transformations, accompanied by profound changes to the social and spatial organization of Cairo, signaled the beginning of the end of Muḥammad 'Alī Street's significance within the Cairene entertainment landscape. These changes will be explored in detail in the next chapter.

Shifting Spaces within the Cairo Entertainment Landscape

In the early twentieth century, downtown Cairo, with its concentration of entertainment halls, and neighboring Muḥammad 'Alī Street, as the primary hub for the background business of professional entertainment, eclipsed all other spaces that had previously figured significantly in Cairo's entertainment landscape. The changes to the physiognomy of Cairo over the course of the nineteenth century and into the twentieth did not diminish the centrality of Azbakīyah and vicinity in Cairene life, nor did they erase the meanings that had been deeply inscribed into it. Rather, the establishment of formalized venues for professional entertainment in the landscape west of the old Khalīj reified its association with entertainment, recreation, and leisure and re-inscribed its heterotopic nature.

On the other hand, the physical transformations of Azbakīyah meant that the important annual festivals that had been centered there—specifically, the Nile flood celebration and the Mūlid al-Nabī—had to be relocated. These festivals continued to be celebrated, but without the deep attachments to certain spaces that had characterized them in prior centuries. Detached from the spaces with which they had long been associated, the nature of these celebrations was destined to change.

The celebration of the Nile flood, already impacted by the filling in of Cairo's lakes and ponds, was changed forever with the disappearance of the Khalīj. Without the canal, there was no dam, and without the dam, there was no need for a ceremony to open it. The flood celebration continued to be observed for a time at Fum al-Khalīj. However, in the early twentieth century, even this observation was scaled back. McPherson (1941: 11) notes:

> A decade or so ago, the evening celebrations, tashrifa, fireworks, and the rest were all together at the Fum el-Khalig, and there was a certain *Gemutlichkeit* about it which was quite lost when the reception tents were erected in a special enclosure on Roda Island, and the populace, not provided with special tickets, prevented by mounted police from crossing the bridge to it, and only able to hear the bands and see the fireworks from the other side of the water.

The completion of the first Aswan dam in 1902 (Raymond 2000: 324) meant the eventual disappearance of the annual Nile flood, an event that had defined the Egyptian year for millennia, and the Nile flood celebration gradually faded into irrelevance.

Already pushed to the west by Ismā'īl's developments in Azbakīyah, Cairo's Mūlid al-Nabī celebrations became increasingly decentralized. McPherson (1941: 35) writes:

> Even the greatest Cairene (and Islamic) moulid, that of the Nebi is not so typical, *qua moulid*, as those of Sidna Husein, Barsum el-Aryan, Sidi Bayumi and most of the others listed below because it does not centre round any spot specially hallowed by the Prophet. Even in my time it has been held in at least three different places. It is a general rather than local feast.

In the early twentieth century, the primary festivities were relocated several times: first to Fum al-Khalīj, later to locations in and around 'Abbāsīyah, to the northeast of the Fatimid city core (McPherson 1941: 264–265). 'Abbāsīyah was also the site of the *maḥmal* processions (*ibid.*,

264, 323–324), which continued for several more decades until disappearing around mid-century. Over the course of the twentieth century, the Mūlid al-Nabī became increasingly detached from any specific physical location.

Cairo's many other *mawālid* remained firmly tied to the shrines and tombs of their associated saints, and weekly *ziyārah* to shrines and cemeteries continued to be a popular practice. However, the increasingly residential character of the city cemeteries over the course of the twentieth century diminished their role as hubs within the Cairene entertainment landscape. While residential infrastructure had been a feature of the cemeteries for centuries, since it was necessary to accommodate both the resident caretakers and guardians of tombs and shrines as well as visitors, the influx of new residents throughout the twentieth century effectively transformed large portions of the cemeteries into lower-class residential neighborhoods (see El Kadi and Bonnamy 2007: 255–268).

Consequently, though the celebration of *mawālid* continued in these spaces, the carnivalesque atmosphere that they created was temporary. That is, outside of the time of the festival, these spaces were experienced as residential neighborhoods, rather than the persistently ambiguous and liminal zones they had been in prior centuries. Nevertheless, *mawālid* continued to impart meaning to the spaces in which they took place (Madoeuf 2006; Schielke 2006, 2009). Schielke (2009: 105), describing *mawālid* in the present day, writes:

> *Mulids* are among the few occasions when subaltern classes can exert a power of definition over the city. A *mulid* is an alternative way to organize urban space and time, one in which anyone can have his or her share. For the duration of the festival, this utopian order is a reality standing in open competition with other urban realities.

Within the temporal framework of the *mawālid*, Cairo's shrines and cemeteries continued to embody the heterotopic qualities that had characterized them in prior eras, but the ambiguity and liminality that the festival created was ephemeral and largely vanished upon its completion: after the *mūlid*, the space went back to being an ordinary residential neighborhood. Festive practice in the city's cemeteries and shrines was also impacted by increasingly heavy-handed government regulation of *mawālid*. McPherson (1941: 48) notes:

> Apart from supernatural intervention, the dominating influence most potent in determining the ultimate date of a moulid is that of the Ministry of Interior. Its permission must be obtained, and any limitations or postponement it may impose must be complied with. Occasionally it withholds permission altogether.

Such regulation would continue throughout the twentieth century and into the present day.

Nevertheless, professional entertainers, including both male and female belly dancers, were a common sight at these celebrations, and their presence contributed to the heterotopic nature of the *mawālid* festivities. At larger *mawālid*, there were tent theaters that featured variety entertainment, including belly dancers. At the 1934 *mūlid* of Ḥusayn, for example, the *ghawāzī* could be seen in a mile-long line of tent theaters neighboring the saint's shrine in Fatimid Cairo (McPherson 1941: 220). Male belly dancers like Ḥusayn Fu'ād were equally popular (McPherson 1941: 84–85). The transgressive nature of the dancers' performances prompted the intervention of the authorities, which the entertainers found creative ways to evade. McPherson (1941: 84) offers this colorful anecdote:

> When a few years ago, the city fathers (or grandmothers) or whoever it is who arbitrates somewhat arbitrarily on the matters of Terpsichore, vetoed the ancient "danse de ventre," and the public so clamoured for it, monotonous though it be, that the artistes, who moreover knew nothing else, lapsed into it, strange evasions were resorted to. On one occasion this dance was interrupted by a lad (set to watch), announcing that police were approaching the entrance. The première danseuse with great presence or mind, and imitated at once by the others, turned the other side towards the door, and danced with the muscle of that. There being no legislation against "la danse de lune" that was not deemed a contravention.

Belly dancers would remain a regular feature of popular *mawālid* until roughly the 1990s.

Conclusion

The story of Cairo's entertainment landscape in the era of the British occupation is the story of downtown Cairo and nearby Muḥammad 'Alī Street. The ascendance of Azbakīyah, 'Imād al-Dīn, and vicinity in the early twentieth century was the culmination of centuries of meaning making in the zone west of the old Khalīj. From the Fatimid period onward, this was an area firmly associated with entertainment, leisure, and vice in the popular imagination. It was also a zone of ambivalence and liminality, where the normal social and spatial boundaries of Egyptian society were blurred, challenged, or upended as diverse populations engaged in behaviors and activities that defied or disrupted the social order. Contrary to "dual-city" narratives that characterize Cairo's turn-of-the-century downtown as a fundamental break from the city's past, the landscape west of Khalīj Street carried forward these long-established meanings even through decades of extensive urban development and foreign occupation.

The entertainment halls which proliferated in Azbakīyah, 'Imād al-Dīn, and vicinity imbued a new physicality to these meanings. These venues tangibly reified the association of this part of Cairo with professional entertainment and reinforced the centrality of this area in the city's landscape of entertainment. As embodiments of ambivalence and liminality, these entertainment halls were physical manifestations of the area's heterotopic qualities. The ubiquity of belly dancers within their walls and on their stages ensured the ongoing connection of these professional entertainers to the zone west of the old Khalīj, and the presence of these marginal figures served to re-inscribe the heterotopic nature of the spaces where they lived and worked.

From the turn of the century, downtown Cairo, with its many entertainment halls, and neighboring Muḥammad 'Alī Street, home to the background business of professional entertainment, overshadowed other spaces that had once figured prominently in Cairo's entertainment landscape. Muḥammad 'Alī Street's easy proximity to the entertainment venues of Azbakīyah, 'Imād al-Dīn, and vicinity, together with the existing associations of nearby spaces with professional entertainment, attracted both professional entertainers and businesses with ties to the entertainment trades. Together, downtown Cairo and Muḥammad 'Alī Street formed the heart of Cairo's landscape of entertainment. This situation would hold true until the middle of the twentieth century: the beginning of a period of profound changes to Cairo's landscape of entertainment, as well as to the circumstances of professional entertainers.

Five

Revolution and Restructuring

In the 1930s and 1940s, the ongoing interference of the British in Egyptian administrative, fiscal, and political matters was a source of growing resentment among the Egyptian populace. Some steps were taken toward a more fully-realized independence. In 1936, shortly after the young King Farouk ascended to the throne, Egypt and Britain signed the Anglo-Egyptian Treaty (Vatikiotis 1991: 293). This agreement stipulated that the British would withdraw all their troops from Egypt, with the exception of those necessary to secure the Suez Canal zone. The following year, the Montreux Convention set in motion the abolition of the Capitulations, an action that would at long last bring foreigners under the jurisdiction of Egyptian law (*ibid.*).

Yet, the 1936 treaty contained provisions for an expanded British military presence during wartime, and with the onset of World War II, Egypt became an important base for Allied operations. The war exacerbated popular unrest at the ongoing British presence in the country, and anti-British sentiment led some in Egypt, including the king, to sympathize with the Axis Powers (Vatikiotis 1991: 345). Some Egyptians were drawn to extremist anti-Western, anti-secular political movements, such as al-Ikhwān al-Muslimūn (the Muslim Brotherhood, established in 1928) and Young Egypt (founded in 1933), adding to the climate of instability. In 1942, in an attempt to leverage the general popularity of the Wafd Party toward broader support for the war effort, the British pressured Farouk to form a Wafd government headed by Muṣṭafā al-Naḥḥās (Vatikiotis 1991: 350–351). Farouk acceded to the British demands, and the Wafd-controlled government was formed. This plan backfired, however, as the apparent complicity of the Wafd with the British led to the widespread popular rejection of the party.

Distrust of both the monarchy and the Wafd government festered within the Egyptian military. From 1882 to 1948, seditious elements had been unable to take root due to the tight control exerted by the British

(Vatikiotis 1991: 375). The old Egyptian army had been effectively disbanded in 1882, after the ʿUrābī revolt. After independence, attempts by the Egyptian government to expand and strengthen the army were stymied by the British, who invoked the national defense provisions agreed upon in 1922 and 1936. However, by 1948, all British troops had withdrawn to the Suez Canal zone, and the army was largely free of British influence and control. In this environment, anti-monarchical and anti-elite sentiment began to grow, particularly in the wake of the 1942 incident. With the army's disastrous defeat in the Palestine War in 1948–1949, many within the military began to advocate for radical change in Egypt's government. A group of young Egyptian officers, all from middle-class backgrounds, began to meet in 1949. Calling themselves the Free Officers, they began to actively recruit others to their cause.

In 1951, the Wafd-controlled government, perhaps under the assumption that it could win back popular support, unilaterally abrogated the Anglo-Egyptian Treaty. However, this action led many in the Egyptian public to the conclusion that any British military presence in Egypt was now illegal, and that British troops and installations were open to attack.

> Egyptian labour (between 60,000 and 100,000 strong) at the instigation of various political groups and organizations refused to work in British camps. Egyptian railways delayed or plainly refused to transport British supplies and personnel. Egyptian customs officials delayed clearance of goods destined for British bases; so did longshoremen and stevedores. Egyptian contractors and suppliers of British troops broke their contracts; tradesmen withdrew their services and businesses [Vatikiotis 1991: 370].

Simultaneously, guerrilla squads clashed with British troops, and demonstrations broke out in the cities and towns of the canal zone. The violence spread to urban Cairo: on January 26, 1952, most of downtown Cairo was set ablaze. In the midst of the chaos, the Free Officers made their move, and on July 23, 1952, the Egyptian monarchy was overthrown.

Amidst dissent within the Revolutionary Command Council, Gamal Abdel Nasser rose to power, ousting his fellow revolutionary Muhammad Naguib to become Egypt's second president in the wake of the 1952 coup. Nasser's socialist policies, including the nationalization of the Suez Canal in 1956, effectively ended foreign influence in Egypt, and Egyptian nationalism was tied to a broader vision of pan-Arab unity. Simultaneously, Nasser's regime improved the lives of ordinary Egyptians by legislating higher wages, shorter working hours, and better working conditions, as well as through the establishment of social services. These improvements came at a cost, however. Nasser was quick to consolidate his power, cracking down ruthlessly on dissent. Civil liberties were drastically curtailed; the Egyptian press was nationalized in May 1960 (Vatikiotis 1991: 397).

Still, Nasser was a widely popular figure in Egypt, owing in large measure to his personal charisma, and the public's loyalty enabled him to wield virtually single-handed control of the Egyptian state. Vatikiotis writes:

> The stability Nasser provided in Egypt by his charismatic personal rule stood in sharp contrast to the instability of the institutions he experimented with. During his rule he produced five parliaments with an average life of two years. He promulgated six constitutions. His cabinets had on average a lifespan of thirteen months. Even on the ideological front, Nasser exhibited successive changes in his commitment. The stability of his sixteen-year rule derived from his charismatic autocracy, or caesarist despotism. The President became the linch-pin of the new Egyptian political order. He had the right to interfere in all areas of national, political, social, economic and cultural life of the country.

Undoubtedly, Nasser's public image was carefully crafted to cultivate the affection and loyalty of the public, and the regime was effective at leveraging state media to this purpose. Nevertheless, it is telling that when he announced his intention to resign after the disastrous Six Day War of 1967, multitudes of Egyptians took to the streets to demand that he stay in office.

Anwar Sadat, one of the original Free Officers, assumed the presidency after Nasser's death, and to the surprise of many, he reversed course on much of his predecessor's agenda. At the outset of his presidency (1970–1981), he purged Nasserites from the government. Severing the ties with the Soviet Union that had been cultivated under Nasser, he instead sought to build Egypt's relationship with the United States. To the outrage of much of the Arab world (and many Egyptians), after the Arab-Israeli War of 1973, Sadat was instrumental in negotiating a peace deal with Israel in 1978, culminating in the peace treaty of 1979.

One of the most striking transformations of Egypt under Sadat was the dramatic rollback of Nasser's socialist economic policies. In an attempt to revive the private sector of the Egyptian economy, Sadat instituted an economic policy of *infitāḥ* (openness), which relaxed government controls over the Egyptian economy and encouraged private investment. Egypt experienced a temporary economic boom, thanks to an influx of foreign investment and international aid, as well as money sent home from Egyptian expatriates working in the Gulf States. However, boom quickly turned to bust, as the rapid influx of capital led to rampant inflation and real estate speculation (see El Kadi and Bonnamy 2007: 261–262, Raymond 2000: 349–350). The overall result of *infitāḥ* was to further widen the gap between the rich and the poor. Austerity measures were ill-received by the Egyptian public: cuts to government food subsidies resulted in the "bread riots" of 1977 (Vatikiotis 1991: 397).

While wielding largely authoritarian power, Sadat reintroduced a limited multi-party system, and reestablished some of the civil liberties that had been curtailed under Nasser. At the same time, he adopted a more tolerant attitude towards extremist Islamist organizations such as the Muslim Brotherhood, releasing many of the activists who had been imprisoned under Nasser. This decision proved to be fateful, however. Sadat's negotiations with Israel, together with his cultivation of closer ties to the West, were widely despised within these groups. Violence and rioting in the wake of the 1979 treaty, as well as increasing clashes between Muslims and Christians, led Sadat to implement a harsh crackdown on religious dissidents and other opposition forces. Viewing Sadat's actions at home and abroad as a betrayal, Islamist extremists conspired to assassinate Sadat, and on October 6, 1981, they succeeded.

Although Sadat took measures toward liberalism and democratization during his administration, the government of Egypt was far from democratic, and the legacy of autocracy that was established under Nasser would be more firmly entrenched under Sadat's successor, Hosni Mubarak (1981–2011). From the 1952 revolution until 2005, there were no presidential elections in Egypt; rather, the president was confirmed though a referendum. The election of 2005, touted as Egypt's first multi-candidate presidential election, was met with widespread allegations of fraud and intimidation by the Mubarak regime (Williams and Wright 2005). Autocratic rule was enforced by means of Egypt's Emergency Law. The Emergency Law, implemented after the war of 1967 but lifted in 1980, was reinstituted after the assassination of Sadat and remained in effect throughout Mubarak's presidency (Williams 2006). The Law enabled a variety of repressive practices, including indefinite detention without trial, the hearing of civilians by military tribunals, and censorship, and placed extensive limits on free speech and association.

The repression and abuses of the regime, as well as Mubarak's personal corruption and nepotism, contributed to popular discontent and resentment. Compounding these issues was the economic situation. From Sadat, Mubarak had inherited a legacy of inflation, rampant national debt, a bloated bureaucracy, and high unemployment. Throughout his presidency, Mubarak was largely unsuccessful in grappling with these problems. Egypt's population explosion in the latter half of the twentieth century exacerbated the strain on the economy, as millions of young Egyptians came of age in an environment offering them few opportunities for a stable livelihood. On January 25, 2011, popular protests erupted throughout the country—Egypt's third revolution in the span of 100 years—ultimately culminating in the resignation of Hosni Mubarak on February 11, 2011.

Egypt's Supreme Council of the Armed Forces maintained control of the country in the wake of the 2011 revolution, vowing to hand over power once parliamentary and presidential elections had been completed. Presidential elections were held in June 2011, and the winner was Muhammad Morsi, of the once-outlawed Muslim Brotherhood. In a prescient statement, Vatikiotis (1991: 445) writes: "In October 1981 the armed forces, and particularly the officer corps, still represented the most important constituency of the regime, and therefore of any Egyptian president. (One could even suggest that for some time to come, the Presidents of Egypt—and therefore the Vice-Presidents—will be military or ex-military men.)"

Indeed, just one year after Morsi took office, widespread public protests regarding the Islamist direction of the new regime provided the pretense for military intervention. On July 3, 2013, General Abdel Fattah El-Sisi, appointed as Defense Minister under Morsi, announced Morsi's removal from office and the suspension of the constitution (*BBC* 2020). Shortly thereafter, the military moved against the Muslim Brotherhood, resulting in the bloody massacres of Brotherhood supporters and other opponents of the military coup at Rābi'ah al-'Adawīyah and al–Nahḍah Squares. The following year, Sisi was elected to the presidency. As president, Sisi quickly clamped down on dissent. His landslide victory in the 2018 presidential contest, an election widely viewed as corrupt, was reminiscent of the Mubarak era. The words of Sisi provide an ominous hint at times to come: "Be warned, what happened seven or eight years ago will not be repeated in Egypt," he said in 2018. "You don't seem to know me well enough. No, by God, the price of Egypt's stability and security is my life and the life of the army" (*BBC* 2020).

Cairo After 1952

The population of Cairo, which by 1947 was already increasing at an unprecedented rate, more than doubled in the twenty year period from 1947 to 1966, and continued to grow (Raymond 2000: 339). The staggering growth was a result of both natural increase and rural-to-urban migration. The two factors were interrelated: Egypt's rapid demographic growth at mid-century far outpaced the resources available in rural areas, making internal migration inevitable. Rural Egyptians were drawn to the capitol by the prospects of employment and better living conditions, particularly during the period of Nasser's industrial and social reforms. From 1960 to 1966, Cairo absorbed 80 percent of Egypt's internal migrants (Raymond 2000: 342).

The city struggled to accommodate its new residents. Under Nasser, a number of urban planning projects were undertaken in an attempt to grapple with the rising population. Residential construction on the west bank of the Nile led to the emergence of middle-class neighborhoods such as al-Duqqī and al-Muhandisīn. Satellite cities, most notably Madīnat Naṣr, were planned outside the city boundaries. Housing for workers was constructed in Shubrā al-Khaymah, Ḥilmīyat al-Zaytūn, and Ḥilwān. New transportation infrastructure was established, including a number of bridges and the Ṣalāḥ Sālim highway. Alongside these planned urban developments were the spontaneous settlements that emerged at the city's periphery, and the city cemeteries, which were steadily transforming into residential neighborhoods. Some neighborhoods expanded upwards, as residents added additional floors to existing buildings.

The government's efforts were inadequate, however. Government spending was insufficient to keep up with the housing demand, and the neediest were often left by the wayside. For example, to accommodate the residents displaced by the construction of the Ṣalāḥ Sālim highway, the government established a public housing project in the cemetery of Imām al-Shāfiʿī. However, the residents evicted from the nearby unplanned settlements, "being eligible for neither compensation nor rehousing, found refuge in the cemeteries or went to build new homes, illegally, on the Muqattam hills, thus founding the new, unplanned settlement of Manshiyat Nasir" (El Kadi and Bonnamy 2007: 261).

The housing crisis was exacerbated under Sadat's *infitāḥ*. Real estate speculation surged, and land costs rose (El Kadi and Bonnamy 2007: 261–262, Raymond 2000: 349–350). Though housing was constructed (much of it without building permits), it was financially out of reach for the Egyptians who needed it the most. As a result, unplanned settlements mushroomed, particularly in the late 1970s and early 1980s. From the 1990s onward, these unplanned settlements have been referred to as *ʿashwāʾiyāt* (random things).

The Egyptian government has "pathologized" the *ʿashwāʾiyāt* (Singerman 2009, Dorman 2009). That is, beginning in the 1980s and 1990s, state-sanctioned discourse has characterized the *ʿashwāʾiyāt* as sites of backwardness, disorder, and criminality. Such discourse serves to "other" these communities (see Singerman 2009), presenting them as marginal aberrations to the city of Cairo, when in reality these neighborhoods have come to house well over half the city's population (Dorman 2009: 272). The state has approached these neighborhoods as a threat to order and security, particularly as anti-government Islamist movements have taken root within them. Yet, with a few exceptions, the Egyptian government has been largely unsuccessful in efforts to clear *ʿashwāʾiyāt*.

As Dorman notes, the state's inability to remove these communities had been due not only to the government's lack of material capacity and local resistance to state intervention: "...any comprehensive approach to urban informality requires giving such neighborhoods a measure of legal recognition and allowing them to develop a measure of social autonomy." Such an approach has not been imaginable under the regimes of Mubarak and Sisi, since providing a degree of legitimacy to the interests and agendas of these communities would constitute a threat to their centralized ideological and political control of the Egyptian state.

Government-planned settlements also began to emerge in the late 1970s, among them the desert towns of al-'Āshir min Ramaḍān (10th of Ramadan) and Sittah Uktūbar (6 October). These towns were initially intended to alleviate Cairo's population density and to promote industrial growth and employment (Raymond 2000: 354). However, Cairo's satellite towns have also served as a destination for middle and upper class Egyptians fleeing the city core. Since the mid–1990s, expensive gated communities have blossomed, both within the satellite desert towns, as well as along the Ring Road (Denis 2006). Cairo's elites have retreated to these exclusive havens, creating an exurban landscape that is radically distinct and detached from the realities of Cairo proper. The gated communities are characterized by an array of amenities that are removed spatially and socially from the vast majority of ordinary Cairenes: golf courses, malls, amusement parks, and private universities and hospitals. Denis (2006: 50) writes:

> At the center of this new way of life are Egypt's elites, themselves connecting together the archipelago of micro-city communities that they administer as if they were so many experimental accomplishments of a private democracy to come. The gated communities, like a spatial plan, authorize the elites who live there to continue the forced march for economic, oligopolistic liberalization, without redistribution, while protecting themselves from the ill effects of its pollution and its risks.

As these "private democracies" have thrived, ordinary Egyptians have continued to experience broad-scale repression and disenfranchisement.

Today, the well-to-do who remain in the city core isolate themselves in elite bastions such as Zamālik. In these elite zones, Egyptians who can afford to do so have embraced aspects of Western leisure culture, patronizing shopping malls and coffee shops—the latter not to be confused with the traditional Egyptian coffee houses that abound in lower-class neighborhoods (Abaza 2006, De Koning 2006). Although located within the city of Cairo, these elite neighborhoods are as socially distant from the lived experiences of most ordinary Cairenes as the gated communities far off in the desert.

Taken together, these massive demographic shifts, together with the frantic ongoing urban development (both planned and unplanned) to accommodate these new realities, have drastically altered the social and spatial make-up of the city. The organization that characterized the city throughout the developments of the late nineteenth and early twentieth centuries—the Fatimid core to the east of the old Khalīj, the newly-developed zone to its west, and suburban expansions pushing to the north, west, and south—has been utterly transformed. The city has metamorphosed into a whole that is diverse and disjointed; as Raymond (2000: 361) writes: "The faces of the city blur; its centers are many and mobile." These many centers are sorted as either *rāqī* (classy or refined) or *baladī/sha'abī* (popular or lower-class) according to the socioeconomic class of their residents, the principal business activities, land costs, population density, and the quality of local infrastructure. Fundamentally, Cairo's present-day organization reflects the massive and ever-widening gulf between rich and poor.

State Intervention versus *Private Enterprise: Implications for Cairo's Entertainment Landscape After 1952*

The social, political, and economic transformations that have convulsed Egypt since 1952, together with the changes to the social and spatial organization of Cairo described above, have had profound ramifications for the city's landscape of entertainment. The Egyptian government's interventionist approach to arts and entertainment since the Nasser era has been unprecedented, leading to the state's direct involvement in changes to music, dance, and other types of professional entertainment. Simultaneously, the liberalization of the Egyptian economy since Sadat has drastically altered the entertainment market, with serious and lasting implications for professional entertainers and the spaces where they have plied their trades. These factors, as well as the structural reorganization of the city since the 1950s, have resulted in a restructuring of the entertainment landscape.

The Revolution of 1952 was rooted in a militant Egyptian nationalism that was firmly anti-Western and anti-elite. The post-revolutionary government emerged under the banner of "Egypt for Egyptians," and with the disruption of the wealth and power of the ruling class and foreign interests, the regime appeared to be taking the first steps toward a more equitable Egyptian society. Yet, the autocratic tendencies that have characterized the Egyptian government until the current day were already present, manifesting as early as the late 1950s in the state's approach to ideological and cultural matters. Early on, Nasser recognized the importance of centralized and controlled ideological messaging for maintaining the authority and legitimacy of the regime, and mobilized the government and the media toward this end.

In "culture"—that is, in cultural expressions such as the fine arts, literature, music, theater, and folk dance—the Egyptian government found an important mechanism for propagating its vision of Egyptian nationhood. This was an ideology of popular unity that celebrated the "ordinary folk" of Egypt, including the lower classes and the rural peasantry. Yet, the policies and messaging of the regime were driven by the interests and agendas of urban, educated, middle- and upper-class Egyptians, and though the Egyptian "masses" were key to its construct of "authentic Egyptiannness," the government found it necessary to elevate them to an enlightened modernity. As Armbrust (1996: 39) writes: "Even during the Nasserist period, however, 'peasant culture' was something to be transcended." Accordingly, though ostensibly celebrating the folk culture of the masses, the state was careful to "sift" Egypt's heritage of folk culture, assigning value to that which fit within the state's vision and rejecting as "vulgar" or "backward" that which did not.

The regime assigned many activities and institutions related to culture to the Ministry of National Guidance, which was reorganized in 1958 as the Ministry of Culture and National Guidance, later simply the Ministry of Culture (Winegar 2009). The Ministry of Culture was based on French and Soviet models—the latter, in particular, providing the model for centralized messaging. Shortly after the creation of the Ministry, the government established its network of *qusur thaqafa* (culture palaces) throughout the country, which served to enact the policies of the Ministry at the local level. The state also began subsidizing a number of entertainment venues throughout Cairo, including many of the city's theaters. With the Ministry of Culture, the Egyptian government assumed a direct and intrusive role in the definition of Egyptian cultural and national identity by means of arts and entertainment: "The major goals at the time remain central to the Ministry's mission today: to define the nation and national identity; to protect cultural patrimony; and to uplift the so-called masses by exposing them to the arts" (Pahwa and Winegar 2012).

The Ministry of Culture, though scaled back under Sadat, was ramped up under Mubarak (Pahwa and Winegar 2012). In 1989, the General Authority of Cultural Palaces was created. As a result, hundreds of additional cultural palaces and cultural houses were established. The Mubarak era introduced an explicitly secularist orientation to the Ministry, no doubt a reaction to Egypt's Islamic revival. Ministry officials complained of what they viewed as a loss of Egyptian cultural identity, a loss which they framed as both cause and effect of the Islamic revival.

> Clearly, Egyptian Ministry of Culture officials and secularist intellectuals have decided that the rise in public piety and religious activism require them to instrumentalize culture in order to civilize certain Egyptians, and Islamic religious practice in particular.... Elites seek to train Egyptians in what they see as enlightened Islam: interpretations and practices that do not challenge their privilege, their ideology of the good society, or the state's aim to create national citizen-subjects [Winegar 2009: 196].

This secularist trend has persisted under the current regime, with the Ministry of Culture utilized as an important tool in combating Islamic extremism while simultaneously promoting a state-sanctioned vision of moderate Islam (*Ahram Online* 2022, Croitoru 2015). Today, the Ministry continues in its foundational goal of propagating the state's ideology of nationhood through the production and dissemination of culture. As was the case under Nasser, "culture" remains a potent tool for supporting the interests of the present regime.

> This, then, seems to reveal the battle plan chosen by the Field Marshal. TV, theatre, music, and literature—these are the weapons, and the battlefield is the minds of Egyptians. With canned book fairs and empty theatres, Egypt will convince the world that everything is fine and that everyone loves Sisi.... The Minister of Culture said that this is 'no time for democracy' while songs celebrating Sisi and calling on him to run for president blare across TV screens. With every national event, we find theatrical celebrations filled with stars singing to Sisi, with Sisi then remarking, "Don't you know that you're the light of our eyes?" [Naji 2014]

The numerous cultural palaces and cultural houses, together with state-subsidized entertainment venues, continue to provide the physical manifestations of the regime's ideology, penetrating the social and spatial reality of Egyptians in Cairo and beyond.

In addition to the Ministry of Culture, the Egyptian government has leveraged its influence over professional syndicates in order to propagate state-sanctioned "culture." Though ostensibly voluntary and democratic bodies designed to protect the professional interests of members, the on-the-ground reality of these trade unions is much different (see Ramadan 2021). With regard to the three syndicates of performing artists—al-Naqābat al-Mihan al-Mūsīqīyah (the Musicians' Syndicate), al-Naqābat al-Mihan al-Tamthīlīyah (the Theatrical Professions Syndicate), and al-Naqābat al-Mihan al-Sīnimā'īyah (the Cinema Syndicate)—membership has been effectively weaponized as a means to regulate cultural production. Individuals must acquire a permit from the appropriate syndicate in order to practice their respective trades. Yet, a syndicate may refuse or revoke permits to individuals deemed "unfit" according to the union's standards. The artistic syndicates have been increasingly cooperative with the agendas and interests of the regime; recently, the syndicates were accorded judicial authority over individuals falling under their purview (Essam El-Din 2021). Ramadan (2021) notes:

> Coordination has increased in recent years between artistic syndicates and security authorities on the one hand and regulatory agencies on the other hand. This was evident in the position of the musicians syndicate, headed by Hany Shaker, when it launched a fierce media and security campaign to ensure the implementation of the ban on Mahraganat (festival) singers. The syndicate filed complaints against a number of those singers, either for singing in public places or for releasing new music videos online.

Notably, professional belly dancers do not have their own trade union; rather, they are included within the Theatrical Professions Syndicate. Though they are required to register with the union (and pay dues), their permits stipulate that they are not entitled to the same protections and benefits afforded to other union members (Farah Nasri, personal communication, December 20, 2022).

As discussed in Chapter One, the state's direct involvement in the arts and entertainment industry has had a dramatic impact on the trajectories of traditional professional entertainment genres, particularly belly dance. The Egyptian government since 1952 has sanctioned and supported cultural expressions that fit within its broader vision of Egyptian nationhood, such as theatrical folk dance, with its quaint portrayals of rural folk life. Simultaneously, the state has rejected and marginalized cultural expressions that deviate from the accepted vision, such as the various form of belly dance. Belly dance, with its frequent transgression of gender norms and its lower class associations, has been deemed vulgar, an unfit representation of Egyptian culture. Meanwhile, the government's steady push towards professionalization and institutionalization in arts and entertainment by means of the Ministry of Culture has meant that traditional forms of entertainment, which generally lack formalized training or credentialing methods, are pushed further into the margins.

The effects of state interventionism on belly dance have been exacerbated by the economic liberalization policies that began under Sadat. While the temporary economic boom brought on by Sadat's *infitāḥ* ensured that there was abundant work and high pay, it also initiated an influx of outsiders into the trade—that is, individuals with no prior connection to the entertainment trades who were drawn to the prospect of steady employment and high income. As boom turned to bust, belly dancers found themselves in an oversaturated market with declining demand.

As noted in Chapter One, the mass inflow of these outsiders disrupted the traditional networks that had been cultivated by professional entertainers in Cairo for centuries. Female dancers began to lose control over their trade, as individual dancers increasingly aligned with male impresarios. In the present day, male impresarios continue to exert a high degree of control in booking performances, setting fees, and other aspects of the business.

The short-lived economic boom under Sadat also prompted a proliferation of nightclubs and cabarets catering both to local big-spenders as well as to foreign tourists. Many of these venues were situated within tourist-oriented sites, such as five-star hotels and Nile cruise boats. Sahin (2018: 68) writes:

> Due to Egypt's independence and opening of the economy, a boom of stratified venues opened that regularly featured raqs sharqi performances. Five-star hotels began springing up, particularly along the Nile, featuring nightclubs that began hosting regular raqs sharqi shows as a way to keep affluent guests spending within the hotel rather than outside of it in an upscale and family-friendly atmosphere. On the heels of the five-star hotels, Nile cruising dinner ships began regularly featuring a packaged entertainment deal of tourist-oriented and family friendly live music, raqs sharqi, and tanoura as the entertainment portion of a 2-hour cruise.

Others began to spring up along Haram Street, a long boulevard extending southwest from Cairo University to the Giza necropolis. In more recent times, cabarets and nightclubs have emerged within a number of permanently-docked boats along the Nile.

Importantly, many of the entertainment venues that have appeared in Cairo since the mid-twentieth century have emerged *outside* the traditional entertainment zones of the city. This marks an enormous departure from the past. From their first appearance in Cairo, venues dedicated to professional entertainment, such as theaters and music halls, were clustered in the area to the west of the old Khalīj. Initially centered in and around Azbakīyah, Cairo's entertainment halls eventually migrated west, with most situated along 'Imād al-Dīn Street and its cross streets. From the mid-twentieth century onward, entertainment venues were unmoored from this space. Many cabarets and nightclubs were tucked away inside hotels and boats, allowing them to exist in neighborhoods far removed from the zones that had so long been associated with professional entertainment. In the present day, many of these venues are situated in the most affluent and privileged areas of the city, such as Zamālik, Heliopolis, and the like, and are financially out of the reach of the vast majority of Cairenes.

Morley (2023: 63–67) provides an excellent overview of the differently classed venues that exist at the present moment, as well as their general locations throughout the city. While venues catering to different social classes certainly existed in the past, recent years have seen a proliferation of venues targeted toward an elite clientele, and the current wealth gap between Egypt's moneyed elites and the rest of the population means that nightclubs and cabarets are far less accessible to ordinary Egyptians than in past decades.

The net result of these factors has been the transformation of Cairo's entertainment landscape in a manner that intersects with the massive structural changes to the city of Cairo since the 1960s: the traditional organization that developed over the course of many centuries has disintegrated into a diverse and many-centered patchwork. From the mid-twentieth century onward, Muḥammad ʻAlī Street and downtown Cairo have declined precipitously from their roles as anchors within the Cairo entertainment landscape. These neighborhoods of Cairo are now generally classed as *baladī/shaʻabī* (popular or lower-class) and, therefore, undesirable. Simultaneously, professional entertainment has diffused into locations scattered throughout the city. These include government-subsidized venues such as the culture palaces and the various theaters that present state-sanctioned forms of arts and entertainment (such as theatrical folk dance), cinemas, a few independent theaters, and the innumerable nightclubs and cabarets, many of which continue to feature belly dance as their main attraction.

Yet, even as Cairo's entertainment landscape has fragmented, the meanings embedded in certain spaces have persisted. Some of these spaces, such as Muḥammad ʻAlī Street, continue to be firmly associated with professional entertainment in the popular imagination, in direct contradiction to present-day realities. Others, such as the streets neighboring the old Azbakīyah Gardens, have largely lost their association with professional entertainment, but continue to be perceived with ambivalence nonetheless.

Downtown Cairo: Continuity and Change

As detailed in the previous two chapters, the changes to the city of Cairo that took place in the late nineteenth and early twentieth centuries did not erase the meanings that had been inscribed into the Cairo entertainment landscape since the Fatimid era. The "dual city" characterization of Cairo west of Khalīj Street as "modern" and/or "colonial" Cairo ignores the pre-existing relationship between these two areas of the city and how that relationship was reified even as urban development projects altered the face of the city. The idea that this "modern" Cairo represented a fundamental break from the past disregards the manner in which long-established meanings persisted throughout the extensive urban developments of Ismāʿīl, the throes of occupation, and the influx of foreigners into the city.

From the Fatimid era onward, the zone to the west of Cairo's old Khalīj had been established as a heterotopic space, a space "outside of all places." This area of Cairo had long existed "outside" the rest of the city: not just in terms of geography, but in terms of its very nature. This was a zone of ambivalence and liminality, where the normal social and spatial boundaries of Egyptian society were blurred, challenged, or even upended as people from radically different social contexts converged, engaging in carnivalesque behaviors and interactions. From the late nineteenth century until the mid-twentieth century, this part of Cairo continued to be characterized by its heterotopic qualities. It remained a zone of confluence among diverse populations, all brought together in a space firmly associated with entertainment, leisure, and vice.

The entertainment halls which proliferated here in the late nineteenth and early twentieth centuries imbued a new physicality to these meanings. The formalized entertainment venues of Azbakīyah and vicinity tangibly reified the association of this part of Cairo with professional entertainment and reinforced the centrality of this area within Cairo's landscape of entertainment. As embodiments of the ambivalence and liminality that had long characterized Cairo west of the old Khalīj, these entertainment halls were physical manifestations of the area's heterotopic qualities. The widespread presence of belly dancers within these venues ensured their ongoing connection to the landscape west of the Khalīj, and the presence of these marginal figures served to re-inscribe the heterotopic nature of the spaces where they lived and worked.

From the turn of the century onward, this area constituted Cairo's downtown, encompassing the neighborhoods of Azbakīyah, Tawfīqīyah, and Ismāʿīlīyah. Describing downtown Cairo in the early decades of the twentieth century, Ryzova (2015: 9) writes:

> This is where the elites, both national and foreign, lived and where modern businesses, services and institutions were located. It was an area of upscale shopping and leisure establishments. While in many ways exclusive, Downtown was also always heterogeneous and predicated on drawing in publics from all over the city, even if temporarily. Middle-income Egyptians flocked there to partake of the many pleasures it had to offer. Downtown's grand magasins catered equally to solvent outsiders, and middle-income families otherwise labelled as "traditional" came here for their seasonal shopping. Cabarets and cinemas along Emad ElDin Street, the city's prime

> entertainment district, catered to a variety of audiences, including provincial youth visiting the brothels on its fringes; and of course many a middling youth, efendi student from near or far, came here simply to wander, window shop and check out the next movie on lobby cards.

The social and spatial centrality of downtown in Cairene life would persist even through significant changes to the resident population there from the 1930s through the 1950s. This period witnessed a large-scale exodus of foreigners from downtown Cairo (and from Egypt in general), and their departure enabled the influx of upwardly mobile Egyptians into the neighborhood. This demographic shift was in process even before the anti-British demonstrations that culminated in the Cairo fire of 1952. Although the fire devastated much of downtown, including its popular entertainment venues, the area quickly rebounded (Figure 28). For example, the grand Casino Opera, which had been gutted by the fire, was soon back in business.*

The influx of new Egyptian residents resulted in a brief florescence of downtown and its centrality to Egyptian narratives of national modernism at mid-century. Though well-to-do Egyptians eventually began to abandon downtown in favor of upscale suburban and exurban neighborhoods, it remained a popular destination for shopping and entertainment throughout the 1970s and 1980s, even among middle and upper-middle class Egyptians who resided elsewhere.

However, in the wake of Sadat's *infitāḥ* policies and the ever widening gulf between the haves and have nots in Egyptian society, downtown began a slow and inexorable decline. While high-end shopping centers, cinemas, and theaters began to emerge to serve the well-to-do populations of fashionable neighborhoods, downtown became a marketplace for cheap (and black market) goods and a destination for budget entertainment (Figure 29). As downtown increasingly attracted the poorer segments of Cairene society for shopping and leisure, Cairo's elites rejected it in favor of the shopping centers and entertainment venues situated within the comfort of their own neighborhoods and gated communities (Puig 2006: 532). By the end of the twentieth century, it was commonplace to hear downtown referred to as a *baladī/sha'abī* area (Armbrust 2006: 418).

Indeed, downtown Cairo—particularly 'Imād al-Dīn Street and the streets to its west and southwest—remains a popular leisure and entertainment destination for lower and lower-middle class Cairenes, lending to its ongoing perception as a space of entertainment, albeit lower class (Figure 30). Budget cinemas remain fairly common along 'Imād al-Dīn Street and

* It is briefly visible in British Pathé footage of Cairo night life in 1964, along with an array of other venues in downtown Cairo and on Haram Street (*Cairo* 1964).

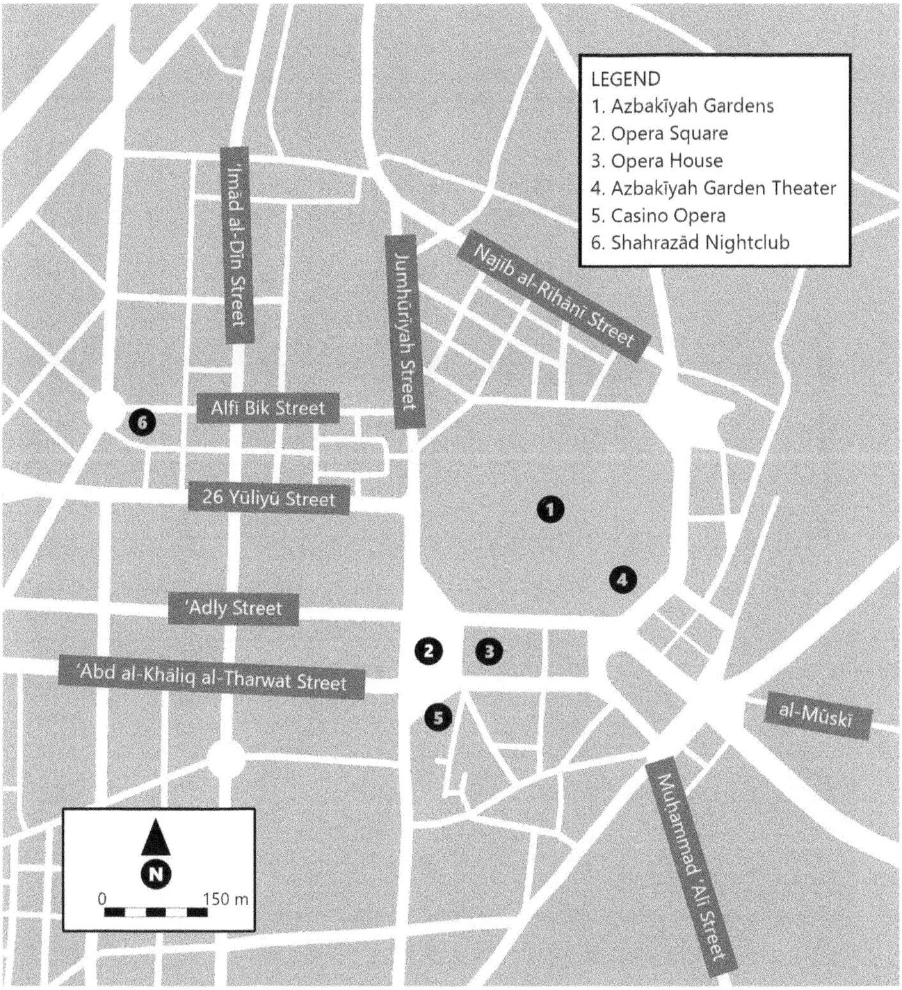

Figure 28: Downtown Cairo in the mid-to-late 1950s, showing some of the main thoroughfares and several sites mentioned in the text (map by the author).

vicinity; there are a few theaters as well. A handful of downtown Cairo's old nightclubs remain, and belly dancers continue to be featured on their stages. One of these is the Shahrazād, located on Alfī Bik Street. Shahrazād began its life in the 1910s as a music hall called the Abbaye des Roses. Just across the street, the New Arizona cabaret continues to function. These spaces ensure the continued presence of female professional belly dancers in downtown Cairo and contribute to downtown's ambiguous reputation.

Nevertheless, Azbakīyah and 'Imād al-Dīn Street no longer form the heart of Cairo's entertainment landscape. Rather, downtown's remaining

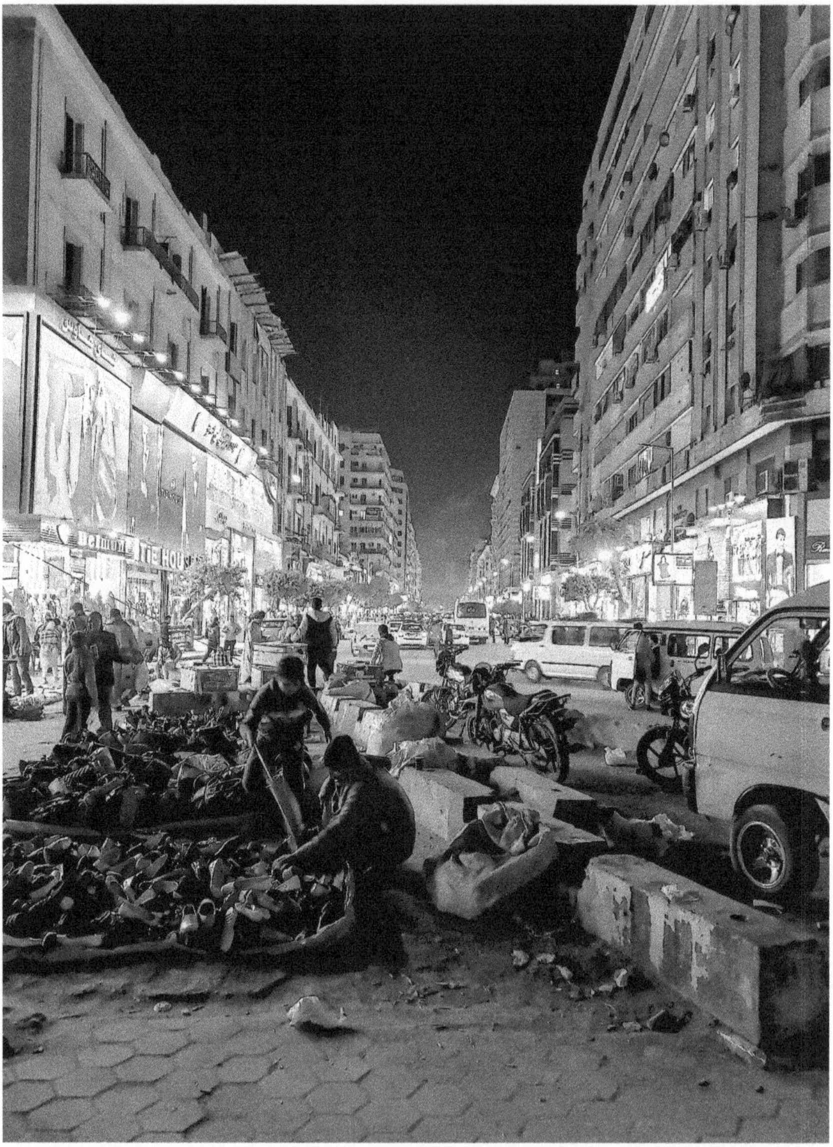

Figure 29: 26 July Street, looking west (photo taken by the author in 2022).

cinemas, theaters, nightclubs and bars vie with a seemingly countless array of such destinations now scattered throughout the city. The latter are found along Haram Street, in boats on the Nile (some permanently docked, others cruising), within the confines of hotels and malls, and at various other locations throughout Cairo. Still, it is noteworthy that in

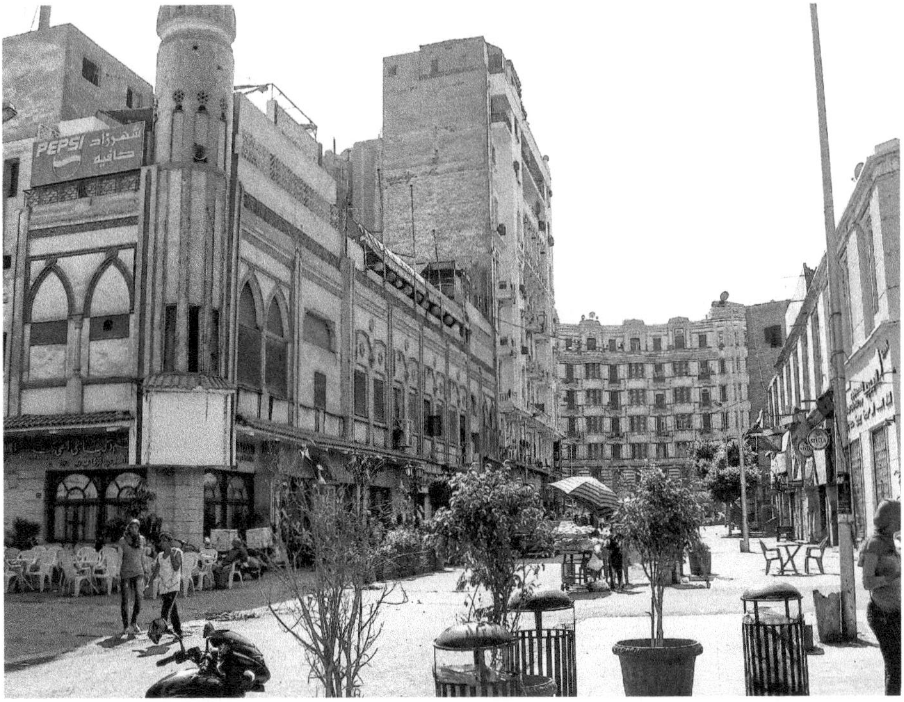

Figure 30: Alfī Bik Street, where the Shahrazād and New Arizona cabarets continue to function (photo taken by the author in 2014).

spite of all these changes, this part of Cairo retains its centuries-long association with entertainment, leisure, and vice.

Also striking is the persistence of this area's heterotopic features. Cairo's downtown remains a space of ambivalence and liminality. Particularly in the evenings and during holidays, when people converge along the wide boulevards to stroll, shop, and socialize, downtown Cairo is a space where social norms are blurry and ambiguous. Armbrust (2006: 421) writes:

> In its leisure mode downtown is also a place where one can be anonymous. Few of the people who go downtown for leisure purposes actually live there. Downtown at night is neutral territory removed from the eyes of elders, and out of the grasp of social institutions. This means that social norms are at least partially relaxed, and that the young people who frequent the area can engage in a certain amount of experimental behavior that may conflict with the social patterns of everyday life.

Downtown's ambiguity and liminality also make it a space where counter-hegemonic narratives have been able to thrive (see Ghannam 2016, Meital 2007, Ryzova 2015). Though Ryzova focuses on downtown

Cairo's non-hegemonic turn following the demographic and economic shifts of the 1970s and 1980s (see Ryzova 2015: 18), it is important to bear in mind that this part of Cairo has long been a site of transgressive and counter-hegemonic discourse. One need only look to the acts presented on the stages of Cairo's early twentieth-century entertainment halls to find examples of discourse that has interrogated and challenged the existing social order (see Fahmy 2011, Gitre 2019). Moreover, these acts were informed by a long historical legacy of transgressive popular entertainment: shadow plays, puppet shows, dance performances, and raunchy comic skits, all performed and enjoyed for centuries in the heterotopic zone west of the old Khalīj.

The Decline of Muḥammad 'Alī Street

As already noted, the influx of outsiders into the entertainment trades in the 1970s disrupted the traditional networks of Muḥammad 'Alī Street's professional entertainers and spurred the rise of the male impresario system for female dancers. These factors, together with the waning significance of downtown within Cairo's entertainment landscape and the dispersal of professional entertainment to locations throughout the city, ensured the street's rapid decline as an entertainment hub. Puig (2006: 520) writes:

> The marginalization of the street has not benefited any other area in particular. The less geographically concentrated and distinctive new spatial organization of the music industry in town reflects the diversity of aesthetic styles and artistic waves that also arose in the 1970s. The sprawling urban recomposition of Cairo and the increased mobility of all classes have also influenced the town's musical spaces. These urban changes are accompanied by a renewing of centralities and a polylocalization of cultural practices.

The street could not maintain its centrality in the diverse and disjointed entertainment landscape that emerged in the latter half of the twentieth century. Muḥammad 'Alī Street became home to an array of small businesses catering to the domestic needs of nearby residents; furniture shops replaced musical instrument sellers along the northern half of the street. As Puig notes, the street has "contracted on itself and its direct surroundings—the districts of Darb al-Ahmar, 'Abdîn and Muskî" (Puig 2001). Today, Muḥammad 'Alī Street, like these neighboring districts, is recognized as a *baladī/sha'abī* area (Puig 2006: 521).

Rather than clustering on or near Muḥammad 'Alī Street, the residences and businesses of professional entertainers came to be dispersed throughout the city, pulled toward new and emerging entertainment centers, such as the cabarets and nightclubs of Haram Street. In the present day, Cairo's professional belly dancers reside in neighborhoods all over the city. Those who perform in high-end venues, such as five-star hotels and elite nightclubs, can afford to reside in fashionable neighborhoods like Zamālik and al-Maʿādī. Manufacturers and sellers of musical instruments, dance costumes, and other items necessary to the entertainment trades are similarly scattered throughout the city. Dance costume manufacturers and vendors, for example, are currently found in locations as disparate as the Khān al-Khalīlī market (in the heart of Fatimid Cairo) and Giza (at the extreme southwest of the present city). Only a handful of musical instrument workshops and sellers remain on Muḥammad ʿAlī Street, and the last costumer on the street, Aḥmad Ḍiyāʾ al-Dīn, recently passed away.

As the cafés of Muḥammad ʿAlī Street gradually closed, the street's musicians increasingly gathered at the coffee houses of the Tawfīqīyah and Ismāʿīlīyah neighborhoods and vicinity (Puig 2001). These cafés, previously the province of musicians specializing in Western instruments, now accommodate a wide array of traditional entertainers. They are located in close proximity to the remaining nightclubs and cabarets of downtown, as well as to the Musicians' Syndicate headquarters. During a November 2022 visit to one such café, Cafeteria Jilābū, I met musicians who specialized in a variety of instruments, including *ṭablah* (the goblet-shaped Egyptian hand drum), electronic drums, accordion, and saxophone. Most of these men were originally from Muḥammad ʿAlī Street.

In spite of its decline as an entertainment hub, Muḥammad ʿAlī Street remains firmly associated with music, song, and dance in the Egyptian popular imagination (Figure 31). Puig (2001) writes:

> The Avenue represents a period, a lifestyle, an artistic form, a specific atmosphere that have disappeared, and the insistence on evoking the place shows all the nostalgia it carries. The latter evokes as much an identity that has now been reworked—especially for strategic purposes in the world of musicians—as a way of life suddenly abandoned in favor of new urban practices and new places.

The persistent image of Muḥammad ʿAlī Street in its heyday has continued to manifest in Egyptian popular culture, in spite of the current state of the street. Such was the case in the 1990s stage musical *Shāriʿ Muḥammad ʿAlī*, with its depiction of a thriving neighborhood of popular entertainers, even as the actual street was being overtaken with furniture stores. Today, many of the people who live and work on Muḥammad ʿAlī Street, unless they have personal connections to the entertainment trades, have little to

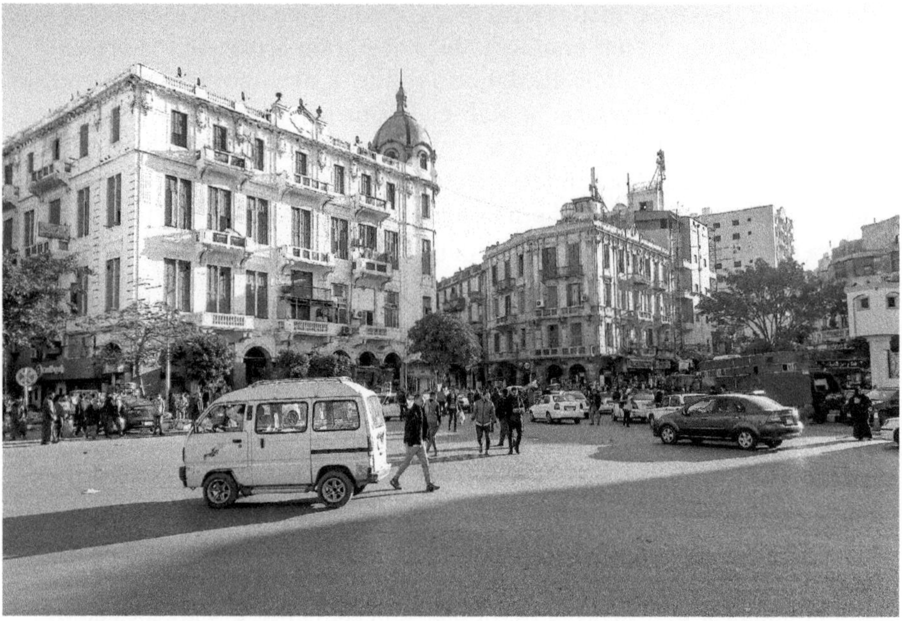

Figure 31: ʻAtabah Square, facing the entrance to Muḥammad ʻAlī Street (photo taken by the author in 2022).

no knowledge of the histories and traditions of the professional entertainers who once populated the street.

For the few remaining professional entertainers who grew up on or near Muḥammad ʻAlī Street, there are costs and benefits to acknowledging their past or present association with the street and with the entertainment trades that were once centered there. For Muḥammad ʻAlī Street musicians, popular nostalgia for the street's past has worked somewhat to their advantage. For example, a 2015 episode of the popular Egyptian television program *Ṣāḥibat al-Saʻādah* (Her Excellency) focused on Muḥammad ʻAlī Street and featured a number of musicians from the street, including a Ḥasab Allāh band (notably, no dancers were interviewed on the program). On the other hand, their association with female professional belly dancers (particularly the *ʻawālim*) and their tendency to work in lower-class settings such as street weddings serve to diminish the reputations of Muḥammad ʻAlī Street musicians in the eyes of their institutionally trained peers. Sayyid Ḥankish, though renowned and respected among the community of Muḥammad ʻAlī Street entertainers, encountered dismissive attitudes among staff at Cairo's Arab Music Institute, who felt that someone who "belongs to the ʻawalim" was not a suitable candidate for training there (Van Nieuwkerk 2019: 71). Still, Muḥammad ʻAlī

Street musicians point out that they possess a cultural and musical dexterity that institutionally trained musicians do not: that is, their traditional background has equipped them with the ability to improvise and adapt to a wide variety of performance settings and audiences (Puig 2006: 524–525).

For many of Egypt's female professional belly dancers, upon retirement, there is a tendency to distance themselves from their former trade, and such is certainly the case with the dancers who grew up on or near Muḥammad 'Alī Street. It is challenging to find any of the remaining *'awālim* who are willing to be interviewed about their work. Family members of dancers are equally reluctant to discuss the trade. In the course of my research, I located a daughter of the *'ālmah* Nazlah al-'Ādil, and I was particularly eager to interview her about her famous mother. As of 2014, the daughter was working at Cairo's Balloon Theater, one of the state-subsidized theaters and host to performances by both the Firqat Riḍā and Firqat al-Qawmīyah theatrical folk dance ensembles. Nazlah's daughter refused all of my attempts to interview her, simply stating that she did not wish to discuss the past. Some of the Muḥammad 'Alī Street musicians that I have interviewed are married to former dancers, but their wives' former careers are never discussed—moreover, it would be a grave insult even to raise the subject with them.

The Rise and Fall of Haram Street

The long thoroughfare known as Haram Street (Pyramid Street) was constructed in the era of Ismā'īl (Figure 32). Completed shortly before the opening of the Suez Canal, this boulevard was intended to facilitate the transport of important visitors from Cairo to the Giza necropolis (Van Nieuwkerk 1995: 47–48). Beginning in the 1940s, the street began to figure more prominently as an entertainment destination. The establishment of Egypt's first large-scale filmmaking studio in Giza undoubtedly contributed to Haram Street's growing significance within Cairo's landscape of entertainment. Studio Miṣr, created by Egyptian businessman Ṭal'at Ḥarb, opened to great acclaim in 1935, and soon many of Egypt's most celebrated film stars took up residence on or near Haram Street (el-Charkawi 1963: 11–12, Cormack 2021: 262–263). Nightclubs and cabarets began to appear, such as the famed l'Auberge des Pyramides (established in 1943) (Hassan 2001). However, the real heyday of Haram Street was in the 1970s and 1980s. Nightclubs and cabarets mushroomed along the length of the boulevard, spurred by the temporary economic boom under Sadat and the influx of Gulf Arab tourism.

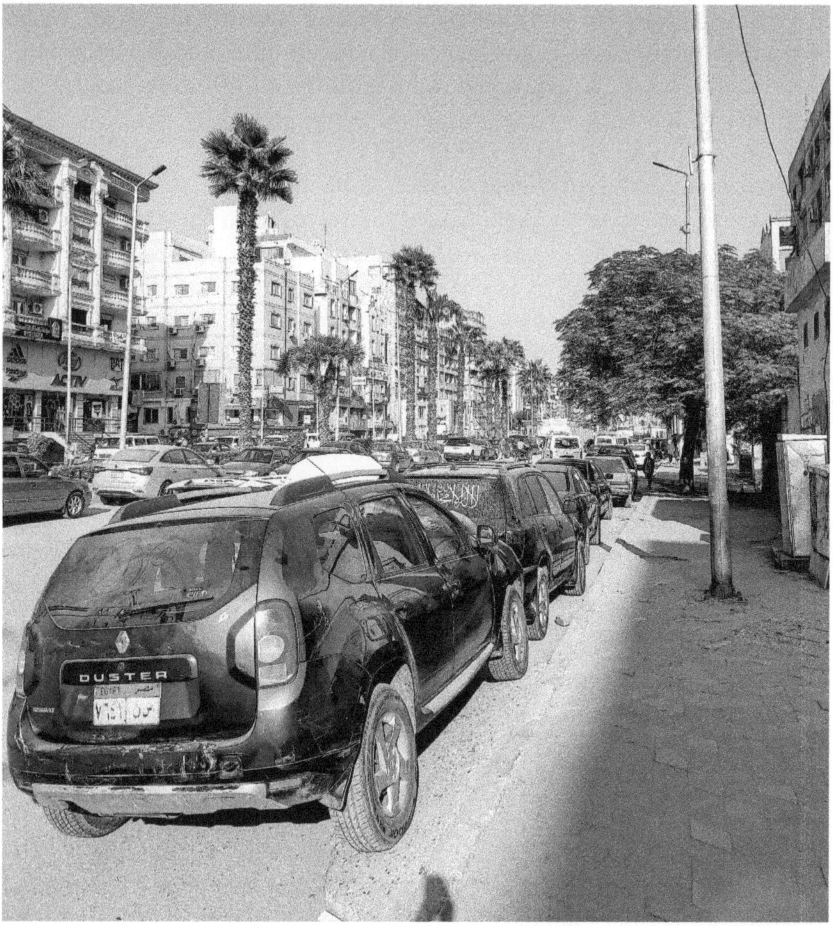

Figure 32: Haram Street, facing northeast (photo taken by the author in 2022).

There are some parallels between the life cycles of Haram Street and Azbakīyah. Like Azbakīyah, Haram Street was originally positioned outside the bounds of the city of Cairo. This made the street an attractive location for cabarets and nightclubs, ambivalent and liminal spaces where Egyptians engaged in activities and behaviors that challenged normal social and spatial boundaries. Much like its older counterpart, Haram Street became a space where diverse populations converged in search of the pleasures it afforded. In essence, Haram Street from the 1940s onward could be characterized as a heterotopic space. Over time, the street and its environs were increasingly urbanized; in the Nasser era, residential settlement of the area began in earnest. Yet, the entertainment venues that proliferated along the length of the street reaffirmed its association with entertainment, leisure, and vice and reasserted its heterotopic qualities. In the present day, Haram Street retains these meanings. In my own experience, well-meaning Egyptian friends—generally middle class, and not involved with the entertainment business—expressed concern for my well-being when I visited there.

The local population's ambivalent attitude towards Haram Street's night spots has periodically manifested in episodes of vandalism and destruction. On various occasions since the 1950s, the street's entertainment venues have become the target of popular ire, variously inspired by rising religious conservatism, economic discontent, and anti-foreign and anti-elite sentiment. A number of the street's nightclubs and cabarets were set alight in 1977 and again in 1986 (*The New York Times* 1977, Ross 1986, Van Nieuwkerk 1995: 64). History repeated itself in the wake of the 2011 revolution, when Haram Street's entertainment venues were once again ransacked and burned (Mikhail 2011).

Like the nightclubs and cabarets of downtown Cairo, the night spots of Haram Street linger on: the street carries forward its association with entertainment, as well as its ambiguous reputation. However, in spite of its rapid rise to prominence in the Cairene entertainment landscape, Haram Street was never destined to overtake downtown as Cairo's new hub of professional entertainment. Rather, the fragmentation of the entertainment landscape since the 1960s has relegated Haram Street, like its downtown counterpart, to one among many entertainment destinations scattered throughout the city.

Festive Spaces: The Persistence of Tradition and Memory

Cairo's entertainment landscape emerged in the Fatimid era. At that time, certain public spaces came to be associated with entertainment and leisure: the canals and ponds of the suburbs, and the city's shrines and cemeteries. Throughout the Fatimid and Mamluk periods, these were important gathering places for Egyptians, particularly on the occasion of popular festivals, including the many popular *mawālid* that emerged in the Mamluk era. While the zone west of the Khalīj remained central to Cairo's landscape of entertainment throughout the urban developments of the late nineteenth and early twentieth centuries, the city's cemeteries gradually transformed into residential neighborhoods. Still, shrines and cemeteries remained focal points for the celebration of the *mawālid*, and within the temporal framework of these popular festivals, they temporarily embodied the heterotopic qualities that had once characterized them.

As Cairo's entertainment landscape has disintegrated into a diverse and many-centered patchwork, and its former hubs have faded into insignificance, Cairo's popular *mawālid* persist. These festivals, and along with them, the street weddings of Cairo's *baladī/sha'abī* neighborhoods, create temporary festive spaces in the Cairo landscape that provide visible reminders of the entertainment landscape as it once was.

Into the present day, *mawālid* serve to temporarily transform mundane neighborhoods into heterotopic spaces. The *mūlid* setting, set apart from ordinary space-time by its vibrant tent fabrics, strands of colored lights, and music blaring from amplifiers, plays host to a contradictory mélange of sacred and secular activities. In the atmosphere of ambiguity and liminality generated by the festival, disparate groups intermingle, and activities and behaviors that transgress Egyptian social norms abound:

> Many deeds perpetrated in public remain unknown or are tolerated: they become acceptable under such fleeting moments and within this closed space, the ideal and arguably necessary place for transgression, exception, and deregulation, under cover of religious celebration. Thus, it is possibly to directly accost young girls who may on such occasions be strolling unaccompanied.... The same goes for carnal contact and dance, consumption of alcohol and drugs, choosing fancy dress, and the parody and derision of "institutions" such as marriage, class and state icons, and normative sexual identity [Madoeuf 2006: 482].

The popular weddings that still take place in the streets of Cairo's lower-class neighborhoods have a similar effect. Puig (2006: 515) writes:

> Large red-colored and ornately patterned tapestries delimit the space reserved for the ceremony while leaving a narrow passage for pedestrians, transforming the street into a festive space serving contradictory functions—as a space of transgression on the one hand (where alcohol, marijuana, and scantily-clad women dancers often circulate) and, on the other hand, as a space where the deepest social and community norms are reproduced.

In these temporary festive spaces, one catches a glimpse of what other spaces in the Cairene entertainment landscape must have been like in earlier times: the lively bustle of Azbakīyah observed by Charles Didier in the 1850s (1860: 9–10), or the "perpetual fair" of Rumaylah described by Napoleon's explorers at the dawn of the nineteenth century (Jomard 1829: 438–440).

Yet, though they remain a persistent part of Egyptian popular culture, the character of Egypt's *mawālid* has changed a great deal since the mid-twentieth century. The Egyptian government's interventionist approach to popular culture since the mid-twentieth century has had profound impacts. The Nasser regime implemented an array of reforms and regulations largely aimed at exploiting the festivals for propagandistic purposes, though the effects of these interventions did not really manifest until the 1970s (Schielke 2006: 195–196). Many of the reforms and regulations implemented in the latter decades of the twentieth centuries targeted the more socially transgressive aspects of the *mawālid*. Belly dancers, both male and female, have been banned from the festivals since the 1990s (*ibid.*, 196). The sale of alcohol at *mawālid* has declined precipitously, and prostitution, once commonplace, is now more or less absent. Still, as Schielke notes, the government's success in banning bars and dance tents likely hinged on the increasing conservatism of the *mūl*id-going public following the Islamic revival (*ibid.*, 197).

On the other hand, the disappearance of alcohol, belly dance, and prostitution from the *mawālid* cannot be attributed solely to the heavy hand of government intervention—at least, not in Cairo. Cairenes can seek out these pleasures in the city's present-day landscape of entertainment, in venues dedicated to entertainment, leisure, and vice:

> Furthermore, as mawlids have become marginalised in the public sphere and in the lifestyle and religiosity of the upper and middle classes, the structure of amusements has changed. Mawlids are no longer centres of alcohol, dancing and prostitution partly because these trades and their customers have moved to less conspicuous and more profitable locations, for example Pyramids Road in Cairo [Schielke 2006: 197–198].

Still, it appears that clandestine dance performances may still occur at some *mawālid* (see Parrs 2017: 205). Further, Schielke (2006: 197) notes: "Transvestites are still part of many a festive procession, although their shows now have a burlesque rather than a homoerotic character."

Whither Belly Dance?

Belly dance and its professional practitioners remain a constant in Cairene life. Yet, the circumstances of today's dancers, and how they fit within the landscape of the city, are much different from a few decades ago. The situation of belly dance and belly dancers in the early-to-mid twentieth century was the culmination of centuries of meaning-making in the Cairene landscape of entertainment. The ascendance of Azbakīyah and 'Imād al-Dīn Street in the entertainment landscape, the proliferation of formalized entertainment venues in these spaces, the ubiquity of belly dancers in these venues, and the blossoming of Muḥammad 'Alī Street as a hub for professional entertainers created an environment that enabled belly dance and its professional practitioners to thrive. In the early-to-mid twentieth century, female professional belly dancers were able not only to ascend to the heights of mainstream celebrity, but also to play a fundamental role in shaping the entertainment landscape of Cairo. Many of the most famous dancers of this period were successful entrepreneurs who owned and/or managed venues in the heart of Cairo's entertainment hubs. The central importance of these women in the entertainment business, as well as within the popular *zeitgeist*, paralleled the centrality of Azbakīyah, 'Imād al-Dīn Street, and Muḥammad 'Alī Street in the entertainment landscape at this time. However, the tide began to turn at mid-century, and the repercussions have been felt ever since.

Today, belly dance and its professional practitioners remain common in Cairo's nightclubs and cabarets. Yet these venues are now scattered all over the city, rather than clustered in the former entertainment hubs of Azbakīyah and 'Imād al-Dīn Street. The majority of the nightclubs and cabarets featuring belly dance are now located aboard Nile boats, within hotels and malls, and at various other locations throughout the city. Tucked away inside hotels and boats, these venues can exist in neighborhoods far removed from Cairo's former entertainment hubs. As noted earlier, many of the venues currently featuring belly dance are situated in Cairo's most affluent areas and are prohibitively expensive for the vast majority of the city's residents.

Though performances in certain venues are widely visible on social media (see below), the spaces themselves are highly exclusive: for example, dress codes at these venues generally prohibit certain signifiers of middle or lower class identity, such as the head scarf and *jalābīyah*. In a strange sense, belly dance performances at Cairo's discos and high-end nightclubs evoke the Fatimid-era *majlis*: isolated from the masses in their exclusive enclaves, Egypt's elites are able to freely indulge their worldly appetites, and like *qiyān* of old, belly dancers labor to satiate their desires.

Just as their workplaces are scattered, the residences of dancers are dispersed all over the city. With the decline of Muḥammad 'Alī Street, there is no central space of residence and/or commerce for today's belly dancers. Rather than clustering together in a single neighborhood, dancers live in locations throughout the city. Businesses connected to the trade, such as costume manufacturers and vendors, are similarly dispersed.

Today's belly dancers are highly visible in films, on television, and through social media, yet few have achieved the degree of celebrity and influence that could rival that of their counterparts from the twentieth century. Exceptions exist, such as Dīnā Ṭal'at, whose film and television career has made her a household name. Unlike their predecessors in the early-to-mid twentieth century, few present-day dancers own or manage their own entertainment venues. Again, notable exceptions exist, such as the popular dancer Lucy, who maintains her Parisiana nightclub on Haram Street (Figure 33).

Thus, much like the entertainment landscape, belly dance and its professional practitioners have been scattered and dispersed. Belly dance is everywhere in Cairo, yet it has no real center. There is no Muḥammad 'Alī

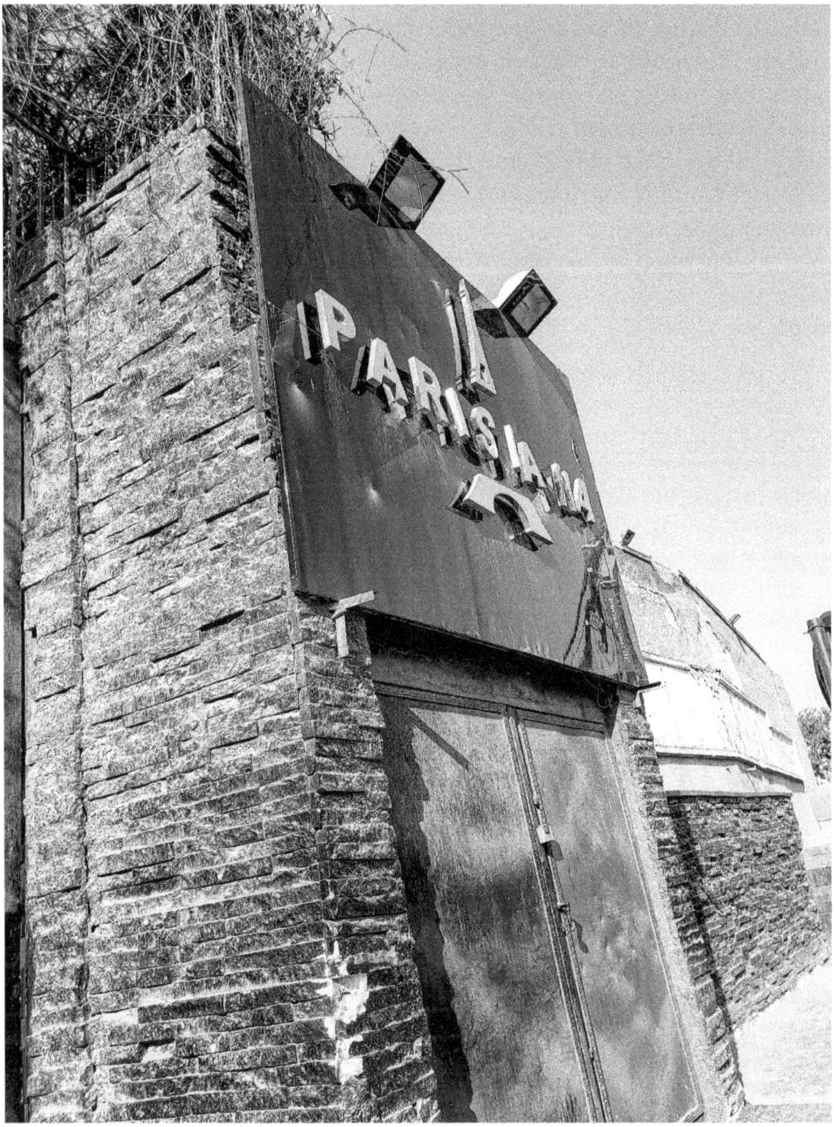

Figure 33: Lucy's Parisiana nightclub on Haram Street (photo taken by the author in 2022).

Street where the majority of the city's dancers live. There is no Azbakīyah dominating the landscape of popular entertainment. Belly dance and its professional practitioners are now more widespread in Cairo than ever before, yet there is no space to which they are really anchored.

As the entertainment landscape has disintegrated and dispersed, many dancers have turned to the virtual landscape of social media in order to further their careers. Indeed, it could be argued that belly dance and its professional practitioners now inhabit a virtual entertainment landscape that is just as real and just as relevant to Egyptian life as the physical entertainment landscape. As noted throughout this work, Egypt's marginal personae have been drawn to inhabit places that make space for their unorthodox lifestyles and behaviors. Increasingly, this is the virtual space of social media.

As Morley (2023) demonstrates, effective use of social media is becoming increasingly crucial for dancers to achieve greater wealth and fame. She writes (2023: 125–126):

> Social media is now indispensable for fame. Dancers of earlier eras became famous, and thereby respectable,* through films and work at prestigious hotels with big theatrical shows. This is no longer a viable career path, as the few remaining theatrical belly dance shows at upscale hotels are only accessible to the upper classes, and photography is prohibited. Dancers can become famous among belly dance fans by dancing in discos and developing their social media presence; only upper-class Egyptians may see their live performances, but at least Egyptians with less money can now see their performances online. But to become a household name, the dancer must leverage the disco fame into work in music videos and movies.

Notably, the discos that sprang up in the wake of the Revolution of 2011 cut costs by hiring DJs instead of live bands, with the result that belly dancers found themselves performing to recorded versions of contemporary hit songs (Sahin 2018: 91). Moreover, since around 2018, Cairo's post-revolutionary discos have permitted audience members to take photos and videos—something previously uncommon in Cairo's cabarets and nightclubs (Morley 2023: 124–125). The resulting performance environment is social media friendly, and belly dancers are now performing for audiences who eagerly capture their dancing on cell phones. Each performance to a popular song carries the potential of "going viral" on social media and launching the dancer into celebrity (and opportunity).

Yet, even as it opens up new possibilities for career advancement and

---

* These dancers certainly achieved a high degree of fame and celebrity. However, as discussed in the Introduction as well as in Chapter One, it is not really accurate to characterize these women as "respectable" according to the norms and attitudes of mainstream Egyptian society.

financial security, social media increasingly forces Egypt's dancers into negotiations with the Eurocentric visual aesthetics prioritized by social media algorithms. As Morley (2023: 124–125) observes:

> The profiles and content of belly dancers on social media are subject to Eurocentric algorithmic logics that prioritize what sells, namely certain brands of sexuality. As elite venues are basing hiring decisions on social media metrics, this contributes to a feedback loop with existing biases in Egyptian society, amplifying the advantages of those deemed sexy and high class (thin, cosmetically- and surgically enhanced, white-passing foreign women) and invisibilizes those deemed unworthy of attention (Egyptian women from the lower classes with larger and minimally modified bodies).

Morley demonstrates that in high-end venues whose marketing is intertwined with social media, dancers must prioritize an aesthetic of visibility. That is, as a dancer's success increasingly depends on the attention she receives on social media, she must tailor her overall presentation—including her face, her body, her costume, and her style of dance—to achieve visibility on social media.

Morley contrasts this aesthetic of visibility with what she terms an "aesthetic of vibration," one that centers sound and affect, and that prioritizes interpersonal interaction and connection. The aesthetic of vibration encapsulates a more traditional Egyptian music and dance aesthetic, in which great value is placed on the performer's understanding of music and of his or her ability to convey and evoke feeling (*iḥsās*) (see Ward 2018: 96–118 for a discussion of aesthetics in Egyptian belly dance). As Morley notes, Cairo venues that "operate away from the eyes of social media" continue to prioritize the aesthetic of vibration (Morley 2023: 90). Notably, this vibrational aesthetic dominates in the nightclubs and cabarets that continue to function in downtown Cairo and on Haram Street, spaces where established meanings regarding belly dance and its professional practitioners persist. In a similar vein, Sahin (2018: 269) observes that these cabaret settings have deep ties to established intracultural meanings; introducing her analysis of present-day Haram Street cabarets, she writes that "the cabaret site was chosen for the final chapter in this ethnography due to how it often requires deepest access into intra-MENA circuitries, bodies, and significations."

Thus, though belly dancers increasingly occupy the virtual landscape of social media, they remain a presence in downtown nightclubs and Haram Street cabarets, contributing to the ongoing role of these spaces as entertainment destinations and their persistent perception as morally ambiguous spaces. Further, some individuals with ties to the entertainment trades still reside and do business in the neighborhood on and around Muḥammad ʿAlī Street, and as noted earlier, some musicians' cafés are located downtown. Their presence ensures that professional entertainment continues to be loosely interwoven in the social and spatial reality of these spaces, in spite of the overall fragmentation of the entertainment landscape.

Conclusion

The 1952 Revolution and its aftermath heralded an era of profound and rapid change, with implications for professional entertainers and the spaces where they have plied their trades. The Egyptian government's interventionist approach to arts and entertainment since the Nasser era, together with the liberalization of the Egyptian economy beginning with Sadat, initiated significant changes in music, dance, and other forms of professional entertainment. Since 1952, the state has sanctioned and supported cultural expressions that fit within its broader vision of Egyptian nationhood, while rejecting and marginalizing those that do not. The Egyptian government's push towards professionalization and institutionalization in arts and entertainment has further relegated certain traditional forms of entertainment—such as belly dance—to the margins. Economic liberalization has exacerbated the adverse impact of these state interventions. The economic policies of Sadat initiated a massive influx of outsiders into the dance trade; this influx, together with ongoing economic uncertainties, contributed to the decline of traditional entertainer networks, as well as the rise of the male impresario system.

Simultaneously, massive demographic shifts, together with frenetic urban development, have drastically altered the social and spatial make-up of Cairo. The organization that continued to characterize the city throughout the developments of the late nineteenth and early twentieth centuries—the Fatimid core to the east of the old Khalīj, the newly-developed zone to its west, and suburban expansions pushing to the north, west, and south—has been transformed. Present-day Cairo is disjointed and many-centered. The city's current organization, above all else, reflects the widening divide between rich and poor.

Taken together, these factors have resulted in the transformation of Cairo's entertainment landscape. The traditional organization that developed over the course of many centuries, and that was described over the last several chapters, has fragmented into a diverse and many-centered patchwork. From the mid-twentieth century onward, Muḥammad 'Alī Street and downtown Cairo have declined precipitously from their roles as entertainment hubs. Simultaneously, professional entertainment, rather than being centered in these traditional zones, has diffused into locations scattered throughout the city. Although Haram Street rapidly rose to prominence as an entertainment destination, the disintegration of the entertainment landscape since the 1960s has relegated this street, like downtown and Muḥammad ʻAlī Street, to one among many entertainment destinations dispersed throughout the city.

While belly dance and its professional practitioners remain a common sight in Cairo's nightclubs and cabarets, these venues are to be found all over the city, rather than in the traditional entertainment hubs of Azbakīyah and ʻImād al-Dīn Street. Though a few cabarets and nightclubs continue to operate in downtown Cairo, and many more can be found along Haram Street, the majority are now located in boats on the Nile, tucked away within the confines of hotels and malls, and at various other locations throughout Cairo. Many of these venues are situated in the most affluent and privileged areas of the city and are financially out of the reach of most ordinary Egyptians. Although belly dance and its professional practitioners are now more widespread in the city of Cairo than ever, there is no space to which they are really bound. Increasingly, dancers must turn to the virtual landscape of social media in order to find their fame and fortune.

Nevertheless, in the popular imagination, downtown Cairo, Muḥammad ʻAlī Street, and Haram Street all retain their connections to professional entertainment—and to belly dance and belly dancers—albeit to varying degrees. Downtown, though no longer the heart of Cairo's entertainment landscape, retains its centuries-long association with entertainment, leisure, and vice. The nostalgic image of Muḥammad ʻAlī Street as a hub of music and dance continues to manifest in Egyptian popular culture, in spite of the current state of the street. And Haram Street, with its nightclubs and cabarets, maintains its infamous reputation.

Epilogue

With this work, I have examined the relationship between belly dance space and belly dancer in the Cairo landscape over the course of the city's history, relying on a theoretical framework informed by Pierre Bourdieu's theory of practice, Michel Foucault's concept of heterotopia, and Mikhail Bakhtin's notion of the carnivalesque. Approaching this relationship as mutually constituting, I have attempted to illustrate how the evolution of Cairo's entertainment landscape from the Fatimid era until the present day has been interwoven with the evolving roles of dance and dancers in Egyptian society. The routine practice of professional entertainers, their audiences, and others have contributed to the production of meaningful spaces in the Cairo landscape.

Conversely, those meaningful spaces have predisposed the individuals moving and acting within them toward certain perceptions and actions. Through this dialectical interplay, the Cairo landscape has been embedded with meanings pertaining to dance and dancers that have been re-inscribed as agents have moved and acted within it. The entertainment landscape of Cairo has emerged from the lived experience of Egyptians, while simultaneously informing the social and spatial reality of Cairenes.

The dialectic between dance space and dancer has served to reify perceptions and behaviors toward dance and dancer in Egyptian society, as well as towards the spaces associated with professional entertainers. For centuries, these men and women have been a liminal and ambiguous presence in Egyptian social and spatial life. Similarly, spaces within Cairo's landscape of entertainment have existed as heterotopic spaces: that is, zones of ambivalence and liminality in the spatial reality of the city. The mutually constituting relationship between the spaces of professional entertainment and professional entertainers has ensured that each has imparted their ambiguous and liminal qualities on the other.

With the foundation of al-Qāhirah in 969, spaces of entertainment came to be woven into the geography of the city, establishing a landscape of entertainment that would continue to develop and elaborate. In the popular imagination, certain public spaces began to have clear associations with entertainment, leisure, and vice: the canals and ponds of the city's suburbs, as well as the city's shrines and cemeteries. By the time the Mamluks assumed control of Egypt, the suburbs of Cairo, as hubs of recreation and leisure, and the city cemeteries, as host to a complex mix of sacred and secular activities, had emerged as heterotopic spaces, where diverse populations converged and interfaced, and where the normal social order was challenged and occasionally upended. Throughout the Mamluk era, the presence and practice of professional entertainers in these spaces contributed to the inscription and re-inscription of heterotopic meanings, and the spaces that constituted Cairo's landscape of entertainment continued to be set apart by their ambiguity and liminality.

Throughout the Ottoman period, Cairo's suburbs and cemeteries carried forward the meanings that had been inscribed within them over previous centuries. The area known as Azbakīyah emerged as the focal point of entertainment and leisure in Cairo's western suburbs. Azbakīyah, together with Rumaylah Square, located adjacent to the Citadel, functioned as the main gathering spaces for the common people. Meanwhile, Cairo's shrines and cemeteries continued to be important spaces of popular entertainment and recreation, particularly during holidays and festivals, until their gradual transformation into residential neighborhoods beginning in the nineteenth century. Important new sites were added to the entertainment landscape, including coffee houses under the Ottomans, and formal theaters under the brief Napoleonic occupation. The urban planning projects of Muḥammad 'Alī Bāshā and his grandson Ismā'īl drastically altered the physiognomy of Cairo, most notably in the zone west of the Khalīj.

In spite of this, spaces like Azbakīyah carried forward their heterotopic qualities, and the association of these spaces with entertainment and its professional practitioners persisted. In these locales, professional entertainers, including professional dancers, found spaces that could accommodate their marginality. Their presence, in turn, served to re-inscribe the heterotopic nature of these spaces. Throughout the Ottoman era, professional entertainers were key to the ongoing re-inscription of heterotopic meaning into Cairo's entertainment landscape.

From the dawn of the British occupation, developments in and around Azbakīyah, already the focal point of the Western suburbs, ensured its centrality in Cairo's landscape of entertainment. Perhaps the most significant development was the emergence of theaters and music halls—dedicated structures for the performance and consumption of professional entertainment—in Azbakīyah and vicinity. The proliferation of formalized entertainment venues in the area reinforced its ties to professional entertainment; these venues embodied the heterotopic qualities long associated with this part of Cairo. Belly dancers thrived in these settings, and by the end of the 1930s, many dancers had achieved celebrity status. Many of Cairo's dancers owned and managed their own venues, enabling them to play a critical role in shaping the early-to-mid twentieth-century Cairo entertainment landscape. Just a short walk from downtown Cairo, Muḥammad 'Alī Street blossomed into a commercial and residential center for belly dancers, singers, musicians, and other entertainment professionals. Together, downtown Cairo and Muḥammad 'Alī Street formed the heart of Cairo's landscape of entertainment, a situation that held true until the middle of the twentieth century.

The mid-twentieth century heralded a period of profound change to Cairo's entertainment landscape, as well as to the circumstances of professional entertainers. The Egyptian government's interventionist approach to arts and entertainment since the Nasser era, together with the liberalization of the Egyptian economy beginning with Sadat, have resulted in significant changes to professional entertainment. At the same time, massive demographic shifts, together with frantic urban development, have dramatically transformed the social and spatial make-up of Cairo. Together, these factors have resulted in the transformation of Cairo's entertainment landscape. The traditional organization centering on downtown Cairo and Muḥammad 'Alī Street has disintegrated into a diverse and many-centered patchwork. While the second half of the twentieth century witnessed the emergence and temporary boom of a new space in the entertainment landscape—Haram Street—this period also saw the gradual decline of downtown Cairo and Muḥammad 'Alī Street. Still, these spaces retain their connections to professional entertainment—and to belly dance and belly dancers—in the popular imagination, and their heterotopic qualities persist.

At the end of this long history, it makes sense to return to where I began. I once again find myself standing outside the 'Atabah Metro station, gazing eastward towards what is left of Azbakīyah Gardens. This space has changed dramatically, even in the last year, let alone in the last one thousand. Yet, the persistence of certain meanings here is remarkable. This part of the city, Cairo's *wusṭ al-balad*, still retains its centuries-long association with entertainment, leisure, and vice: a connection established with the creation of the Fatimid city, when this area was a bucolic countryside dotted with seasonal ponds and royal *manāẓir*. A few hundred years ago, Azbakīyah was a lake, and professional entertainers plied their trades among its pleasure-seekers, both elite and common. The voices of singing women rang out from the elaborate boats skimming across the waters, while their male and female counterparts on the banks sang and danced to entertain the masses gathered there. A century ago, the lake was gone, but the singers and dancers were still to be found—just a short walk away in one of the music halls of 'Imād al-Dīn Street. Even today, they can be seen at the Shahrazād nightclub on Alfī Bik Street: originally a turn-of-the-century music hall, and an emblem of the endurance of meaning in this part of Cairo.

It's not only the persistence of this area's association with entertainment that I find so striking: I am also astonished by the endurance of this area as a heterotopic space. Cairo's downtown remains a space of ambivalence and liminality, a place "outside of all places." Here, the normal social and spatial boundaries of Egyptian society continue to be blurred, challenged, or even upended. Here, disparate groups continue to converge and interface, and in venues like Shahrazād, engage in activities and behaviors that are elsewhere frowned upon. In spite of the fragmentation of the entertainment landscape and the dispersal of belly dance to venues throughout the city, professional belly dancers continue to ply their trade here. As ambiguous and liminal personae whose identities and behaviors situate them outside the mainstream of Egyptian society, dancers have been intimately tied to Cairo's heterotopic spaces like this one for centuries. These settings can accommodate the unorthodox lifestyles and behaviors of professional entertainers, whose regular presence imparts their own marginality into the spatial reality and informs perceptions of the space.

So, as I stand here staring at the last remnants of the Azbakīyah Gardens, listening to the chaos of Cairene life unfolding around me, I find myself amazed by the continuity within all the change. The entertainment landscape that was built over the course of so many centuries quickly disintegrated in the wake of the massive changes that have convulsed Cairo since the 1960s. Cairo's landscape of entertainment is now fragmented, lacking a clear center. Cairo's belly dancers are similarly fragmented and de-centered: there is no single space to which they are now anchored within the city, and dancers are increasingly turning to the virtual landscape of social media in search of fame and success. Yet, their persistent presence in spaces like downtown Cairo speaks to the long historical interconnection between dancers and these places, and the endurance of meanings deeply inscribed, and not easily erased, within the city's landscape.

Bibliography

Text Sources

Abaza, Mona. 2006. "Egyptianizing the American Dream: Nasr City's Shopping Malls, Public Order, and the Privatized Military." In *Cairo Cosmopolitan: Politics, Culture, and Urban Space in the New Globalized Middle East*, edited by Diane Singerman and Paul Amar, pp. 193–220. Cairo: The American University in Cairo Press.

Abbas Hilmi II Papers. Durham, UK: Durham University.

'Abd ar-Rāziq, Aḥmad. 1973. *La Femme au Temps des Mamlouks en Égypte*. Le Caire: Institut Français d'Archéologie Orientale du Caire.

Abou Saif, Laila. 1973. "Najīb al-Rīḥānī: From Buffoonery to Social Comedy." *Journal of Arabic Literature* (IV): 1–17.

About Naemet Mokhtar. n.d. Translation by Priscilla Adum. *All About Belly Dancing, by Shira*. http://www.shira.net/about/naemet-mokhtar.htm.

Abu-Lughod, Janet L. 1971. *Cairo: 1001 Years of the City Victorious*. Princeton: Princeton University Press.

Académie Royale des Sciences, des Lettres et des Beaux-Arts de Belgique. 1870. *Bulletins de l'Académie Royale des Sciences, des Lettres et des Beaux-Arts de Belgique. Ser. 2 T.* 29. Bruxelles: F. Hayez.

Adum, Priscilla. n.d. "Badia Masabni: The Lady and Her Clubs." *All About Belly Dancing, by Shira*. http://www.shira.net/about/badia-lady-and-clubs.htm.

Africano, Giovan Lioni. 1550. "Della Descrittione Dell'Africa et Delle Cose Notabili Che Ivi Sono." In *Delle Navigationi et Viaggi, Primo Volume*, edited by Giovanni Baptista Ramusio, pp. 2–103. Venice: Giunti.

Africanus, Leo. 1896. *The History and Description of Africa*. Translated by John Pory. Edited by Robert Brown. Volume III. London: Hakluyt Society.

Ahl al-Fann. 1955. "Faḍīḥat Mūsīqīyah Rāqiṣah Titagawwil Shawāra' al-Qāhirah." 26 February: 40.

Ahmed, Heba Farouk. 2005. "Nineteenth-Century Cairo: A Dual City?" In *Making Cairo Medieval*, edited by Nezar Alsayyad, Irene A. Bierman, and Nasser Rabbat, pp. 143–172. Lanham, Maryland: Lexington Books.

al-Ahrām. Egyptian daily newspaper. 1891–1931.

Ahram Online. 2022. "Int'l Conference of the Supreme Council for Islamic Affairs to Discuss Climate Change: Egypt Minister." 3 September. https://english.ahram.org.eg/News/475351.aspx.

Alsayyad, Nezar. 2011. *Cairo: Histories of a City*. Cambridge: The Belknap Press of Harvard University Press.

Alsayyad, Nezar, Irene A. Bierman, and Nasser Rabbat, editors. 2005. *Making Cairo Medieval*. Lanham, Maryland: Lexington Books.

And, Metin. 1963. *A History of Theatre and Popular Entertainment in Turkey*. Ankara: Forum Yayınları.

Armbrust, Walter. 1996. *Mass Culture and Modernism in Egypt*. Cambridge: Cambridge University Press.

———. 2001. "Colonizing Popular Culture or Creating Modernity." In *Middle Eastern Cities 1900–1950: Public Spaces and Public Spheres*, edited by Jakob Skovgaard-Petersen and Hans Chr. Korsholm Nielsen, pp. 20–43. Aarhus: Aarhus University Press.

———. 2006. "When the Lights Go Down in Cairo: Cinema as Global Crossroads and Space of Playful Resistance." In *Cairo Cosmopolitan: Politics, Culture, and Urban Space in the New Globalized Middle East*, edited by Diane Singerman and Paul Amar, pp. 415–443. Cairo: The American University in Cairo Press.

Aucoin, Pauline McKenzie. 2017. "Toward an Anthropological Understanding of Space and Place." In *Place, Space and Hermeneutics*, edited by Bruce B. Janz, 395–412. Cham, Switzerland: Springer International Publishing.

BBC. 2020. "Egypt President Abdul Fattah al-Sisi: Ruler with an Iron Grip." 1 December. https://www.bbc.com/news/world-middle-east-19256730.

Badawi, M.M. 1988. *Early Arabic Drama*. Cambridge: Cambridge University Press.

Badia Masabni in 1966 Television Interview. n.d. Translation by Priscilla Adum. *All About Belly Dancing, by Shira*. http://www.shira.net/about/badia-interview-1966.htm.

Baedeker, Karl. 1878. *Egypt, Handbook for Travellers. Part First: Lower Egypt, with the Fayûm and the Peninsula of Sinai*. Leipsic: K. Baedeker; London: Dulau and Co.

———. 1885. *Egypt, Handbook for Travellers. Part First: Lower Egypt, with the Fayûm and the Peninsula of Sinai. 2nd Edition, Revised and Augmented*. Leipsic, London: K. Baedeker.

———. 1898. *Egypt: Handbook for Travellers. 4th Remodelled Edition*. Leipsic: K. Baedeker.

Baer, Gabriel. 1964. *Egyptian Guilds in Modern Times*. Jerusalem: The Israel Oriental Society.

Bakhtin, Mikhail. 1984. *Rabelais and His World*. Translated by Helene Iswolsky. Bloomington: Indiana University Press.

———. 1998. "Carnival and the Carnivalesque." In *Cultural Theory and Popular Culture: A Reader*, 2nd Edition, edited by John Storey, pp. 250–259. Harlow, England: Pearson.

Beeston, A.F.L., translator. 1980. *The Epistle on Singing Girls of Jāḥiz*. Warminster: Aris and Phillips Ltd.

Behrens-Abouseif, Doris. 1985. *Azbakiyya and Its Environs: from Azbak to Ismā'īl, 1476–1879*. Cairo: Institut Français d'Archéologie Orientale.

———. 1997. "The *Maḥmal* Legend and the Pilgrimage of the Ladies of the Mamluk Court." *Mamlūk Studies Review* 1: 87–96.

———. 2012. "A Bronze Tambourine-Player." In *Metalwork and Material Culture in the Islamic World: Art, Craft and Text*, edited by Venetia Porter and Mariam Ross-Owen, pp. 217–222. London: I.B.Tauris.

Blanc, Charles. 1876. *Voyage de la Haute Égypte: Observations sur les Arts Égyptien et Arabe*. Paris: Librairie Renouard.

Bloom, Jonathan M. 2007. *Arts of the City Victorious: Islamic Art and Architecture in Fatimid North Africa and Egypt*. New Haven: Yale University Press.

Blount, Sir Henry. 1636. *A Voyage into the Levant*. The Second Edition. London: I. L. for Andrew Crooke.

Bocthor, Ellious. 1828. *Dictionnaire Français-Arabe*. Paris: Chez Firmin Didot.

Bourdieu, Pierre. 1977. *Outline of a Theory of Practice*. Translated by Richard Nice. Cambridge: Cambridge University Press.

———. 1989. "Social Space and Symbolic Power." *Sociological Theory* 7(1): 14–25.

———. 1996. "Physical Space, Social Space and Habitus." Vilhelm Aubert Memorial Lecture, Institutt for Sosiologi og Samfunnsgeografi, Universitetet i Oslo, *Rapport* 10.

———. 2003. "The Berber House." In *The Anthropology of Space and Place: Locating Culture*, edited by Setha M. Low and Denise Lawrence-Zúñiga, pp. 131–141. Malden, Massachusetts: Blackwell Publishing.

———. 2018. "Social Space and the Genesis of Appropriated Physical Space." *International Journal of Urban and Regional Research* 42(1): 106–114.

The Brooklyn Daily Eagle. 1927. "Mrs. Palmer Sees New Day for Women Dawning in Egypt." 23 April: 3.

Brunyate, W.E. 1906. "Egypt." *Journal of the Society of Comparative Legislation* 7(1): 55–65.

al-Būlāqī, Maḥmūd Ḥamdī. 1904. *Mufriḥ al-Jins al-Laṭīf wa-Ṣuwwar Mashāhīr al-Raqqāṣīn*. Second Edition.

Burckhardt, John Lewis. 1830. *Arabic Proverbs; or, the Manners and Customs of the Modern Egyptians Illustrated from Their Proverbial Sayings Current at Cairo*. London: J. Murray.

Carlton, Donna. 1994. *Looking for Little Egypt*. Bloomington: IDD Books.

Caswell, Fuad Matthew. 2011. *The Slave Girls of Baghdad: The Qiyān in the Early Abbasid Era*. London: I.B. Tauris.

Chabrol, Gilbert Joseph Gaspard de. 1826. "Essai sur les Moeurs des Habitans Modernes de l'Égypte." In *Description de l'Égypte*. Tome Dix-Huitième, Partie 1. État Moderne. Paris: Imprimerie de C.L.F. Panckoucke.

Chalcraft, John T. 2005. *The Striking Cabbies of Cairo and Other Stories: Crafts and Guilds in Egypt, 1863–1914*. Albany: State University of New York Press.

el-Charkawi, Galal. 1963. *The Present Situation and Trends of the Arab Cinema*. UNESCO Report. Paris: UNESCO.

Charmes, Gabriel. 1883. *Five Months at Cairo and in Lower Egypt*. London: Bentley.

Clot-Bey, A.B. 1840. *Aperçu Général sur L'Égypte*. Tome Deuxième. Paris: Fortin, Masson et Cie

Cormack, Raphael. 2021. *Midnight in Cairo: The Divas of Egypt's Roaring '20s*. New York: W.W. Norton and Company.

Cortese, Delia, and Simonetta Calderini. 2006. *Women and the Fatimids in the World of Islam*. Edinburgh: Edinburgh University Press.

Croitoru, Joseph. 2015. "Culture Policy in Egypt: The Soothing Power of Culture." *Qantara.de*. 19 June. https://en.qantara.de/content/culture-policy-in-egypt-the-soothing-power-of-culture.

al-Damurdāshī, Aḥmad. 1991. *Al-Damurdashi's Chronicle of Egypt, 1688–1755*. Translated and annotated by Daniel Crecelius and 'Abd al-Wahhab Bakr. Leiden: Brill.

Danielson, Virginia. 1991. "Artists and Entrepreneurs: Female Singers in Cairo during the 1920s." In *Women in Middle Eastern History: Shifting Boundaries in Sex and Gender*, edited by Nikki R. Keddie and Beth Baron, pp. 292–309. New Haven: Yale University Press.

———. 1997. *The Voice of Egypt: Umm Kulthūm, Arabic Song, and Egyptian Society in the Twentieth Century*. Chicago: University of Chicago Press.

———. 1999. "Moving Toward Public Space: Women and Musical Performance in Twentieth Century Egypt." In *Hermeneutics and Honor: Negotiating Female "Public" Space in Islamic/ate Societies*, edited by Asma Afsaruddin, pp. 116–139. Cambridge: Harvard University Press.

Dankoff, Robert and Sooyong Kim. 2011. *An Ottoman Traveller: Selections from the Book of Travels of Evliya Çelebi*. London: Eland Publishing Limited.

De Koning, Anouk. 2006. "Café Latte and Caesar Salad: Cosmopolitan Belonging in Cairo's Coffee Shops." In *Cairo Cosmopolitan: Politics, Culture, and Urban Space in the New Globalized Middle East*, edited by Diane Singerman and Paul Amar, pp. 221–233. Cairo: The American University in Cairo Press.

Delmas, Émile. 1896. *Égypte et Palestine*. Paris: Fischbacher.

Denis, Eric. 2006. "Cairo as Neoliberal Capital? From Walled City to Gated Communities." In *Cairo Cosmopolitan: Politics, Culture, and Urban Space in the New Globalized Middle East*, edited by Diane Singerman and Paul Amar, pp. 47–71. Cairo: The American University in Cairo Press.

Didier, Charles. 1860. *Les Nuits du Caire*. Paris: Hachette.

Dinning, Hector William. 1920. *Nile to Aleppo, with the Light-horse in the Middle-East*. London: George Allen & Unwin Ltd.

Dorman, W.J. 2009. "Of Demolitions and Donors: The Problematics of State Intervention in Informal Cairo." In *Cairo Contested: Governance, Urban Space, and Global Modernity*, edited by Diane Singerman, pp. 269–290. Cairo: The American University in Cairo Press

Dougherty, Roberta L. 2005. "Dance and the Dancer in Egyptian Film." In *Belly Dance:*

Orientalism, Transnationalism, and Harem Fantasy, edited by Anthony Shay and Barbara Sellers-Young, pp. 145–171. Costa Mesa, California: Mazda Publishers, Inc.
Duff Gordon, Lucie, Lady. 1875. *Last Letters from Egypt*. London: Macmillan.
Dunn, Michael Collins. 2011. "Historical Discursus for April 2: The First Battle of the Wasa'a or Wozzer." *Middle East Institute Editor's Blog: A Blog by the Editor of the Middle East Journal*. http://mideasti.blogspot.com/2011/03/historical-note-for-april-2-first.html.
Early, Evelyn A. 1993. *Baladi Women of Cairo: Playing with an Egg and a Stone*. Boulder, Colorado: Lynne Rienner Publishers.
Ebers, Georg. 1887. *Egypt: Descriptive, Historical, and Picturesque*. Trans. Clara Bell. London: Cassell & Co.
The Egyptian Directory and Advertising Company, Limited. 1907. *The Egyptian Directory (l'Annuaire Égyptien)*. Sixth Edition (1908). The Directory Printing Office: Cairo.
Essam El-Din, Gamal. 2021. "Egypt's Parliament to Grant Art-Centric Syndicates Judicial Powers to Crack Down on 'Substandard Artists.'" *Ahram Online*. 29 November. https://english.ahram.org.eg/News/443488.aspx
Fahmy, Farida. 1987. "The Creative Development of Mahmoud Reda, a Contemporary Egyptian Choreographer." Unpublished MA thesis, University of California, Los Angeles.
Fahmy, Ziad. 2011. *Ordinary Egyptians: Creating the Modern Nation through Popular Culture*. Stanford: Stanford University Press.
Fairchild Ruggles, D. 2015. "The Geographic and Social Mobility of Slaves: The Rise of Shajar al'Durr, A Slave-Concubine in Thirteenth-Century Egypt." *The Medieval Globe* 2(1): 41–55.
Fogle, Nikolaus. 2011. *The Spatial Logic of Social Struggle: A Bourdieuian Topology*. Lanham, Maryland: Lexington Books.
Fonder, Nathan Lambert. 2013. *Pleasure, Leisure, or Vice? Public Morality in Imperial Cairo, 1882–1949*. Unpublished PhD dissertation, Harvard University, Cambridge.
Foucault, Michel. 1986. "Of Other Spaces." *Diacritics* 16: 22–27.
Fraser, Kathleen. 2002. "Public and Private Entertainment at a Royal Egyptian Wedding: 1845." *Habibi* 19(1). http://thebestofhabibi.com/vol-19-no-1-feb-2002/royal-egyptian-wedding.
______. 2015. *Before They Were Belly Dancers: European Accounts of Female Entertainers in Egypt, 1760–1870*. Jefferson, North Carolina: McFarland.
Ghannam, Farha. 2016. "The Rise and Decline of a Heterotopic Space: Views from Midan al-Tahrir." *Jadaliyya*. 25 January. https://www.jadaliyya.com/Details/32895.
Giffin, Etta Josselyn. 1911. "Report of the International Congress for the Amelioration of the Lot of the Blind, Held at Cairo, Egypt, February, 1911." In *Eleventh Convention of the American Association of Workers for the Blind*, pp. 37–40. Philadelphia: American Association of Workers for the Blind.
Gitre, Carmen M. K. 2019. *Acting Egyptian: Theater, Identity, and Political Culture in Cairo, 1869–1930*. Austin: University of Texas Press.
Gordon, Matthew S. 2017. "Abbasid Courtesans and the Question of Social Mobility." In *Concubines and Courtesans: Women and Slavery in Islamic History*, edited by Matthew S. Gordon and Kathryn A. Hain, pp. 27–51. New York: Oxford University Press.
Habeiche, Joseph J. 1890. *Dictionnaire Français-Arabe. Première Édition*. Le Caire: Imprimerie du Journal "al-Mahroussa."
al-Hakim, Tawfiq. 2019. *Return of the Spirit*. New York: Penguin Books.
Hanna, Nabil Sobhi. 1982. "Ghagar of Sett Guiranha: A Study of a Gypsy Community in Egypt." *Cairo Papers in Social Science* 5(1).
Hanna, Nelly. 2002. "The Urban History of Cairo around 1900: A Reinterpretation." In *Historians in Cairo: Essays in Honor of George Scanlon*, edited by Jill Edwards, pp. 189–201. Cairo: The American University in Cairo Press.
Hassan, Fayza. 2001. "Now the Party's Over." *al-Ahram Weekly*. 23 August. https://www.masress.com/en/ahramweekly/23988.
Hawthorn, Ainsley. 2019. "Middle Eastern Dance and What We Call It." *Dance Research* 37(1): 1–17.

Heynen, Hilde. 2008. "Heterotopia Unfolded?" In *Heterotopia and the City*, edited by Michiel Dehaene and Lieven De Cauter, pp. 311–323. London: Routledge.
al-Ḥifnī, Ratībah. 2001. *al-Sulṭānah Munīrah al-Mahdīyah wa al-Ghinā fī Miṣr Qablahā wa fī Zamānihā*. al-Qāhirah: Dār al-Shurūq.
al-Hilāl. 1894. "Abṭāl al-Raqṣ." 1 August: 729.
Hopkinsville Kentuckian. 1899. "In an Arab Music Hall." 30 May: 7.
Hugonnet, Léon. 1883. *En Égypte: le Caire, Alexandrie, les Pyramides*. Paris: C. Lévy.
Ibn Baṭṭūṭah. [as Ibn Battúta.] 1953. *Travels in Asia and Africa 1325–1354*. Translated and selected by H. A. R. Gibb. Third impression. London: Routledge and Kegan Paul Ltd.
Ibn Taghrībirdī, Abū al-Maḥāsin Yūsuf. 1929–1972. *al-Nujūm al-Zāhirah fī Mulūk Miṣr wa al-Qāhirah*. al-Qāhirah.
al-Ibrashy, May. 2005. "The Cemeteries of Cairo and the *Comité de Conservation*." In *Making Cairo Medieval*, edited by Nezar Alsayyad, Irene A. Bierman, and Nasser Rabbat, pp. 235–256. Lanham, Maryland: Lexington Books.
Irwin, Robert. 2004. "Futuwwa: Chivalry and Gangsterism in Medieval Cairo." *Muqarnas* 21: 161–170.
al-Jabartī, ʿAbd al-Raḥmān. [as El Djabarti, Cheikh Abd-El-Rahman.] 1888–1896. *Merveilles Biographiques et Historiques, ou Chroniques Du Cheikh Abd-El-Rahman El Djabarti*. Traduites de l'Arabe par Chefik Mansour Bey, Abdulaziz Kahil Bey, Gabriel Nicolas Kahil Bey, et Iskender Announ Effendi. Le Caire: Ministère de l'Instruction Publique.
______. 1904. *ʿAjāʾib al-Athār fī al-Tarājim wa al-Akhbār*. al-Qāhirah: al-Maṭbaʿah al-ʿĀmirah al-Sharafīyah.
______. ʿAbd al-Raḥmān. 2006. *Napoleon in Egypt: al-Jabartī's Chronicle of the French Occupation, 1798*. Translated by Shmuel Moreh. Princeton: Markus Wiener Publishers.
Jankowski, James. 1991. "Egypt and Early Arab Nationalism, 1908–1922." In *The Origins of Arab Nationalism*, edited by Rashid Khalidi et al., pp. 243–270. New York: Columbia University Press.
Jollois, Jean-Baptiste Prosper. 1826. "Notice sur la Ville de Rosette." In *Description de l'Égypte*. Tome Dix-Huitième, Partie 1. État Moderne. Paris: Imprimerie de C.L.F. Panckoucke.
Jomard, Edme-François. 1829. "Description de la Ville et de la Citadelle du Kaire." In *Description de l'Égypte*. Tome Dix-Huitième, Partie 2. État Moderne. Paris: Imprimerie de C.L.F. Panckoucke.
El Kadi, Galila, and Alain Bonnamy. 2007. *Architecture for the Dead: Cairo's Medieval Necropolis*. Cairo: The American University in Cairo Press.
Kahle, Paul, editor. 2015. *Three Shadow Plays by Muḥammad Ibn Dāniyāl*. Cambridge: Gibb Memorial Trust.
Kaptein, N.J.G. 1993. *Muḥammad's Birthday Festival*. Leiden: Brill.
Karayanni, Stavros Stavrou. 2004. *Dancing Fear and Desire: Race, Sexuality and Imperial Politics in Middle Eastern Dance*. Waterloo, Ontario: Wilfrid Laurier University Press.
Kennard, Adam Steinmetz. 1855. *Eastern Experiences*. London: Longman, Brown, Green, and Longmans.
Khosrau, Nassiri. 1881. *Sefer Nameh. Relation du voyage de Nassiri Khosrau*. Publié, traduit et annoté par Charles Schefer. Paris: E. Leroux.
Klunzinger, C.B. 1878. *Upper Egypt: Its People and Its Products*. London: Blackie and Son.
Knox, Thomas Wallace. 1879. *The Oriental World; or, New Travels in Turkey, Russia, Egypt, Asia Minor, and the Holy Land*. San Francisco: Hawley, Rising, and Stiles.
Lagrange, Frédéric. 1994. "Musiciens et Poetes en Egypte au Temps de la *Nahda*." Unpublished PhD dissertation, Universite de Paris VIII a Saint-Denis.
______. 2009a. "L'Adīb et l'Almée: Images de la Musicienne Professionnelle chez Nagīb Maḥfūẓ et Tawfīq al-Ḥakīm." *Annales Islamologiques* 43: 337–375.
______. 2009b. "Women in the Singing Business, Women in Songs." *History Compass* 7/1: 226–250.
Lane, Edward. 1860. *An Account of the Manners and Customs of the Modern Egyptians*. Fifth Edition. London: John Murray.
______. 2005 [1836]. *Manners and Customs of the Modern Egyptians*. New York: Cosimo Classics.

Lane-Poole, Sophia. 1846. *The Englishwoman in Egypt: Letters from Cairo. (Second Series).* London: Charles Knight and Co.
Lawrence, Denise L., and Setha M. Low. 1990. "The Built Environment and Spatial Form." *Annual Review of Anthropology* 19: 453–505.
Leeder, S.H. 1913. *Veiled Mysteries of Egypt and the Religion of Islam.* New York: Charles Scribners' Sons.
______. 1918. *Modern Sons of the Pharaohs.* London, New York: Hodder and Stoughton.
Leland, Charles. 1873. *The Egyptian Sketch Book.* London: Strahan and Co., Trubner and Co.
Lewicka, Paulina B. 2005. "Restaurants, Inns and Taverns That Never Were: Some Reflections on Public Consumption in Medieval Cairo." *Journal of the Economic and Social History of the Orient* 48 (1): 40–91.
Linden, J. 1884. *L'Illustration Horticole.* V. 31. Gand, Belgium: Compagnie Continentale D'Horticulture (Société Anonyme).
Loewenbach, Lothaire. 1908. *Promenade Autour de l'Afrique, 1907.* Paris: Ernest Flammarion.
Lorius, Cassandra. 1996. "'Oh Boy, You Salt of the Earth': Outwitting Patriarchy in *Raqs Baladi.*" *Popular Music* 15/3: 285–298.
Low, Setha M., and Denise Lawrence-Zúñiga, editors. 2003. *The Anthropology of Space and Place: Locating Culture.* Malden, Massachusetts: Blackwell Publishing.
Lutfi, Huda. 1991. "Manners and Customs of Fourteenth-Century Cairene Women: Female Anarchy versus Male Shar'i Order in Muslim Prescriptive Treatise." In *Women in Middle Eastern History: Shifting Boundaries in Sex and Gender,* edited by Nikki R. Keddie and Beth Baron, 99–121. London, New Haven: Yale University Press.
Madkour, Mona. 2008. "Male Belly Dancers Apply for Permits in Egypt." *Al Arabiya.* 11 May. https://www.alarabiya.net/articles/2008/05/11/49679
Madoeuf, Anna. 2006. "Mulids of Cairo: Sufi Guilds, Popular Celebrations, and the 'Roller-Coaster Landscape' of the Resignified City." In *Cairo Cosmopolitan: Politics, Culture, and Urban Space in the New Globalized Middle East,* edited by Diane Singerman and Paul Amar, pp. 465–487. Cairo: The American University in Cairo Press.
Mahfouz, Naguib. 2001. *The Cairo Trilogy.* New York: Alfred A. Knopf.
al-Maqrīzī, Taqī al-Dīn. [as Maqrizi.] 1895. *Description Historique et Topographique de l'Égypte* Traduit par U. Bouriant. Première Partie. Paris: E. Leroux.
______. [as Makrizi.] 1906. *Description Historique et Topographique de l'Égypte.* Traduit par Paul Casanova. Troisiéme Partie. Le Caire: Imprimerie de l'Institut Français d'Archéologie Orientale.
______. 1906–1908. *Kitāb al-Khiṭaṭ al-Maqrīzīyah; al-Musammāh bi-al-Mawā'iẓ wa-al-I'tibār bi Dhikr al-Khiṭaṭ wa-al-Āthār.* al-Qāhirah: Maṭba'at al-Nīl.
______. [as Makrizi.] 1920. *Description Historique et Topographique de l'Égypte.* Traduit par Paul Casanova. Quatrieme Partie. Le Caire: Imprimerie de l'Institut Français d'Archéologie Orientale.
Marsh, Adrian. 2000. "Gypsies and Non-Gypsies of Egypt: The Zabaleen and Ghagar Communities of Cairo." *KURI Journal* 1(3).
McPherson, J.W. 1941. *The Moulids of Egypt (Egyptian Saints-Days).* Cairo: N.M. Press
Meital, Yoram. 2007. "Central Cairo: Street Naming and the Struggle over Historical Representation." *Middle Eastern Studies* 43(6): 857–878.
Al-Messiri Nadim, Nawal. 1979. "The Concept of the Ḥāra. A Historical and Sociological Study of al-Sukkariyya." *Annales Islamologiques* 15: 313–348.
Mestyan, Adam. 2017. *Arab Patriotism: The Ideology and Culture of Power in Late Ottoman Egypt.* Princeton: Princeton University Press.
Meyers Sawa, Suzanne. 1987. "The Role of Women in Musical Life: The Medieval Arabo-Islamic Courts." *Canadian Women's Studies* 8 (2): 93–95.
Michaud, Joseph François. 1833–1835. *Correspondance d'Orient, 1830–1831.* Paris: Ducollet.
Mikhail, Alan. 2007. "The Heart's Desire: Gender, Urban Space and the Ottoman Coffee House." In *Ottoman Tulips, Ottoman Coffee: Leisure and Lifestyle in the Eighteenth Century,* edited by Dana Sajdi, pp. 133–170. London: Tauris Academic Studies.
Mikhail, Sarah. 2011. "Egypt Turmoil Hits Cairo Nightlife." *Reuters.* 6 April. https://

www.reuters.com/article/uk-egypt-nightlife/egypt-turmoil-hits-cairo-nightlife-idINLNE73504820110406

Morley, Margaret L. 2023. "From Vibration to Visual Aesthetics: Political Economies of Attention in Cairo's Contemporary Belly Dance Industry." Unpublished PhD dissertation, Indiana University.

Morren, Edouard. 1881. *La Belgique Horticole. V. 31.* Liége, Belgium: A La Direction Générale, Boverie 1.

Moseley, Sydney A. 1917. *With Kitchener in Cairo.* New York: Cassell and Company.

al-Muṣawwar. 1958. "Dawlat al-'Awālim fī Miṣr." 28 October: 25–29.

al-Muwayliḥī, Muḥammad. 2015. *What 'Īsā Ibn Hishām Told Us, or, A Period of Time.* Two Volumes. Edited and translated by Roger Allen. New York: New York University Press.

Myrne, Pernilla. 2017. "A *Jariya's* Prospects in Abbasid Baghdad." In *Concubines and Courtesans: Women and Slavery in Islamic History,* edited by Matthew S. Gordon and Kathryn A. Hain, pp. 52–74. New York: Oxford University Press.

Naji, Ahmed. 2014. "Culture in the Age of Sisi: The Continued Propaganda of Illusions." *The Tahrir Institute for Middle East Policy.* https://timep.org/commentary/analysis/culture-in-the-age-of-sisi/

Nearing, Edwina. 1993. "Ghawazi on the Edge of Extinction." *Habibi* 12(2). http://thebestofhabibi.com/2-vol-12-no-2-spring-1993/ghawazi

______. 2004a. "Khairiyya Mazin Struggles to Preserve Authentic Ghawazi Dance Tradition." *The Gilded Serpent.* 3 January. http://www.gildedserpent.com/articles25/edwinakhairiyyastruggles.htm

______. 2004b. "Sirat al-Ghawazi." *The Gilded Serpent.* 11 February. http://www.gildedserpent.com/articles25/edwinaghawazich1.htm

Nerval, Gérard de. 1884. *Voyage en Orient. Volume I.* Paris: C. Lévy.

The New York Times. 1977. "Cairo Eases Prices, But Rioting Goes On." 20 January. https://www.nytimes.com/1977/01/20/archives/cairo-eases-prices-but-rioting-goes-on.html

______. 2008. "Making a Comeback: Male Belly Dancers in Egypt." 2 January. https://www.nytimes.com/2008/01/02/world/africa/02iht-letter.1.8984242.html

Newbold, Capt. 1856. "The Gypsies of Egypt." *Journal of the Royal Asiatic Society of Great Britain and Ireland* 16: 285–312.

Niebuhr, Carsten. 1792. *Travels through Arabia, and Other Countries in the East. Vol. I.* Translated by Robert Heron. Edinburgh: R. Morison and Son.

Nielson, Lisa. 2017. "Visibility and Performance: Courtesans in the Early Islamicate Courts (661–950 CE)." In *Concubines and Courtesans: Women and Slavery in Islamic History,* edited by Matthew S. Gordon and Kathryn A. Hain, pp. 75–99. New York: Oxford University Press.

Pahwa, Sonali, and Jessica Winegar. 2012. "Culture, State and Revolution." *Middle East Report* 263. https://merip.org/magazine/263/.

Parrs, Alexandra. 2017. *Gypsies in Contemporary Egypt: On the Peripheries of Society.* Cairo: The American University in Cairo Press.

Penfield, Frederic Courtland. 1899. *Present-Day Egypt.* London: Macmillan.

Pococke, Richard. 1743. *A Description of the East, and Some Other Countries.* Vol. I. London: W. Bowyer.

Poffandi, Stefano G. 1896. *1897 Indicateur Égyptien Administratif et Commercial.* Alexandria: Imprimerie Générale, L. Carrière.

______. 1901. *1902 Indicateur Égyptien Administratif et Commercial.* Alexandria: Imprimerie Générale A. Mourés et Cie.

______. 1904. *1904 Indicateur Égyptien Administratif et Commercial.* Alexandria: Imprimerie Générale A. Mourés et Cie.

Popper, William. 1954. *History of Egypt, 1382–1469 A.D. Part I, 1382–1399 A.D.* Translated from the Arabic annals of Abu l-Maḥâsin Ibn Taghrî Birdî. Berkeley: University of California Press.

______. 1957. *History of Egypt, 1382–1469 A.D. Part III, 1412–1422 A.D.* Translated from the Arabic annals of Abu l-Maḥâsin Ibn Taghrî Birdî. Berkeley: University of California Press.

______. 1958. *History of Egypt, 1382–1469 A.D. Part IV, 1422–1438 A.D.* Translated from the Arabic annals of Abu l-Maḥâsin Ibn Taghrî Birdî. Berkeley: University of California Press.

Pradines, Stephane, and Sher Rahmat Khan. 2016. "Fāṭimid Gardens: Archaeological and Historical Perspectives." *Bulletin of the School of Oriental and African Studies* 79 (03): 1–30.

Prokosch, Erich. 2000. *Kairo in der Zweiten Hälfte des 17. Jahrhunderts*. Istanbul: Simurg.

Puig, Nicolas. 2001. "Le long Siècle de l'Avenue Muhammad 'Alî." *Égypte/Monde Arabe* [En Ligne] (4–5). https://journals.openedition.org/ema/879.

———. "Egypt's Pop-Music Clashes and the 'World-Crossing' Destinies of Muhammad 'Ali Street Musicians." In *Cairo Cosmopolitan: Politics, Culture, and Urban Space in the New Globalized Middle East*, edited by Diane Singerman and Paul Amar, pp. 513–536. Cairo: The American University in Cairo Press.

The Queenslander [Brisbane, Queensland, Australia]. 1886. "Our Cairo Letter." 27 February: 336.

Ramadan, Sarah. 2021. "A Closed Door: A Paper on Membership as an Entry Point for Independent Artistic Syndicates in Egypt." *Association for Freedom of Thought and Expression*. 22 March. https://afteegypt.org/en/research-en/research-papers-en/2021/03/22/21293-afteegypt.html.

Rapoport, Yossef. 2007. "Women and Gender in Mamluk Society: An Overview." *Mamlūk Studies Review* 11(2): 1–47.

Raymond, André. 1957. "Une Liste des Corporations de Métiers au Caire en 1801." *Arabica* T. 4 (Fasc. 2): 150–163.

———. 1973. *Artisans et Commerçants au Caire au XVIIIe Siècle*. Tome I. Damas: Institut Français de Damas.

———. 1974. *Artisans et Commerçants au Caire au XVIIIe Siècle*. Tome II. Damas: Institut Français de Damas.

———. 1980. "The Rab': A Type of Collective Housing in Cairo during the Ottoman Period." In *Architecture as Symbol and Self-Identity*, edited by Jonathan G. Katz, pp. 55–62. Philadelphia: Aga Khan Award for Architecture.

———. 2000. *Cairo*. Translated by Willard Wood. Cambridge: Harvard University Press.

Reynolds, Dwight F. 2017. "The *Qiyan* of al-Andalus." In *Concubines and Courtesans: Women and Slavery in Islamic History*, edited by Matthew S. Gordon and Kathryn A. Hain, pp. 100–123. New York: Oxford University Press.

Reynolds-Ball, Eustace A. 1898a. *The City of the Caliphs; a Popular Study of Cairo and its Environs and the Nile and its Antiquities*. Boston, London: Estes and Lauriat, T. Fisher Unwin.

———. 1898b. *Cairo of To-Day: A Practical Guide to Cairo and Its Environs*. London: Adam and Charles Black.

Richardson, Kristina. 2009. "Singing Slave Girls (*Qiyan*) of the 'Abbasid Court in the Ninth and Tenth Centuries." In *Children in Slavery through the Ages*, edited by Gwyn Campbell et al., pp. 105–118. Athens, Ohio: Ohio University Press.

———. 2022. *Roma in the Medieval Islamic World: Literacy, Culture, and Migration*. London: I.B. Tauris.

Romer, Isabella Frances. 1846. *A Pilgrimage to the Temples and Tombs of Egypt, Nubia, and Palestine, in 1845–6*. Vol. II. London: R. Bentley.

Ross, Michael. 1986. "Egypt Security Unit Revolt Spreads; 15 Reported Slain." *Los Angeles Times*. 27 February. https://www.latimes.com/archives/la-xpm-1986-02-27-mn-12081-story.html.

Roushdy, Noha. 2009. "Femininity and Dance in Egypt: Embodiment and Meaning in al-Raqs al-Baladi." *Cairo Papers in Social Science* 32 (3).

Rowson, Everett K. 1991. "The Effeminates of Early Medina." *Journal of the American Oriental Society* 111: 671–93.

———. 1997. "Two Homoerotic Narratives from Mamlūk Literature: al-Ṣafadī's Law'at al-Shākī and Ibn Dānyāl's al-Mutayyam." In *Homoeroticism in Classical Arabic Literature*, ed. J. W. Wright, Jr., and Everett K. Rowson, pp. 158–91. New York: Columbia University Press.

———. 2003. "Gender Irregularity as Entertainment: Institutionalized Transvestism at the

Caliphal Court in Medieval Baghdad." In *Gender and Difference in the Middle Ages*, edited by Sharon Farmer and Carol Braun Pasternack, pp. 45–72. Minneapolis: University of Minnesota Press.

Ryzova, Lucie. 2015. "Strolling in Enemy Territory: Downtown Cairo, its Publics, and Urban Heterotopias." In *Divercities: Competing Narratives and Urban Practices in Beirut, Cairo and Tehran*, edited by Nadia von Maltzahn and Monique Bellan. Beirut: Orient Institut.

Sadgrove, P.C. 1996. *The Egyptian Theatre in the Nineteenth Century (1799–1882)*. Berkshire: Ithaca Press.

Sahin, Christine M. 2018. "Core Connections: A Contemporary Cairo Raqs Sharqi Ethnography." Unpublished PhD dissertation, University of California, Riverside.

Said, Edward W. 1979. *Orientalism*. New York: Vintage Books.

St. John, James Augustus. 1834. *Egypt and Mohammed Ali*. Vol. I. London: Longman, Rees, Orme, Brown, Green & Longman.

Saleh, Magda Ahmed Abdel Ghaffar. 1979. "A Documentation of the Ethnic Dance Traditions of the Arab Republic of Egypt." Unpublished PhD dissertation, New York University.

Salmon, W.H. 1921. *An Account of the Ottoman Conquest of Egypt in the Year A.H. 922 (A.D. 1516)*. Third impression. London: The Royal Asiatic Society.

Sanders, Paula. 1994. *Ritual, Politics, and the City in Fatimid Cairo*. Albany: State University of New York.

Sandys, George. 1673. *Sandys Travels*. The Seventh Edition. London: J. Williams Junior.

Savary, Claude-Étienne. 1785. *Lettres sur l'Égypte*. Tome 1. Paris: Onfroi.

Sawa, George Dimitri. 2018. *Musical and Socio-Cultural Anecdotes from Kitāb al-Aghānī al-Kabīr*. Leiden: Brill.

al-Sayyid Marsot, Afaf Lutfi. 1995. *Women and Men in Late Eighteenth-Century Egypt*. Austin: University of Texas Press.

Schielke, Samuli. 2006. "Snacks and Saints: Mawlid Festivals and the Politics of Festivity, Piety and Modernity in Contemporary Egypt." Unpublished PhD dissertation, University of Amsterdam.

———. 2009. "Policing *Mulids* and Their Meaning." In *Cairo Contested: Governance, Urban Space, and Global Modernity*, edited by Diane Singerman, pp. 83–110. Cairo: The American University in Cairo Press.

Scott, James Harry. 1908. *The Law Affecting Foreigners in Egypt. Revised Edition*. Edinburgh: William Green and Sons.

Shafik, Viola. 2006. *Popular Egyptian Cinema: Gender, Class, and Nation*. Cairo: The American University in Cairo Press.

el-Sharkawy, Youssra. 2017. "Male Belly Dancers Break Taboos in Egypt." *Al-Monitor*. 13 February. https://www.al-monitor.com/pulse/originals/2017/02/egypt-male-belly dancer-break-taboos.html.

Shay, Anthony. 2002. *Choreographic Politics: State Folk Dance Companies, Representation, and Power*. Middletown, Connecticut: Wesleyan University Press.

———. 2014. *The Dangerous Lives of Public Performers: Dancing, Sex, and Entertainment in the Islamic World*. New York: Palgrave Macmillan.

Shiloah, Amnon. 1962. "Réflexions sur la Danse Artistique Musulmane au Moyen Âge." *Cahiers de Civilisation Médiévale, 5e Année* (20): 463–474.

———. 1995. *Music in the World of Islam: A Socio-Cultural Study*. Detroit: Wayne State University Press.

Shoshan, Boaz. 1993. *Popular Culture in Medieval Cairo*. Cambridge: Cambridge University Press.

Singerman, Diane. 2009. "The Siege of Imbaba, Egypt's Internal 'Other,' and the Criminalization of Politics." In *Cairo Contested: Governance, Urban Space, and Global Modernity*, edited by Diane Singerman, pp. 111–144. Cairo: The American University in Cairo Press

Sladen, Douglas. 1911. *Oriental Cairo: The City of the "Arabian Nights."* Philadelphia: J.B. Lippincott Company.

Société Anonyme Égyptienne de Publicité. 1912. *The Egyptian Directory (l'Annuaire*

Égyptien). 27ne Année (1913). Imprimerie de la Société Anonyme Égyptienne de Publicité: Cairo.
Spiro, Socrates. 1897. *An English-Arabic Vocabulary of the Modern and Colloquial Arabic of Egypt*. Cairo: al-Mokattam Printing Office.
______. 1923. *Arabic-English Dictionary of the Modern Arabic of Egypt*. Second Edition. Cairo: Elias Modern Press.
Star [Canterbury, New Zealand]. 1902. "The Ghawazee of Cairo: The Picturesque Dancing Women of Egypt." Issue 7512. 20 September: 2.
Taylor, Christopher S. 1999. *In the Vicinity of the Righteous: Ziyāra and the Veneration of Muslim Saints in Late Medieval Egypt*. Leiden: Brill.
Thomas, C.F. 2000. "Dom of North Africa: An Overview." *KURI Journal* 1(1).
Tietze, Andreas. 1975. *Muṣṭafā ʿĀlī's Description of Cairo of 1599: Text, Transliteration, Translation, Notes*. Vienna: Österreichischen Akademie der Wissenschaften.
Toledano, Ehud R. 1990. *State and Society in Mid-Nineteenth-Century Egypt*. Cambridge: Cambridge University Press.
Tolmacheva, Marina A. 2017. "Concubines on the Road: Ibn Battuta's Slave Women." In *Concubines and Courtesans: Women and Slavery in Islamic History*, edited by Matthew S. Gordon and Kathryn A. Hain, pp. 163–189. New York: Oxford University Press.
Tucker, Judith E. 1985. *Women in Nineteenth-Century Egypt*. Cambridge: Cambridge University Press.
Van Nieuwkerk, Karin. 1995. *A Trade Like Any Other: Female Singers and Dancers in Egypt*. Austin: University of Texas Press.
______. 2019. *Manhood Is Not Easy: Egyptian Masculinities through the Life of Musician Sayyid Henkish*. Cairo: The American University in Cairo Press.
Vatikiotis, P.J. 1991. *The History of Modern Egypt: From Muhammad Ali to Mubarak*. Fourth Edition. Baltimore: The Johns Hopkins University Press.
Villoteau, Guillaume André. 1826. "De l'État Actuel de l'Art Musical en Égypte." In *Description de l'Égypte*. Tome Quatorzième. État Moderne. Paris: Imprimerie de C.L.F. Panckoucke.
Von Kremer, Alfred. 1864. "The Gipsies in Egypt." *The Anthropological Review* 2(7): 262–267.
Ward, Heather D. 2013. "Desperately Seeking Shafiqa: The Search for the Historical Shafiqa el Qibtiyya." *The Gilded Serpent*. 3 October. http://www.gildedserpent.com/cms/2013/10/03/nisaa-desperately-seeking-shafiqa/
______. 2018. *Egyptian Belly Dance in Transition: The Raqs Sharqi Revolution, 1890–1930*. Jefferson, North Carolina: McFarland
Warner, Charles Dudley. 1900. *My Winter on the Nile*. Boston: Houghton, Mifflin and Company.
Wehr, Hans. 1976. *A Dictionary of Modern Written Arabic*. Third Edition. Ithaca: Spoken Language Services, Inc.
Wilkinson, Sir John Gardner. 1847. *Hand-Book for Travellers in Egypt*. London: John Murray, 1847.
Williams, Caroline. 1983. "The Cult of ʿAlid Saints in the Fatimid Monuments of Cairo Part I: The Mosque of al-Aqmar." *Muqarnas* 1: 37–52.
______. 1985. "The Cult of ʿAlid Saints in the Fatimid Monuments of Cairo Part II: The Mausolea." *Muqarnas* 3: 39–60.
Williams, Daniel. 2006. "Egypt Extends 25-Year-Old Emergency Law." *Washington Post*. 1 May. https://www.washingtonpost.com/wp-dyn/content/article/2006/04/30/AR2006043001039.html
Williams, Daniel, and Robin Wright. 2005. "Controversy Swirls Over Egypt Vote." *Washington Post*. 9 September. https://www.washingtonpost.com/wp-dyn/content/article/2005/09/08/AR2005090800151.html.
Winegar, Jessica. 2009. "Culture is the Solution: The Civilizing Mission of Egypt's Culture Palaces." *Review of Middle East Studies* 43 (2): 189–197.
Worrell, W.H. 1920. "Kishkish: Arabic Vaudeville in Cairo." In *The Moslem World*, Volume X, edited by Samuel M. Zwemer, pp. 134–137. New York: Missionary Review Publishing Co.

Yiḥyā, Muḥammad. 2017. *al-Manaṣṣah*. 13 August. https://almanassa.com/ar/story/5341.
Zirbel, Katherine E. 2000. "Playing It Both Ways: Local Egyptian Performers between Regional Identity and International Markets." In *Mass Mediations: New Approaches to Popular Culture in the Middle East and Beyond*, edited by Walter Armbrust, pp. 120–145. Berkeley: University of California Press.
al-Zuhūr. 1913. "al-Raqṣ al-Miṣrī." November: 357–362.

Films and Audio

Anā al-Duktūr. 1968. 'Abbās Kāmal, director. Egypt.
The Bellydancers of Cairo. 2006. Natasha Senkovich, director. NS Enterprises. Los Angeles.
Cairo. 1964. British Pathé. London. https://www.britishpathe.com/video/cairo
Dancers. 2007. Celame Barge, director. Atef Hetata, producer. Egypt.
Fatāt al-Sīrk. 1951. Ḥusayn Fawzī, director. Egypt.
In Our Own Words: The Cairo Dance Scene Explained. 2020. Sara Farouk, director. Francesca Sullivan, producer. Egypt.
al-Khamsah Jinīh. 1946. Ḥassan Ḥilmy, director. Egypt.
La Nuit, Elles Dansent. 2011. Isabelle Lavigne and Stéphane Thibault, directors. Les Films du Tricycle. Canada.
Qaṣr al-Shūq. 1966. Ḥassan al-Imām, director. Egypt.
Raqṣ Shafīqah. 1908. Performed by Bahiyah al-Maḥallāwīyah. Odéon 45032.
The Romany Trail. 1992. Jeremy Marre, director. Shanachie Records. Newton, New Jersey.
Wa'd. 1954. Aḥmad Badrakhān, director. Egypt.
al-Zawjah al-Thāniyah. 1967. Ṣalāḥ Abū Sayf, director. Egypt.

Maps

Description de l'Égypte. 1809. Pl. 15—Plan Général de Boulâq, du Kaire, de l'île de Roudah, du Vieux Kaire et de Gyzeh and Pl. 26—Plan Particulier de la Ville from État Moderne, Planches, Tome Premièr. Paris: l'Imprimerie Royale.
Dufour, Adolphe Hippolyte. 1838. *Le Kaire*. From *Abrégé de Géographie*. Troisième Édition. Paris: Jules Renouard et Cie.
Goad, Charles E. 1905. *Insurance Plan of Cairo, Egypt*. London: Chas. E. Goad.
Kāmil, Khalīl. 1953. *Cairo Tourist Map (al-Qāhirah: Kharīṭah Siyāḥīyah)*. al-Qāhirah: Maṣlaḥat al-Siyāḥah.
———. 1959. Cairo: The City of Minarets (Cairo Tourist Map). Cairo: United Arab Republic Tourist Administration.
Popper, William. 1955. Various maps of Cairo from *Egypt and Syria under the Circassian Sultans, 1382–1468 A.D.: Systematic Notes to Ibn Taghrî Birdî's Chronicles of Egypt*. Berkeley: University of California Press.
Survey of Egypt (Maṣlaḥat al-Misāḥah). 1920. *General Map of Cairo*. Cairo: Survey of Egypt.
Wagner and Debes. 1885. *Cairo*. From *Egypt, Handbook for Travellers. Part First: Lower Egypt, with the Fayûm and the Peninsula of Sinai. 2nd Edition, Revised and Augmented*. Leipsic, London: K. Baedeker.
Wagner and Debes. 1911. *Cairo*. From *The Mediterranean: Seaports and Sea Routes*. Leipzig: Karl Baedeker.

Index

www.ingramcontent.com/pod-product-compliance
Ingram Content Group UK Ltd.
Pitfield, Milton Keynes, MK11 3LW, UK
UKHW030825211224
452747UK00004B/188

9 781476 690308